SURGEONS, SAINTS AND PSYCHOPATHS

The Epic Story of Heart Surgery

STEPHEN WESTABY

MENSCH PUBLISHING

Mensch Publishing
51 Northchurch Road, London N1 4EE, United Kingdom

First published in Great Britain 2024

A catalogue record for this book is available from the British Library

ISBN: HB: 978-1-91291460-9; eBook: 978-1-912914-61-6

The illustrations in this book were sent to the author
by the pioneers themselves during the early 1990s.
Many were originally published in the textbook,
Landmarks in Cardiac Surgery.

Dedication

The notion that the family comes first never did apply to heart surgeons but we all live to regret that. This book is for my children, Gemma and Mark, and my granddaughters, Alice and Chloe. Needless to say I couldn't have achieved what I did without Sarah, a fine Accident and Emergency nurse in her own right.

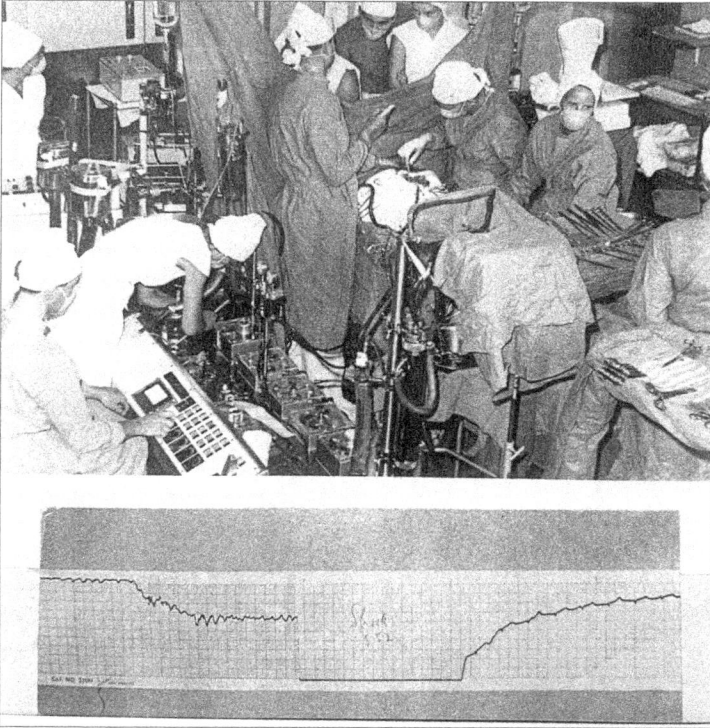

Photograph taken in the operating theatre during Christiaan Barnard's first heart transplant in Cape Town. The electrocardiographic trace beneath records the organ dying in the donor Denise Darvall, and being resurrected by renewed blood flow in the recipient, Louis Waskansky.

Contents

Preface

It is not a dangerous operation.
We have never lost a surgeon doing it!
—Mark M Ravitch

In 1896 Dr Stephen Paget wrote in his masterful textbook *Surgery of the Chest* that 'operations on the heart have already reached the limits set by nature. No new method and no new discovery can overcome the natural difficulties that attend a wound to the heart.' Barely anything had changed when I was delivered into the world, or should I say into the backstreets of a northern steel town, more than half a century later. For practical purpose there was no cardiac surgery.

One sunny summer's morning in July my darling mother cradled me from the delivery suite, pink, warm and wailing loudly from a fine pair of newly-expanded lungs. A robust 8lb baby boy genetically programmed to survive and thrive. But for the unfortunate girl in the cot next to me it was a different story. At least her mother didn't have a perineal tear because the baby was small. And it came with a whimper not a roar. All babies are blue when they first greet the light of day, but as they scream and object to the battering in the birth canal their lungs take in air for the first time and expand. The inhaled oxygen renders their blood corpuscles bright red and their little body soon 'pinks up'. This one didn't.

The veteran midwife was quick to recognise the problem. 'It's a beautiful baby girl,' she murmured, 'but I need to call the doctor.' Minutes seemed like hours as they waited. And when he came it wasn't reassuring.

'Sorry but it's a blue baby' was all the medic said as he gently placed the little mite into her mother's arms. The poor woman didn't realise the significance of the term 'blue baby'. Why would she? 'What does that mean?' she asked with pleading eyes whilst my own joyful mother tried not to listen.

'It means that there is a blockage preventing blood from reaching the lungs and probably a hole in the heart,' he explained in a matter-of-fact way as the midwife stared at the ceiling. As the mother listened intently she could see me suckling and her own nipples were already leaking colostrum. Naturally enough she tried to offer it to her precious purple offspring but attempts to feed proved too much. The infant whimpered, gurgled then choked on the milk turning a sinister shade of grey. Hours later as the sun descended behind the blast furnaces the little girl fell silent and limp in her mother's arms. The midwife took her away in a shoe box. Mother cried. My mother wept too. The father never arrived to greet his daughter into the world. He was working a late shift in the steelworks. There was no time off for childbirth in those days. It was 1948 the year Britain's National Health Service (NHS) came about.

How did I learn about this? It happened that every year on my birthday during the school holidays, my mother would buy flowers then take me on a bus across town to deliver them on the sad woman's doorstep. Eventually I asked why. The poor woman watched me grow up but never had any children of her own. The first attempt had been too traumatic for her.

In my formative years we lived in a council house directly across the street from my maternal grandparents. I spent a considerable time with them because mother worked as a cashier in the Trustees Savings Bank on the High Street. My grandfather soon recognised that I was ambidextrous and taught me to draw and paint. He had been the local air raid warden during World War II and like all men of that era he smoked and worked in the smoggy haze of the steel mills.

I was eight when I first witnessed him suffer chest pain as we walked the dog in the park. He would find an excuse to stop and wipe the perspiration from his forehead. Inclines made things worse and in retrospect it was classic angina pectoris. Not enough blood flow to the heart muscle.

Then one day it was different. He suddenly clutched his chest in agony, felt faint, and sank to his knees. Aged 59 this was a full-blown heart attack. A ruptured atheromatous plaque had occluded a vital coronary artery and a billion muscle cells were dying as I struggled to bring him home.

The family doctor came to the house in a black Austin Healey and told my grandfather to stay in bed. Over the next weeks a large patch of dead muscle changed into scar tissue, but fibrous tissue doesn't contract. It stretches. The left ventricle dilated and contracted poorly so he became breathless with swelling of the legs and abdomen. Tablets didn't help. There was only digoxin from the foxglove plant in those days and no effective water pills. Soon his bed had to be brought downstairs in front of the fire but he couldn't lie flat without gasping for air. It was more comfortable to sit bolt upright in an armchair all night. What else could be done? 'Nothing', we were told. Life with heart failure was unbearable for him and interminably grim for the family to witness. Soon kidney failure followed as it always does.

One cold December afternoon as I walked home from school, I saw the Austin Healey parked outside the house again. The curtains were drawn this time, but not sufficiently that I couldn't peer through them. There were my devastated mother and grandmother on either side of the bed each clasping a cold sweaty hand. Grandfather's face was grey and contorted as bloodstained froth poured from his nose and mouth. The kindly GP was in the process of injecting a hefty dose of morphine fully intending 'to put an end to his suffering'. It did. A simple act of kindness from a caring doctor for a dying patient in a bygone era when nothing else could be done. Within days of Christmas this was not a tableau I would easily forget. Indeed it stayed with me for my whole career. If you could help someone in that situation why wouldn't you?

It wasn't just coronary and congenital heart disease that caused heart failure in those days. Many healthy young lives were destroyed by a simple streptococcal throat infection followed by rheumatic fever. Normal heart valves were damaged by the immunological process becoming leaky or narrowed. And syphilis was rife during World War II which also caused valve disease and aortic aneurysms. None of these conditions responded to medication so despairing and sceptical physicians eventually turned to surgeons to find a solution.

To distract us from grandfather's miserable death my parents bought their first television set. The screen was black and white and only nine inches wide but a single documentary was about to change my life. In February 1958 *Your Life in Their Hands* showed an early heart operation from the Hammersmith Hospital. Surgeons were peering intently into the chest and the camera gave us a brief glimpse of the sick heart beating away in its fibrous sac. They were about to take over the patient's circulation with something called a heart-lung machine and I remember thinking: 'Why couldn't this have been done years ago?' The scenes were quite revealing for the time since for the most part cardiac surgery remained an unknown entity to the general public. To increase awareness was the point, of course, but such revelations didn't go down well in certain circles. So much so that it prompted a heated debate in Parliament the following day.

> *Hansard* February 28th 1958 – Sir Ian Clark Hutchinson challenged the Postmaster General, Mr Marples with the fact that 'many doctors considered the morbid programme *Your Life in their hands* to have a bad effect upon viewers. So would he kindly instruct the BBC to refrain from showing similar again?'

> The Postmaster General responded by informing the House that 'the BBC had consulted the Royal College of Surgeons, the Royal College of Physicians and the College of General Practitioners beforehand to gain their approval.'

> Mr Henry Morrison MP supported the graphic presentation. 'Is the right honourable gentleman aware that I saw this programme last night? It dealt with an operation on the heart and I thought it was done very carefully and respectfully; it was educational and conducted in cooperation with the local hospital authorities. May I ask the Postmaster General not to be unduly influenced by his honourable friend?'

But I was influenced. It was then at the age of nine that I decided to be a heart surgeon.

Twenty years later I was performing heart surgery with that same team at the Hammersmith hospital and twenty years after that I made a *Your Life in Their Hands* episode myself. I implanted a revolutionary new type of artificial heart at the Royal Brompton Hospital for a heart failure patient that bore many similarities to my unfortunate grandfather. 'What goes around, comes around', as they say. I expect he would be proud of me.

Why was it so difficult and controversial to perform surgery on that one organ?

Let's begin with some facts about the magnificent machine I spent my whole career with. What the heart does is awfully simple. It pumps. But should the pump fail, life becomes simply awful. Crushing chest pain, severe breathlessness, fluid retention and crippling fatigue are the hallmarks of heart disease which can affect all age groups. The healthy adult heart weighs in the vicinity of 11 ounces. My school biology classes taught it has four parts, two thin-walled collecting chambers called the right and left atria, then two thicker pumping chambers, the right and left ventricles.

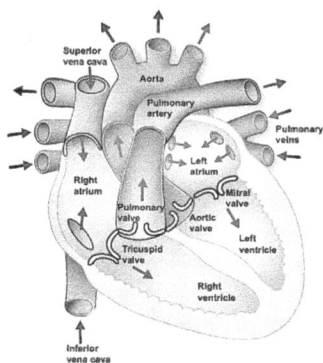

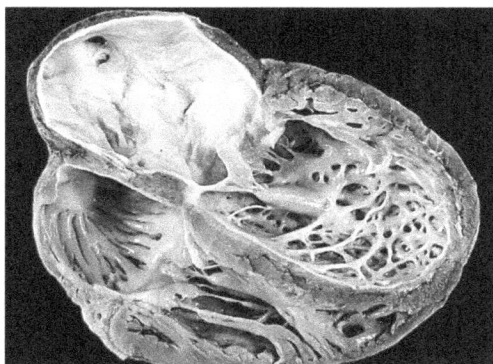

Schoolbook diagram in contrast with the terminally sick heart as I knew it.

That was a trifle misleading because the atria pump too. As well as being at risk of stroke from turbulence and blood clots people with the common rhythm problem atrial fibrillation, have less energy because atrial contraction is lost. Diagrams in textbooks suggest that the chambers are side by side but that is wide of the mark too. My analogy is of the heart as a house with two bedrooms upstairs above a kitchen and sitting room below. Why? Because the ventricles are very different from one another. Nor are they left and right. More front and back.

The thicker and more powerful left ventricle is conical in shape with circular muscle bands that vigorously constrict and rotate the chamber. There are five billion individual cells comprising the left ventricle, more than half of which are the contractile units known as cardiomyocytes. Each of these muscle cells is intimately connected to its neighbours by cell membrane junctions which provide an integrated electrical network throughout the heart. Within the cardiomyocyte are carefully organised protein molecules that slide over each other causing shortening and muscular contraction.

Both ventricles must generate strong and rapid force to propel blood through an extensive network of arteries, capillaries and veins. Then they relax abruptly causing the chambers to refill after every beat. There are around seventy beats per minute at rest but this rises as far as 180 beats on strenuous exercise. The responses to nervous and hormonal stimulation deliver a range of between five to twenty litres of blood to the body's 75 trillion cells each minute. Extrapolate from there and the figures are staggering. One hundred thousand beats distribute 7600 litres of blood every day. This amounts to thirty-five million beats in a year and 2.5 billion in an average lifetime. In 24 hours a red blood corpuscle will travel 12,000 miles through the vascular system, four times the distance across the USA. And despite those billions of beats in a lifetime, half of the cardiomyocytes present at birth will still be present when you die, having consumed enough energy to drive a truck to the moon and back. Only 1% of them are exchanged each year in younger age groups. Contrast these hard working 'forever' cells with those which line the gut and live for less than a week.

Contraction and relaxation are not as simple as they sound. As the left ventricle pumps in 'systole' the cavity both narrows and shortens to eject blood. This flows through the outlet valve into the aorta and around the body amounting to an astounding one million barrels of blood during an average lifetime. Enough to fill more than three supertankers. During relaxation, or the 'diastolic' phase, the chamber recoils, both widening and lengthening. The negative pressure created sucks in blood from the left atrium via the mitral valve, so called through its resemblance to a bishop's mitre. Whilst an apt description others preferred the likeness to a lady's corset with suspenders!

The right ventricle works in an entirely different way serving to pump the same volume of blood through the pulmonary valve to the lungs at lower pressure and resistance. With a thinner wall, it is crescentic in shape and wrapped around the front of the left ventricle. The left ventricular wall between the two chambers is called the interventricular septum and given its 'New moon' shape the right ventricle pumps like a bellows. Thus the efficiency of the two cavities is very much dependent upon each other and the integrity of their indigenous electrical wiring system. The heart's cycle is a veritable Argentine tango but with one difference. Each carefully synchronised beat takes less than one second and the dance goes on forever.

The exquisitely coordinated rhythm is orchestrated by two specialised nests of pacemaker cells called the sinoatrial node situated in the wall of the right atrium, and the atrioventricular node strategically situated between collecting and pumping chambers. Electrical signals are propagated by a continually fluctuating current across the outer membranes of the pacemaker cells in contrast to the ordinary cardiomyocyte which beats only when prompted. These electrical currents form the basis for an important investigation – the electrocardiogram or ECG – which reveals many aspects of the heart's integrity. From rhythm to wall thickness, heart attack to muscle disease.

Sick hearts don't like to be handled, hence the difficulty in operating on them. They object by interrupting their carefully synchronised motion, firing off extra, or ectopic beats, adopting runs of rapid rhythm or even squirming uncontrollably in what we call ventricular fibrillation. Without an urgent electric shock, fibrillation is a terminal event and defibrillators were only introduced in the 1950s. In the event of cardiac arrest, flow ceases abruptly throughout the 60,000 miles of blood vessels, instantly depriving the tissues of oxygen and vital nutrients. The toxic metabolites carbon dioxide and lactic acid rapidly accumulate and in time the cells are destroyed. Game over.

Heart muscle is remarkably adaptive. When we exercise our arms and legs vigorously the skeletal muscle gets tired and stiff through accumulation of lactic acid. Not so the cardiomyocyte. These cells have the extraordinary capacity to beat between 70 to 150 times each minute for a lifetime without tiring. Only a compromised blood supply or heart muscle disease can impact this scenario. The heart itself receives just 5% of the body's blood flow through three tiny coronary arteries. Contrast that with the 20% taken by the brain, an organ of nerve cells that lies completely within its box. With age these vessels may clog with fatty atheromatous plaques that accumulate calcium. Certain diets and smoking predispose to this 'furring up' of the pipes. Should the heart's own arteries become obstructed, the increased flow needed for exercise cannot happen and lactic acid will accumulate in response. This causes the gripping chest pain we call angina. Stop exercising and the pain will subside. At least we hope it will.

Even the healthy organ can change dramatically. After regular intensive training an athlete's heart becomes 20% to 30% thicker, not through multiplication of cells but from their enlargement. In contrast the left ventricular cavity can double its volume during the circulatory overload of pregnancy, only to shrink down by as much as 40% within ten days of birth. All this happens in response to mechanical stress and adaptation in the cardiomyocyte's shape and size, not an increased number of cells.

In contrast a full-blown heart attack is a catastrophic event unless treated in the catheter laboratory within an hour. When those hard-working muscle cells are abruptly deprived of blood flow and oxygen through complete coronary artery occlusion, disaster ensues. Individual cardiomyocytes accumulate toxic chemicals causing many to burst spilling their contents through ruptured cell membranes. This causes severe pain and as many as two billion cells will die as a result. A small proportion of the remainder may replicate but nowhere near sufficient to repair the damage. Instead the fibroblast cells which constitute the structural framework around the cardiomyocytes, proliferate rapidly to produce scar tissue. This prevents the heart from rupturing, though not always, in which case the patient dies suddenly a few days afterwards. Sudden ventricular fibrillation is nonetheless the commonest cause of death after a heart attack through loss of stability within the complex electrical network.

Can this lethal sequence of events be prevented? Yes it can but only by skilled interventional cardiologists. They will pass a catheter through the aorta into the blocked artery to dilate the occluded segment and insert a stent to keep it open. The dying muscle is then re-perfused and rescued but all this depends upon rapid access to a cardiac hospital and the availability of a specialist. Not everyone has that benefit and unfortunately less so in the NHS. The trade-off between heart muscle and scar tissue after heart attack is a measure of quality of care.

These problems all had evolving surgical solutions during the second half of the twentieth century.

Unfortunately scar tissue is not stable. Under relentless pressure within the cavity of the left ventricle it stretches. The wounded chamber then begins to dilate and under the laws of physics, the pressure on the wall increases as the cavity enlarges. Then the mitral valve begins to leak and the pressure in the left atrium and veins from the lungs rises. That causes breathlessness. As the heart fails, progressively other organs suffer too. The kidneys don't work as well and the whole body retains water. The legs and belly eventually swell with fluid and the liver stretches as the pressure rises within the veins draining blood from the lower body. Relentless misery that I was well familiar with.

How long do other organs survive if the heart stops? That is the critical question that underpins the process of organ transplantation. Death occurs gradually through the metabolic mayhem which follows the discontinuation of oxygen and glucose delivery to the tissues. What we know is that the thoracic organs, both heart and lungs, will remain viable outside the body for four to six hours. The liver can survive for twelve hours and the kidneys for up to thirty-six hours. Needless to say, those tissues with a low metabolic rate including skin, tendons, heart valves and corneas can last much longer. But what about the brain?

Whilst the brain accounts for just 2% of overall body weight it consumes approximately 20% of the oxygen made available through the circulation. The nerve cells also require a generous supply of glucose for their energy requirements. In conditions of low oxygen delivery known as hypoxia, the ability to metabolise the glucose is rapidly lost and nervous function fails. Therefore after a couple of minutes of circulatory arrest consciousness fades. By five minutes, or just three hundred missed heart beats, irreversible neurological damage is thought to occur and breathing efforts will cease. It doesn't require complete cardiac arrest to cause hypoxia. Severe rhythm disturbances or very low blood pressure prove problematic too.

What happens in the mind during cardiac arrest is a cause for curiosity. An electroencephalogram (EEG) is the brain's electric monitoring equivalent to the heart's electrocardiogram. Doctors in the USA were undertaking an EEG on an 87-year-old man who needed brain surgery to release a blood clot after head trauma. Coincidentally the man suffered a heart attack and died whilst the investigation was in progress, but the team continued the brain's imaging for fifteen minutes after death. When the electrical traces were scrutinised the findings were fascinating. Focusing on the thirty seconds before and after cardiac arrest, they observed the very same changes in electrical wave patterns observed in people who are either dreaming, experiencing flashbacks or processing memories. The brain waves recorded during the cardiac arrest and immediately afterwards implied that accelerated memories of the patient's life were occurring analogous to those frequently reported after near death experiences.

Reporting the findings in the journal *Frontiers in Aging Neuroscience*, the authors wrote: 'The human brain may possess the capacity to generate coordinated activity during the process of dying. And indeed, similar findings in controlled rat experiments supported the suggestion.' This fits well with many stories I heard from patients later in my career. The brain and the heart are inseparable bedfellows so to speak, but the descent into death may not be as rapid as we once thought. Contrary to previous notions that brain cells die within five to ten minutes evidence now suggests that when left alone, neurones die slowly over a period of many hours or even days after the heart stops and the patient dies. Paradoxically it is the reintroduction of oxygen during resuscitation that causes the cells to die much more rapidly. This is what we call re-perfusion injury. The longer someone has been left in cardiac arrest, the more profound is the cell injury process.

Someone with fewer than five minutes without blood flow to the brain has a much higher probability of rescue and recovery than someone who experiences more prolonged hypoxia. Common sense really; and all down to oxygen free radicals.

As a junior doctor in a large teaching hospital in London I always volunteered for the cardiac arrest team. There were three of us on standby day and night and more often than not, we were veterans of the first XV rugby team. Two were resident house physicians because the surgeons were usually committed to theatre during the daytime. The third was a trainee anaesthetist whose job it was to secure the airway with an endotracheal tube and pump oxygen into the lungs. Athletics was a key part of the role. When the crash call came we would dash down the corridors, sprint up the stairs and whizz through the wards at top speed eventually converging on the patient. Time was of the essence. Whilst the clock ticked, the blood deprived-brain was dying, but we knew nothing of free radicals.

Picture the ward nurse kneeling astride the victim's belly on the bed, palms crossed over the breast bone pumping away rhythmically but in timid fashion. Whilst Grim Reaper perches on the bedhead, timid doesn't cut it. So in dives the rugby team for what amounts to a brutal business. Crunch, crunch, crunch, crunch. Frantic compressions slam the sternum against the thoracic spine squeezing the motionless heart between them. Even in vigorous mode external cardiac massage only achieves 20% of the heart's normal output. Simultaneously, the forced displacement of the rib cage sucks, then expels air from the lungs so, in effect, mouth-to-mouth respiration is unnecessary.

When the resuscitation nurse arrived she brought me a syringe of adrenaline on a long lumbar puncture needle. Pausing the compressions I would drive that needle through the chest wall aiming for the cavity of the left ventricle. With the powerful stimulant installed it was crunch, crunch, crunch, again to deliver the drug into the coronary arteries. That would even provoke a rhythm even in those who had flat-lined. Either that or transform slow agonal ventricular fibrillation to brisk electrical mayhem more susceptible to a powerful shock. Zap. The patient's back muscles contract violently in response, arching the spine and lifting the body into the air. By then the anaesthetist would have a cannula in place and would give a dose of sodium bicarbonate to neutralise the acid in the blood.

In essence there was rarely a heart we couldn't re-start. It would often re-fibrillate in disgust at the abuse, but we would zap it again. More often than not it would have some sort of productive rhythm as it returned to the mattress. That was the moment to leave the battered organ alone to get its act together.

We took pride in restoring the circulation and resurrecting the dead, but it came at a price. Many of the ribs would be dislocated or fractured from the breastbone by then. Were our efforts in time to prevent catastrophic hypoxic brain injury? A result that would condemn the live body to a persistent vegetative state. The statistics tell the story. Only one in four patients survived and the majority had brain damage. Some didn't, however, justifying our efforts. Did our sporting resuscitation team think about the corpse in front of us as a person? That wasn't part of the plan. Someone triggered the resus bleep and we answered the call. We went through the motions, but normally we would never see that patient again. They went off to intensive care, we returned to our own wards. There was none of the post-traumatic stress that contemporary articles describe in regard to resuscitation. Just 'on with the next'.

Perhaps surgeons are inherently different. Certainly the physicians regarded us as an inferior species. I stayed with sick hearts and many of my rugby club mates in the resus team became surgeons too. But now comes the obvious question. If the brain is critically injured by a few minutes of circulatory arrest, how can we possibly perform a complex surgical reconstruction within a sick and irritable heart filled with blood under pressure and in constant rapid motion? There was a solution but it took time. And magnificent men.

The great stimulus towards surgery within the heart occurred during World War II with its penetrating chest injuries and the fellowship between British and American surgeons in Europe as they fought to remove bullets and shrapnel. Cross-fertilisation of ideas between the allies inspired determined young men to return home and pursue more effective surgical solutions for crippling heart deformities. What followed proved epic and shocking for the profession and the layman. Grim Reaper sat on every surgeon's shoulder and the protagonists were labelled as reckless psychopaths. Whilst hidden from the media, many more patients died than survived.

Through both chance and design I became a student, then a colleague of many of the cardiac surgical pioneers on both sides of the Atlantic. Because I found their reminiscences so compelling, I decided to write the definitive textbook on the subject. *Landmarks in Cardiac Surgery* was published in 1997, exactly one hundred years after the first successful repair of a knife wound to the heart in Germany. But stab wounds proved the limit of heart surgery for a further half century and medical treatment was equally primitive. Heart disease remained a death sentence. In his textbook of medicine of 1913, the famous Oxford Professor William Osler summarised the whole of congenital heart disease in four pages. This was his only advice on treatment: 'The child should be warmly clad and guarded from all circumstances liable to cause bronchitis. In the attacks of urgent dyspnoea (shortness of breath) with lividity (blue faces) blood should be let. Saline cathartics are also useful. Digitalis must be used with care; it is sometimes beneficial in the later stages.'

During a career that spanned fifty years I operated on many thousands of sick hearts, more than ten thousand in Oxford alone. Some were tiny and deformed, others huge following months of severe heart failure. Some were fast, some slow, some were fat, some lean. Each different, but in constant rhythmical motion the heart is a mesmerising organ to handle and watch. Guts just wriggle and squirm. Lungs inflate and deflate, but the heart dances. For me it was *Swan Lake* in the chest yet admittedly somewhat faster. I had the privilege to repair it and help the patient towards a better life using techniques developed in my lifetime.

From my personal perspective, the tale of how surgeons strove to operate within the heart ranks as one of the greatest stories ever told. So in these dismal days of 'woke' introspection and defensive medical practice I believe these tales make compelling reading for the general public. From beginning to end the narrative reads like a thriller but with rather more corpses.

The Impossible Dream

Nothing is impossible.
The word itself says, I'm possible.
—Audrey Hepburn

When non-medical visitors enter the cardiac operating theatre and tentatively peer over the drapes, their reaction is always the same. They are riveted by the spectacle of the heart beating in its glistening fibrous sac between the harsh metal blades of the chest spreader. Most linger, mesmerised by its beauty and rhythm. Fascinated to view the colours of contracting muscle and glistening fat set against blood-stained blue drapes. Some try to work out which chamber is which and wonder at the tiny coronary arteries as they snake their way over the surface. Others don't get that far. They swoon in a heap at the anaesthetist's feet or feel faint and excuse themselves, unnerved by the sights and sounds of this unfamiliar environment. And it goes without saying, a proportion of those who choose to watch soon about-face once the blood starts slopping about.

It was a similar experience for most of our trainees. However much general surgery they had under their belts the prospect of having to place their first stitch through the wall of a tense, pulsating aorta or a quivering right atrial appendage was enough to make them piss their pants. The thought of having to cut into those structures, then control the bleeding was even more worrying. That's the way it is. Heart surgery is different and always has been. It needs a certain character to get involved, and inevitably those who made the first tentative steps had little experience of the heart at the time. They were mostly general surgeons but invariably alpha males. Courageous individuals who encountered dire circumstances where lifesaving intervention was needed. Reckless perhaps because the heart was deemed untouchable from the surgical standpoint, a concept only reinforced by failure.

The heart is not an easy organ to access, sitting as it does between the solid breast bone and spine, then encapsulated by ribs and lungs. Integrity of the chest wall is important. Negative pressure is created within the chest cavity when breathing in and that sucks in air and oxygen through the windpipe. Then the ribs recoil and expel the inhaled gas with its by-product carbon dioxide. Should the chest wall be penetrated by a knife, bullet or scalpel, air enters through the hole on inspiration and the lung collapses. This is called a pneumothorax, as a result of which the patient suffers acute breathlessness, becomes distressed, and is in no position to cooperate. In addition, during the first attempts to operate on wounds to the chest there were no anaesthetic drugs. The patients had to have lost sufficient blood to be cerebrally obtunded or plied with enough alcohol to be well and truly out of it, a situation that I fondly recall from my medical school days.

The optimum exposure of the heart from a surgical perspective is through the breast bone, sweeping aside the remnants of the thymus gland and directly opening the fibrous pericardial sac beneath. This avoids entering the pleural cavity and contact with the lungs. In 1897 Herbert Milton of the Kasr El Aini Hospital in Cairo sent an article to the *Lancet* in which he described his sternum splitting incision.

Milton remarked: 'Heart surgery is still in its infancy but it requires not a great stretch of fancy to imagine plastic operations on its valvular lesions.' Ideally the sternotomy approach required a high-speed oscillating saw but it wasn't available in the early days, so a sharp chisel and mallet had to do. Undoubtedly the easier option was a painful incision through the muscle of the left chest wall with wide spreading of the ribs. Horrendously painful for a conscious patient who becomes acutely short of breath when the lung collapses.

Napoleon's legendary military surgeon Baron Dominique Larrey was well accustomed to inflicting pain. On a single day during the Battle of Borodino in 1812 he performed two hundred limb amputations on alcohol-intoxicated but fully awake wounded soldiers and was not perturbed by attempting to open the chest without anaesthetic. One patient, Bernard Sainte-Ogne, was a 30-year-old foot soldier who tried to stab himself in the heart when accused of a crime he did not commit. The left lung and pericardium were both lacerated but he survived since the knife did not penetrate through into a cardiac chamber. The lung collapsed however and infection followed causing pus to fill the chest cavity.

Faced with the soldier's increasing fever and pain, Larrey used embrocation of camphorated oil followed by scarification of the chest wall as counter-irritation. That had little effect as pus then filled the pericardial sac and began to compress the heart. Sainte-Ogne's condition soon deteriorated inexorably with gross swelling of the legs and abdomen as pressure on the right atrium obstructed the venous blood - cardiac tamponade. Patients can actually survive penetrating wounds to the right atrium or ventricle if the pressure around the heart equates with the pressure within the chambers so that haemorrhage stops. That's why we insist it's dangerous to transfuse such patients before surgery which only serves to promote more bleeding.

Having diagnosed compression of the heart Larrey boldly opened the left chest between the fifth and sixth ribs. Fortunately pus in the chest cavity had caused the lung to adhere to the chest wall so it didn't collapse suddenly with devastating effect on his conscious patient. On incising the pericardium a considerable volume of thick creamy green pus squirted out in synchrony with the heartbeat. Success. For the first few days Sainte-Ogne was markedly improved by the operation but then the chest wound became infected and recurrent signs of cardiac compression became apparent. Undaunted, Larrey operated for a second time but there were no antiseptics or antibiotics in those days so infection was destined to win the day. Poor Sainte-Ogne eventually died more than two months after his self-inflicted wound, and wished he'd never bothered.

Three important advances were needed to improve the performance and safety of chest surgery – they were anaesthetics, antiseptics and antibiotics. Larrey had none of these available to him though he noticed that during bitterly cold winters, intense cold seemed to numb the limbs of those needing amputation. That said, pain relief was of little importance to the 'barber' surgeons of the day. In 1839 Alfred Velpeau wrote: 'The avoidance of pain during operations is a fantasy that should not be indulged in. Cutting instruments and pain are inextricably associated with each other in the mind of patients.' And so they were for many years to come.

In Larrey's book *Surgical Experiences in Military Camps*, published in 1829, he described six survivors from wounds involving the pericardial sac, one of which afflicted a 24-year-old soldier. In preparation for the attempted drainage of blood from around the heart Larrey tested his approach on cadavers. Once confident of his strategy he performed removal of dead and infected tissue from the bullet entry wound, then on visualisation of the distended sac he inserted a gum elastic tube through the membrane to drain fluid. Despite the absence of anaesthetic or antiseptic technique the procedure was successful and the young man recovered.

Of course Britain had its own flamboyant surgeons. Known as 'the fastest blade in the West End', Dr Robert Liston reportedly amputated a patient's infected gangrenous leg in less than two minutes. Unfortunately speed came at the price of precision and the limb came away with two of the assistant's fingers. Days later the patient and wounded apprentice both succumbed to rampant streptococcal infection. Worse still a distinguished surgical observer whose codpiece was slashed as the bloodied knife was withdrawn, fainted then suffered a fatal heart attack. That constituted three hundred percent mortality in a single operation which persists as a record today. Operating with bravado for astonished audiences Liston would wave his sharp blade in readiness murmuring 'time me gentlemen, time me!' On other occasions, whilst operating without anaesthetic, he is known to have inadvertently removed a man's testicles during an above knee amputation then incised an aneurysm in a boy's neck mistaking it for a cyst. Rapid exsanguination followed in spectacular fashion. Nonetheless Liston was a resolute gentleman and the most distinguished surgeon of his time. His fast pace reduced deaths from haemorrhage and shock on the operating table, a factor which would ultimately gain importance when operating on the beating heart.

It was not until fifty years later that the term 'Hertztamponade' was coined by a German surgeon with the typically English name of Edmund Rose. Rose wrote a medical paper describing the characteristic findings of cardiac compression by blood clots found in twenty-three wounded patients, several of whom survived without surgery. The conclusion was that heart wounds were not inevitably fatal as previously believed. The first occasion on which a surgeon deliberately operated on an injured heart was in October 1872 at St Bartholomew's Hospital in the East End of London. After a brawl in a public house the 31-year-old tailor experienced sharp pain in the left chest and could not find a splendidly long needle he normally kept in his coat pocket. The first hospital visit was of no help as x-rays were not yet invented. Nine days later severe pain persisted when he moved his left arm, so this time the hospital admitted him and found a discrete puncture wound.

George Callender, a general surgeon, made an incision between the ribs and eventually located the missing needle which had penetrated the pericardium and was embedded in heart muscle close to the apex of the left ventricle. The needle was withdrawn without bleeding. No stitches were needed and the tailor made an uneventful recovery. Nothing was said about it by the modest Callender and the concept that the heart was untouchable persisted. The myth was largely thanks to the undisputed master of abdominal surgery, Theodore Billroth, who at the 1880 meeting of the Vienna Medical Society stated: 'Any surgeon who wishes to preserve the respect of his colleagues would never attempt to suture (stitch) the heart.'

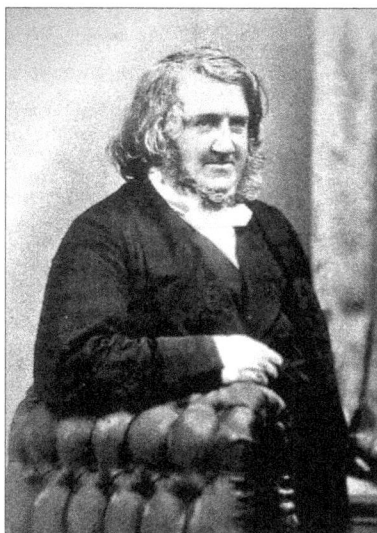

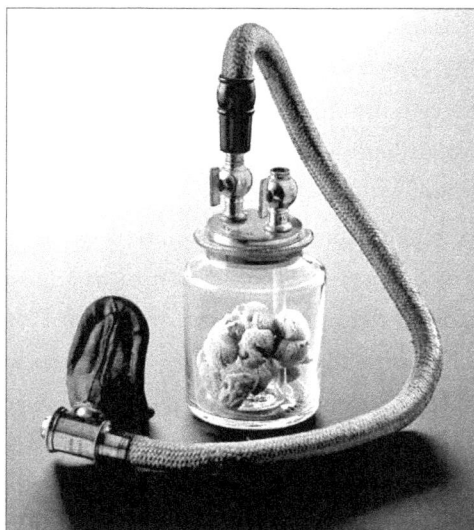

Fig 1.1 A. James Young Simpson. B. The chloroform Inhaler.

Undoubtedly the major advance that promoted surgery as a profession was the advent of anaesthesia. Why? Because the prospect of performing a prolonged and agonisingly painful surgical procedure on a squirming patient was never going to cut it, so to speak. Larrey knew that limb amputations could be performed in minutes but it took several burly assistants to keep the individual still.

Since prehistoric times, alcohol made from fermented fruit juice or grain was used as a sedative to relieve pain. As a medical student I used it on many occasions for toothache or rugby injuries. Herbs such as henbane, deadly nightshade, hemlock, poppy and mandragora were employed in the production of pain-relieving potions and the Chinese surgeon Hua Tuo used the coca-based sedative scopolamine to ease the agony of awake abdominal surgery. An eighth-century manuscript from Monte Casino describes the novel concoction of opium, mangragora, fresh poppy leaves and henbane juice to render patients unconscious. Later in the twelfth century, ivy juice, mulberries, lettuce and sorrel seeds were added to the preparation. Distillation of the combination created a very strong alcoholic liquor which could be soaked up in a sponge, allowed to dry then held over the patient's mouth and nose to render them unconsciousness. Revival was achieved by pouring vinegar into the nostrils. But don't try this at home, however inaccessible health care might seem.

In 1776 the gentleman farmer and chemist Joseph Priestley discovered the gases carbon dioxide and nitrous oxide. At the time a Cornish apothecary Humphrey Davy was in the habit of testing new drugs on himself and discovered that nitrous oxide produced a feeling of euphoria and well-being followed by a migrainous headache. He was nonetheless intrigued that severe pain from a broken tooth soon disappeared on inhaling the gas. There was no practical application of this finding until 1844 when in Hartford, Connecticut a particular fairground entertainment included 'men who could not stop laughing' through breathing nitrous oxide. It happened that a Boston dentist, Horace Wells, was watching the spectacle with a certain amount of disdain when one of the idiots fell from the stage and badly fractured his arm. Wells was intrigued to note that instead of screaming in agony the man burst into uncontrollable laughter somewhat oblivious to the dreadful deformity. And sure enough, laughing gas appeared to relieve the pain of tooth extraction including an intervention on the dentist himself.

Greatly impressed by the discovery Wells arranged a demonstration for neighbouring dentists and surgeons. Sadly, on that occasion the gas was poorly prepared and the disappointed patient roared with pain. When further antics with laughing gas produced mixed and often hilarious results, another Boston dentist William Morton, suggested using the volatile agent, ether, instead. To that end he devised a face mask onto which the liquid ether was poured, causing the vapour to be inhaled.

On October 14th 1846 Morton administered an ether anaesthetic to his patient, Gilbert Abbot, who had a large tumour in his neck.

Abbot lapsed into unconsciousness and remained so whilst the surgeon, John Warren, operated successfully. The following day the technique was repeated for an orthopaedic procedure by Henry Bigelow at Massachusetts General Hospital. The original daguerreotype photograph of the operation still hangs in the Boston Medical Library. General anaesthesia with ether transformed surgical practice, was soon used liberally in the USA and introduced into Europe just two months later.

In November 1847, James Young Simpson, the Professor of Obstetrics in Edinburgh used chloroform vapour for the first time to relieve pain for a woman in labour.

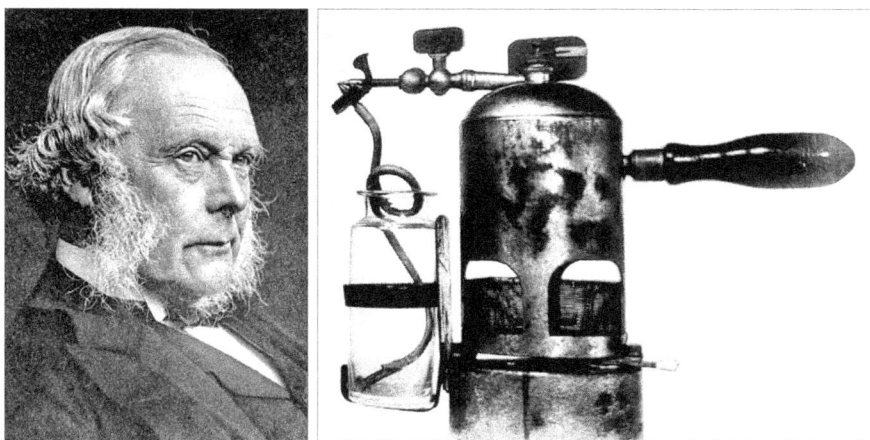

Fig 1.2 A. Joseph Lister. B. Carbolic Acid Diffuser.

Within a month he reported fifty such applications of chloroform in a variety of obstetric procedures causing widespread interest. When Queen Victoria was in an advanced state of pregnancy with her eighth child, Prince Albert was made aware of the benefits of chloroform by the Scottish physician John Snow. The Queen went into labour at Balmoral just two days later, and Snow was summoned as a matter of urgency. Inhaling from a chloroform-soaked handkerchief held over the face, Prince Leopold was born as Victoria lay barely conscious and completely oblivious to pain. This was a complete revelation compared with the noisy previous seven occasions.

News travelled fast and in a couple of weeks both French and English ambulance teams were using chloroform to treat wounded soldiers at the battle of Sebastopol. It was then that the American physician Oliver Wendell Holmes coined the term 'anaesthetic' from the Greek word 'no feeling' – yet all was not straightforward. In January 1848 a 15-year-old girl, Hannah Greener, died suddenly in Newcastle whilst having a toenail removed, and the danger of 'chloroform syncope' became a popular subject for discussion in medical journals. Opinion was divided over the cause. Snow considered heart failure from a toxic concentration of vapour to be the problem whereas Simpson and Joseph Lister suspected respiratory depression to be the fatal element.

Sometimes positive outcomes emerge from adversity. On 3rd July 1849 the surgeon Charles Bleeck removed a cancerous breast from a 42-year-old woman anaesthetised with chloroform. The mastectomy was done in four minutes but with the final slice of the blade the patient appeared to collapse dead onto the floor. Bleeck could not feel a pulse and she was not breathing. There was no response to cold water or ammonia applied to the nose so he instinctively engaged in mouth-to-mouth respiration. On the fourth forceful inspiration the woman gave a convulsive gasp and was revived. Undeterred, the intrepid surgeon proceeded to remove an enlarged lymph node from the axilla during which she roared with pain and complained of his acrid breath. Perhaps that was the ammonia, and whilst this was the first record of resuscitation during anaesthesia, the French *Académie des Sciences* in Paris had recommended mouth-to-mouth resuscitation for drowning victims since 1740.

Soon afterwards an American surgeon James Metcalf presented a similar achievement to the New York Academy of Medicine. 'All at once I applied my lips to those of the patient holding his mouth open with my right hand and closing his nose with my left. I inflated the lungs slowly and gently so as to imitate as much as possible a natural inspiration. After fifteen to twenty breaths the patient gave a feeble gasp and an artery in the surgical wound spurted blood.' Metcalf appropriately recommended artificial respiration for all patients with chloroform syncope, and whilst ether remained preferable on the grounds of safety, chloroform worked faster, seemed more acceptable to the patient and had a lesser somnolent effect on the surgeon.

In time it was apparent that deaths during ether anaesthesia occurred through respiratory depression and responded to crude positive pressure ventilation. In contrast chloroform fatalities were attributed to heart failure and required more spectacular resuscitation efforts. In 1870 Moritz Schiff, the Professor of Physiology in Florence, advocated opening the left chest between the ribs in order to directly massage the heart. He had practised this on dogs. 'One makes rhythmic movements with the hand holding the whole heart,' he wrote. And with remarkable insight for the times Schiff suggested that revival occurred through restoration of coronary blood flow, not just through mechanical stimulation. He even advocated occluding the body's main artery, the abdominal aorta, during cardiac massage so as to ensure that blood was directed preferentially to the brain and heart.

It was another thirty years in 1900 before successful cardiac massage was reported in a patient. On that occasion chloroform had been used to anaesthetise a 43-year-old woman with uterine cancer who at the end of her hysterectomy suffered a cardiac arrest. After unsuccessful mouth-to-mouth respiration the surgeon Christian Igelsond of Tromso, Norway rapidly performed a left thoracotomy and massaged the ventricles between thumb, middle and index fingers. After a minute, with blood flow restored to the heart muscle, the organ stiffened and started to beat. What's more the woman survived the agonising experience with complete recovery.

Two years later in London, Sir William Arbuthnot Lane achieved a second success in a 65-year-old man undergoing bowel surgery. When the heart stopped during ether anaesthesia, Lane thrust his hand into the abdominal incision to compress the heart through the diaphragm and against the breastbone. Together with artificial respiration, that was sufficient to restore the circulation and the patient recovered. The following year, 1903, Dr George Crile reported the first successful use of external cardiac compressions for resuscitation in the United States.

For most of the nineteenth century operations were only undertaken when absolutely necessary, and there was a good reason for that. The link between bacteria and infection had not yet been established. Wound infection with copious pus was considered a normal aspect of the healing process but contributed to exorbitant surgical mortality. So much so that there was talk of actually banning all surgery from many hospitals because of the consequences of sepsis. Sir John Erichsen, President of the Royal College of Surgeons, insisted: 'The abdomen, chest and brain will forever be closed to operations by a wise and humane surgeon.' It was the era when bed linen and laboratory coats were not washed and surgical instruments only cleaned before they were put away for storage. The same metal probe was used to explore pockets of pus in consecutive patients during a ward round. Erichsen believed that inflammation and pus arose from sinister miasmas emanating from the wound itself that became concentrated in the air. He calculated that in a ward of a dozen patients an infected wound in half of them caused saturation of the atmosphere with dangerous gases that caused gangrene. And a gangrenous limb had to come off.

An enthusiastic surgical trainee called Joseph Lister worked for Sir James as a 'dresser'. At just thirty-three years of age, Lister the son of an eminent member of the Royal Society was appointed Professor of Surgery at the University of Glasgow through his early interest and experimentation on inflammation.

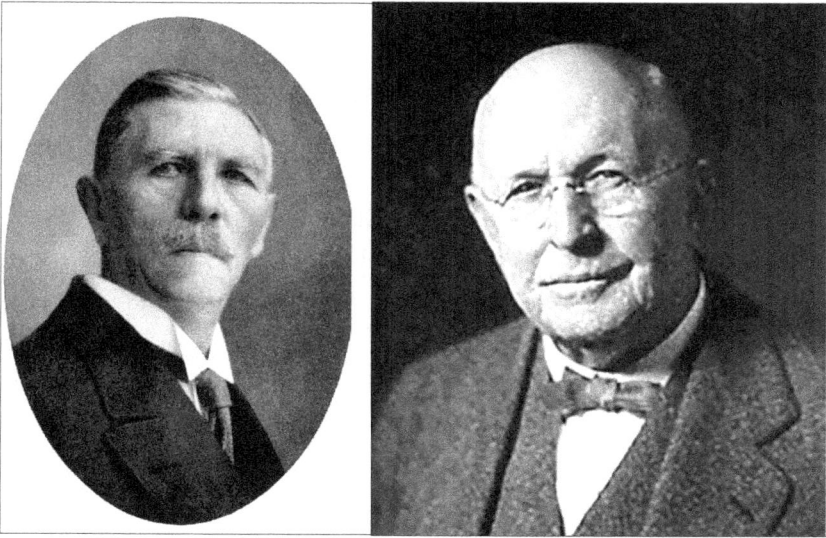

Fig 1.3 A. Ludwig Rehn. B. Luther Hill.

The intellectual breakthrough came when on the advice of the professor of chemistry he read Louis Pasteur's paper *Recherches sur la putrefaction*. This work on the bacterial mechanism of fermentation caused Lister to question whether microorganisms could be involved in the putrefaction of surgical wounds and the development of gangrene after open limb fractures. He postulated that infection occurred through exposure of bone and the subcutaneous tissues to contamination when the protection of the skin was lost, the very issue responsible for a huge difference in survival between patients with open and closed injuries.

Having learned of creosote being used to disinfect sewage Lister applied carbolic acid as an antiseptic agent on skin for the first time. He made efforts to exclude bacteria from the surgical field by cleansing hands and instruments with disinfectant and spraying the air above the operating table. He could then show that it was possible for wounds to heal in the absence of infection which had previously been considered part of the repair process.

In Lister's own words: 'It did not seem right to withhold it longer from the profession generally.'

The findings were originally published in two papers in the *Lancet* in 1867 then discussed at the meeting of the British Medical Association in Dublin that year. He explained to a mesmerised audience that: 'Previous to its introduction (antiseptic technique) the two large wards in which most of my orthopaedic and trauma cases are treated were amongst the unhealthiest in the whole surgical division at the Glasgow Royal Infirmary. Yet since the antiseptic treatment has been brought into full operation my wards have completely changed their character. During the last nine months not a single instance of pyaemia, gangrene or erysipelas has occurred in them.' Just as well, because the discovery of antibiotics was still eighty years away.

Whereas surgeons had previously operated with contaminated, even blood-caked, instruments and topcoats, Lister's principles of aseptic technique rapidly boosted the survival prospects for all surgical patients. Germany led the way followed by the USA and France whilst Britain remained sceptical. Same old story! Perhaps it was a reaction to the fact that Lister was known to be a difficult character. He neglected to share any credit for the discovery with his colleagues, was very much against the introduction of women into surgical practice, and harshly criticised medical teaching south of the border. A typical surgeon from a privileged family who was eventually rewarded with a peerage.

A well-recognised surgical (and general) characteristic is the ability to trumpet success and forget about failures. So it was with the valiant efforts to save patients with wounds to the heart. Some we know about but many we don't. Moreover, suggestions that the romantic fantasy about the heart being 'the seat of the soul' somehow prohibited cardiac surgery are pure nonsense. The fact is that surgeons lacked the confidence to operate on the moving target, as summarised by the American Charles Elsberg: 'We must remember that we have to deal with an organ in constant motion, believed to be very sensitive to the smallest mechanical insult or injury. It was feared that during the slightest manipulation the heart might suddenly stop, that the mere passage of a needle might be followed by the direst of results.' And even before reaching the heart there were problems. Patients having their chests opened were inevitably subject to collapse of the lung with consequent breathing difficulties. So much anaesthetic was needed that the surgeon inhaled a significant dose too.

In 1876 the Hamburg physician Gotthard Bulau began to introduce tubes between the ribs to evacuate collections of blood, air or pus. An important addition to that procedure was the introduction of the underwater seal drainage system which prevented air from entering the chest cavity through the drain. Sitting by the bedside the water-filled bottle allowed intrapleural collections to be evacuated from around the lung without causing collapse and became a standard addition to all chest operations.

In 1895 a young Norwegian surgeon, Axel Cappelen, was confronted with a 24-year-old man who had been stabbed in the left chest. As the patient descended into shock and lost consciousness Cappelen decided that there was nothing to lose by exploring the wound. He soon discovered that the knife had passed through the chest wall beside the breast bone and, on removing the fourth rib, blood spurted through a hole in the pericardium. Beneath was an inch-long laceration of the left ventricle still hosing out briskly with every beat despite the fall in blood pressure. What's more the distal end of a major coronary artery was transected and bleeding separately. Pumped up with his own adrenaline, the intrepid Cappelen proceeded to close the defect with catgut stitches applied carefully into the moving target. Hardly a difficult job but there were no previous cases of successful cardiac suture in the medical literature so he was operating instinctively in stressful circumstances.

Catgut was suited for human guts, but not hearts. Added to that, the tension placed on each knot was critical. It is so easy to overtighten the thread and slice through the traumatised muscle so blood squirts in your face. The heart rhythm would have been disturbed by manipulation and being poked with a needle. Then unfortunately Cappelen had to ligate the squirting coronary artery leaving a substantial area of muscle without a blood supply. There was no blood transfusion in those days so the victim was given an infusion of saline solution to restore the sagging blood pressure. He regained consciousness to the encouragement of his carers, but died of heart failure two days after the operation. Autopsy confirmed a sound closure of the knife wound but revealed an extensive patch of dead muscle in the left ventricle through loss of its blood supply.

Fame eluded Cappelen quite simply because the injury involved a coronary artery. The low-pressure right ventricle is situated directly behind the breast bone and is subject more frequently to stab wounds so it was only a matter of time before someone took the honours. That happened to be the Frankfurt surgeon, Ludwig Rehn. Rehn had already made an important contribution with the astute observation that workers subject to prolonged exposure to the chemical aniline in the dye industry were likely to develop bladder cancer. His trauma patient in September 1896 was a 22-year-old soldier who had been discharged from the army through rheumatic valvular heart disease. During a drunken brawl the man was stabbed directly through the anterior chest wall and into the right ventricle. The wound naturally caused brisk haemorrhage but this slowed as blood accumulated in the pericardium and pressure within the chamber fell. This is a balancing act which often prevents rapid exsanguination in stab wounds, and left Rehn in a 'who dares wins' situation.

Having opened the left chest between the ribs and evacuated a clot from the pericardium, renewed spurting from the defect showed Rehn where his stitches were needed. Just three of them side by side, and the job was done. Encompassing Lister's principles of asepsis, Rehn packed the chest with iodine soaked gauze before closing the incision, and the patient survived. He did develop a collection of pus round the left lung but was known to be alive ten years later.

Did Rehn's success herald the beginning of cardiac surgery as claimed by many historians? Not at all. Over the centuries more patients had survived wounds to the heart without surgery than with it. In his book *Anatomical Observations* published in 1604 Barthelemy Cabrol described a number of hearts examined at autopsy that bore scars from previous penetrating wounds. In Paget's *Surgery of the Chest* published the year after Rehn's triumph, Billroth remained highly sceptical about the repair of cardiac wounds whilst Paget himself advocated 'absolute rest of body and mind, a light diet and in some cases morphine'. If this proved unsuccessful 'the pericardium could be tapped or a small incision made into it to relieve cardiac tamponade'. Of course most of the victims were dead by then.

The first heart operation reported from the United States took place on 14th September 1902. This seems surprisingly late since the American Civil War of the 1860s resulted in some 750,000 deaths, though most occurred through wound infection or dysentery. As it happened the surgeon concerned had trained in Britain with Joseph Lister and, like Rehn, employed his boss's aseptic principles. Luther Hill of Montgomery Alabama was called to the home of a 13-year-old boy who had been stabbed five times in the chest. Hill found him 'gasping for breath, agitated and in shock with barely palpable pulse and inaudible heart sounds'. Recognising cardiac tamponade and in the knowledge of Rehn's success he proceeded to open the left chest under the light of an oil lamp. The best description of events comes from Hill's own article reporting the case in the medical literature.

'The chest wound was about three-eighths of an inch in length and from it came a stream of blood at every systole. I removed the boy from his bed to a table at 1 o'clock at night eight hours after the stabbing and proceeded to cleanse the field of the operation and place the patient in as favourable a condition as my surroundings in the negro cabin would allow. Commencing an incision about half an inch from the left border of the sternum, I carried it along the third rib for four inches. A second incision was started at the same distance and carried along the sixth rib for four inches. A vertical incision along the anterior axillary line was made connecting them. The musculo-osseous flap was raised with the cartilages of the ribs (next to the sternum) acting as the hinges. There was no blood in the pleural cavity, but the pericardium was enormously distended. I enlarged the wound in the pericardium to a distance of two inches and evacuated about ten ounces of blood. The pulse immediately improved (when the tamponade was relieved) as was commented upon by Dr L D Robinson who so successfully and skilfully administered the chloroform. I had my brother Dr R S Hill pass his hand into the pericardial cavity and bring the heart upwards and at the same time steady it sufficiently for me to pass a catgut suture through the centre of the wound in the heart and control the haemorrhage. I cleansed the pericardial sac with a saline solution and closed the opening in it with seven interrupted catgut sutures. The pleural cavity was also cleansed with a saline solution and drained with iodoform gauze.

The operation lasted forty-five minutes. The patient's pulse on reaching his bed was 145 and respiration 56. I injected strychnine hypodermically and employed autotransfusion. On 17th September he commenced to improve and his recovery has been uninterrupted.'

The paper in *Medical Record*, November 29th 1902, also presents a table of thirty-seven other reported cases of emergency surgery for cardiac wounds worldwide between 1896 and 1902 with eleven survivors. Hill concluded that 'any operation which reduces certain mortality by almost 30% is entitled to a permanent place in surgery'. And that 'every wound of the heart should be operated upon immediately'. This was an optimistic departure from Billroth and Paget, yet little changed until World War II. Heart surgery remained on hold pending further improvements in anaesthesia, diagnosis and the management of infection.

Wilhelm Roentgen, Professor of Physics at the University of Würzburg discovered x-rays completely by chance.

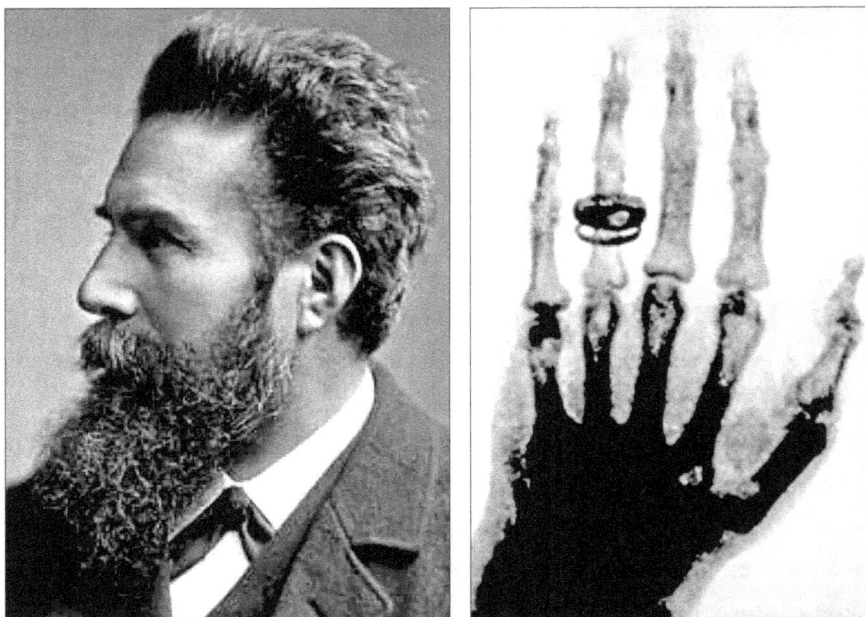

Fig 1.4 A. Wilhelm Roentgen. B. First X-ray ever taken showing his wife's hand.

They were named x-rays through the uncertain nature of the discharge from a cathode ray tube that could pass through the tissues and leave an image on a photographic plate. The first radiological image of a human limb was that of his wife's hand wearing her wedding ring on 29th November 1895. The revelation had a profound effect on the medical world and Roentgen received the Nobel Prize. The first occasion x-rays were used in a diagnostic context was the following year when a drunken sailor was admitted to a London hospital with a knife in his back. He was paraplegic and the x-ray taken of the spine showed the tip of the blade wedged between two vertebrae, encroaching on the spinal canal. After surgery to remove the offending object, the paraplegia resolved.

In 1903 the French surgeon Theodore Tuffier used x-rays to locate a bullet in the chest of a wounded soldier. Already an advocate of thoracotomy for internal cardiac massage, Tuffier identified the missile within the bounds of the heart shadow, and operated to find it amidst inflammatory fibrinous adhesions within the pericardium. The heart itself had not been injured and he was able to remove it with a finger, so the man made an uneventful recovery.

The electrocardiogram emerged at the turn of the century when Willem Einthoven of Leiden modified a string galvanometer and connected electrodes to the chest wall to detect the electrical impulses from the heart. He identified the characteristic P, Q, R and S waves in 1903 and found many changes in the pattern in patients with heart disease. An ink-writing polygraph was coupled with the galvanometer to study the mechanism of heartbeat and rhythm disorders, though it was not until 1919 that the physician James Herrick described the electrocardiographic changes of coronary thrombosis and heart attack in a patient. Conveniently an autopsy confirmed the association soon afterwards.

Imaging within the heart and blood vessels was not far behind, ironically initiated by a urologist. Werner Forssmann's intention was to insert tubes into the bloodstream as a method to deliver stimulant drugs during an emergency on the operation table. What was available to him was a ureteric catheter which he would normally pass through the bladder up into the tube draining the kidney. Having easily reached the right atrium via the arm veins of a cadaver he engaged the help of an assistant with the purpose of catheterising himself. When the assistant's nerve failed, Forssmann proceeded to cut down on a vein in his own left elbow and threaded the fine tube through a wide-bore needle into the bloodstream. Using a mirror positioned so that he could watch the x-ray screen himself, he manipulated the catheter through his arm into the right heart then walked upstairs to the hospital x-ray department to confirm his achievement.

Two years later Forssman obtained a water-soluble iodine contrast medium which he used successfully to image blood vessels in dogs. Unfortunately things didn't go as well when he tried it on himself and suffered a near-fatal allergic reaction. It was 1938 before radiologists in New York used an iodized contrast medium to image the right heart chambers and blood vessels to the lungs. What we call 'angiography' of the left heart chambers and major arteries soon followed providing a tremendous impetus towards investigative cardiology and planned surgical procedures.

One of the most important developments in anaesthesia was the concept of reversible muscle paralysis with curare. This enabled control of breathing through rhythmic inflation of the lungs and in 1910 was combined with insertion of a tracheal tube directly into the windpipe. An instrument called a laryngoscope was designed to visualise the vocal chords and the new method was popularised during World War I when the British anaesthetists, Magill and Rowbotham used endotracheal intubation and positive pressure ventilation for Sir Harold Gillies's plastic surgery patients. With badly-burned or wounded faces, head and neck reconstructive surgery often took many hours, so anaesthesia by face mask was clearly unsuitable.

The next piece in the jigsaw was the emergence of antibiotics, an event that radically changed the whole of medical practice. Penicillin was discovered through a random observation in 1928 when the bacteriologist Alexander Fleming was growing staphylococci bacteria on a culture medium at St Mary's Hospital in London.

The Petri dishes had been left on a workbench for three weeks in the summer whilst his staff went on holiday. Somehow they became contaminated with a mysterious mould, the spores of which had entered through the laboratory window. When Fleming returned he saw that the colonies of staphylococci in contact with the mould had been killed. Whatever the nature of the invader it had the ability to destroy a dangerous source of infection. Out of curiosity Fleming grew more of the mould which he named Penicillium. He then introduced it to other bacteria including streptococci, pneumococci, gonococci, meningococci, and the diphtheria bacillus each of which was responsible for a huge number of fatalities each year. In each case the bacterial colonies were destroyed by contact with penicillin but when given to healthy animals it seemed harmless.

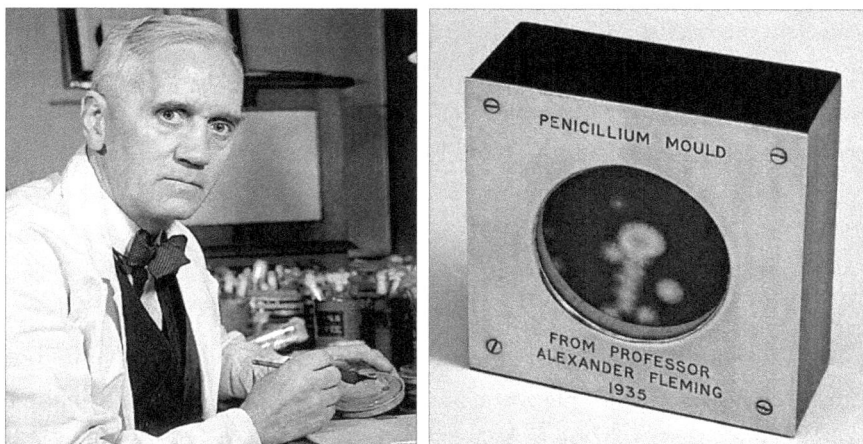

Fig 1.5 A. Alexander Fleming. B. An original Petri Dish.

Eventually Fleming became frustrated by the inability to isolate the active component from the mould and when he mixed it with blood in the test tube the bactericidal effect seemed to disappear. Having written one brief paper on the subject in 1929 he abandoned his investigations, as a result of which many thousands of patients continued to die from simple surgical infections.

And so to Oxford. In 1937 Howard Florey, a bright young Australian graduate, was appointed head of the Dunn School of Pathology. Florey had a keen interest in combating sepsis as war broke out and he hired a Jewish biochemist Ernest Chain who had fled from Nazi Germany. Scouring the literature they discovered Fleming's original report, obtained a sample of penicillin and resumed investigations into its mechanism of action. But it wasn't going to be easy. They experienced the same difficulty in separating the active substance from the mould since less than one part in two million was pure penicillin. Nonetheless a biochemist in the team, Norman Heatley did succeed in purifying it and in May 1940 it was tested for the first time in the laboratory.

Eight mice were infected with a lethal dose of streptococcus bacteria, four of which were then given penicillin by injection. The following day the treated mice were all well and the untreated already dead. It was black and white. The overwhelming importance of the experiment was clear to the Oxford team and on August 24th 1940 they published the manuscript *Penicillin as a chemotherapeutic agent* in the *Lancet*. The potential for penicillin's use in war wounds was readily apparent to Florey, Chain and Heatley who proceeded to produce as much mould as they could in hospital bed pans.

The first human patient to receive penicillin was Elva Ackers, a woman dying from cancer who nobly volunteered to take the first dose. She suffered only minor skin irritation due to impurities after the injection, but no other side effects. Soon afterwards Albert Alexander, a 43-year-old policeman, was dying from cellulitis and sepsis after a simple scratch from a rose thorn. He was given 200mg of penicillin initially followed at three-hourly intervals by a further 100mg. Within 24 hours he experienced a dramatic fall in temperature and general improvement in his moribund condition. Tragically he relapsed and died days later when supplies of the antibiotic ran out despite the team isolating the penicillin from his urine and reusing it. The second infected recipient, a boy of 15 with septicaemia, responded rapidly to treatment and survived.

Encouraged by that first success the team worked tirelessly to produce the drug but staggeringly no funding was forthcoming from the British pharmaceutical industry or the Government. In despair Florey and Heatley crossed the Atlantic and approached the US Government. Soon penicillin manufacture was funded along the same lines as the atomic bomb. Heatley stayed in America where penicillin was produced in sufficient quantities to treat the war wounded. Curiously, Fleming, who had taken no interest in the Oxford work, requested some penicillin from Florey to treat a dying friend. When the man recovered the circumstances were reported in *The*

Times which naturally recounted Fleming's original finding, and implied that he alone was responsible for the wonder drug. Eventually Fleming, Florey and Chain shared the Nobel Prize for their work whilst Heatley was left out in the cold. More antibiotics appeared rapidly and transformed the outlook for bacterial infection.

Wounds of the heart and profuse blood loss go together like strawberries and cream. So for many patients survival depended upon replenishing their circulatory volume. Blood transfusion as we know it began in 1818 when the British Obstetrician James Blundell transfused a woman bleeding after childbirth with blood from her husband. Aspirating an estimated '4 ounces' from the man's arm with a syringe Blundell injected the blood directly into the wife who happily survived. Spurred on by success he repeated the initiative on ten more occasions, judging the process to be beneficial in five. Blood groups were not recognised in those days so there was no such thing as cross matching.

Blundell's pioneering work in obstetrics was followed by a hiatus until the physician Samuel Armstrong Lane at St George's Hospital, began to use whole blood transfusion to treat haemophilia. Again the efforts were successful but no one cared to follow. On the contrary, and perhaps through disasters with blood, physicians in the US began to transfuse milk into bleeding patients. Milk was taken from cows, goats and even women and proved a bloody, or should we say, milky disaster. The process inevitably created severe and often fatal adverse reactions, so in 1884 milk was replaced by salt solution.

In 1900, the Austrian physician Karl Landsteiner identified three blood types which he named groups A, B and C. This was a hugely important though not definitive finding that was revised soon afterwards changing blood type C to group O. Group AB was then characterised after which Landsteiner received the Nobel Prize for his work in 1930. It was Reuben Ottenberg in New York who recognised the inheritance of blood groups within families, identified the universal utility of group O donors, and went on to perform the first transfusion to employ blood typing and careful crossmatching. Cross matching was an enormous contribution which enabled high-volume blood transfusion and greatly increased the safety of trauma resuscitation and complex surgery especially on the heart.

Premature clotting before the donor blood could enter the recipient's circulation remained a serious problem until Richard Lewisohn incorporated the anticoagulant solution sodium citrate. Blood could then be stored in a refrigerator rather than needing to perform direct transfusion from donor to patient. But despite this being an important step it took another decade before sodium citrate was generally accepted. Glucose was then added to the citrate solution and further prolonged the safety of storage for several days after collection. As a result blood banks were established and were used by the British army during World War I. The first hospital blood bank was introduced at the Cook County Hospital in Chicago in 1937 after which the system was rolled out throughout the USA. Landsteiner then defined the Rhesus blood type and recognised it as the cause of most adverse reactions during transfusion.

In 1940 Edwin Cohn, Professor of Biological Chemistry at Harvard Medical School, developed a process to break down blood plasma into separate components. Termed cold ethanol fractionation it allowed the molecules, albumin, gamma globulin and fibrinogen to be isolated and made available for patient use. These steps forward held critical importance during World War II when the United States government established a nationwide appeal for the collection of blood. In response the English chest surgeon Charles Drew of St George's Hospital organised a 'Plasma for Britain' initiative to ship blood and plasma across the Atlantic then on to the European theatre of war. With the help of the American Red Cross more than 13 million units of blood were acquired and used to rescue wounded soldiers after D-Day.

During the Japanese attack on Pearl Harbour, when blood for transfusion ran out, the prominent Philadelphia surgeon Isidor Ravdin treated shock with albumen solution injected directly into the blood stream. There it has a powerful osmotic effect to absorb fluid from surrounding tissues into the blood stream to help sustain pressure. Of course red blood cells were needed to carry oxygen but blood stored in breakable glass bottles proved problematic in a war zone. It wasn't until 1950 that plastic bags were adopted for blood collection and transfusion following which hospital blood banks were created in Britain and Europe. And no specialty would require more blood than cardiac surgery.

During World War II the American military manual *A guide to therapy for medical officers* provided a bland and somewhat optimistic treatment of suspected cardiac wounds. First 'aspirate blood from the pericardium by the costoxiphoid route if possible'. Next 'repeat if there is a recurrence'. And lastly 'if it recurs again perform surgical drainage through an extrapleural exposure'. This essentially cautioned the operator against precipitating collapse of a lung. Dr Paul Samson of the Second Auxiliary Surgical Group in France declared cardiac tamponade to be unusual ostensibly because of the large missile holes in the pericardium. And in reality most casualties died from a cardiac wound. Those that reached a medical centre were not generally diagnosed before opening the chest since tamponade by blood clots had already arrested the bleeding. Of course there was no pre-hospital transfusion to blow the clots off, and even in the middle of the twentieth century most surgeons remained reluctant to place a stitch in a beating heart. Except one that is.

Curiously enough cardiac surgery began in the Cotswold countryside not far from my own home in Woodstock. Some fifteen miles west of Oxford, across the border in Gloucestershire, the historic Stowell Park estate was home to a huge American military hospital. With its own airstrip, the make-do facility was assembled to receive the thousands of casualties from the D-Day landings and the subsequent Operation Overlord, the battle for Normandy in 1944.

The 160th General Hospital of the US Army consisted of hundreds of metal Quonset huts built on a brick base to house wards, operating theatres and basic intensive care units for the treatment of chest injuries. At peak occupation the site housed more than 500 wounded patients with operations undertaken round the clock. On D-Day alone 4,414 British and American soldiers were killed and more than 5,000 injured. Many were flown in to the nearby air force bases at Brize Norton and Little Rissington.

Dwight Harken, a 34-year-old Harvard graduate had trained at the Brompton Hospital with the leading thoracic surgeon Arthur Tudor Edwards.

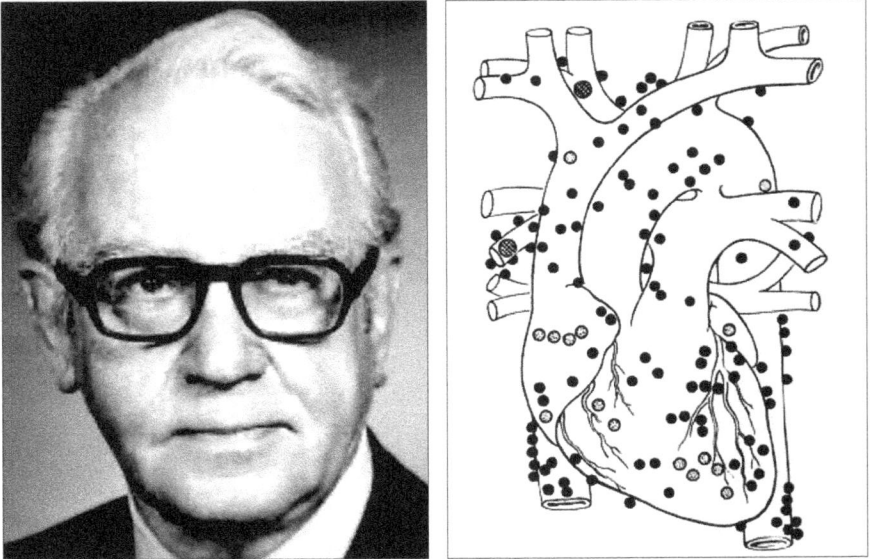

Fig 1.6 A. Dwight Harken. B. Diagram from his publication showing the sites of bullets and shrapnel removed from soldiers' chests.

A tall muscular American football player, he was supported by the experienced anaesthetist Charles Burstein together with generous supplies of penicillin, an x-ray machine and unlimited bottles of blood for transfusion. Nevertheless the operating facilities were primitive. The table sat in the centre of a poorly-insulated metal hut with a corrugated iron roof heated by a small stove in the winter but stiflingly hot under the sun in the summer. The ether anaesthetic gas and odour of antiseptics pervaded a room without air conditioning. Even the lighting was poor. That makes it even more remarkable that he could operate upon 134 patients with bullets or shrapnel in or around the heart without a single death. Dim operating theatre, bright surgeon fortunately.

News of Harken's daring operations in the countryside caused considerable interest around the London hospitals. This prompted delegations of thoracic surgeons, including his old mentor Tudor Edwards to journey out to Gloucestershire to watch him. The case chosen for the first gathering was not an enviable one. The patient, Leroy Rohrbach, was an infantry sergeant who had survived a wound to the chest during the battle for the town of

Saint Lo, shortly after D-Day. Following evacuation to England his chest x-ray revealed a piece of shrapnel situated within the boundaries of the heart's shadow. The Americans at Stowell Park had a new technique known as stereoscopic radiography whereby two images could be combined to give a 3-dimensional picture. So-called fluoroscopy provided moving images to indicate whether a foreign body was being buffeted by the bloodstream within a cardiac chamber. Mobile foreign bodies had the potential to be swept on through the circulation with unpredictable results. And in this case the fluorescent screen showed the inch-long metal fragment to be bobbing around with each heartbeat.

Before the demonstration on 19th February 1945 Harken had already operated on Rohrbach twice in an attempt to remove it but failed when he could not grip the fragment securely within the tips of his forceps. That made it all the more surprising that he should make a third attempt before a distinguished audience. The evening before surgery Harken wrote to his wife explaining his gamble on the reoperation. 'If I kill this man I shall be regarded as foolhardy rather than bold and heart surgery could be set back decades. If I succeed heart surgery may well be on its way.'

Cleary he was determined to make it a success since a film cameraman was perched on a scaffold above the operating table ready to record the procedure for posterity. Harken re-entered the left chest through the previous healed incision and used a Tudor Edwards rib spreader designed by his old boss to expose the heart itself. From the fluoroscopy he expected to find the foreign body resting on the diaphragmatic aspect of the right ventricle because it was too large to pass through the pulmonary valve to the lungs. Sure enough, by palpating the muscle he could feel it within the chamber but to extract it successfully would require a sizeable incision. For safety therefore he inserted two 'purse-string' sutures into the ventricular wall with which his assistant could quickly pull closed the hole to stem the bleeding once the shrapnel was out.

What else might go wrong besides bleeding? The cutting and manipulations might fibrillate the irritable organ and as yet there were no defibrillators. It would be two more years before the emergence of the defibrillator and its application to the heart of a surgical patient. Moreover it took ten years after that in 1957 before an alternating current system was introduced for closed-chest defibrillation. Consequently Burstein's eyes were firmly fixed on the ECG monitor in order to warn Harken of rhythm disturbances.

For an anxious moment all was quiet in that cold Quonset hut they euphemistically called an operating theatre. Then with his left index finger pressing firmly on the metal Harken cut into the right ventricle, introduced a more robust pair of forceps and fastened them around the missile. Pulling gently but firmly the fragment emerged through the muscle followed by a gush of dark red blood and a run of ectopic beats. As Harken described it in the follow-up letter to Anna that same night: 'Suddenly with a pop, as if a champagne cork had been drawn, the fragment jumped out of the ventricle aided by the pressure within the chamber. Blood poured out in a torrent. What's more tightening the purse string sutures didn't close the incision. No matter. A finger on the hole stopped it and bleeding was controlled with a back-up stitch.' The crucial part of the procedure was over in three minutes leaving the distinguished audience mightily impressed. Unfortunately in haste the needle had sewn his rubber glove into the incision too. No matter. Harken and Burstein were ecstatic by then.

Word spread about the courageous young American who made heart surgery look simple. And sure enough surgeons back home could watch and be amazed by the film recording at cardiological conferences. Cardiac surgery had arrived, the organ was no longer off limits and British surgeons wanted to be part of it. Harken went on to become Chief of Thoracic Surgery at Peter Bent Brigham Hospital, Boston and Professor of Surgery at Harvard Medical School. Reflecting on his adventures in Europe he wrote: 'Before World War II I had marvelled at the work of Drs Whipple, Cutler, Churchill, Graham and Mr Tudor Edwards of London, among others. I was confounded by their reluctance to touch, even retract the heart. Some had flirted with the idea of intracardiac surgery, but most efforts were simply pericardiectomy for constrictive pericarditis. When I saw that largely mechanical heart with uniflow valves I wondered about the reluctance of these master surgeons to touch it. It seemed incomprehensible that we surgeons who are technically minded, should not attack this significantly mechanical organ.'

Of course, had the manipulations fibrillated the soldier's heart causing him to die on the operating table, history would have judged the events differently. As it was the 'who dares wins' cliché proved repetitive throughout the pioneering stage of the specialty.

The official report on British surgery in World War II testifies to Harken's 'outstanding success, daring interventions and brilliant results which constitute one of the most striking chapters of surgical achievement in any war'. In that context perhaps the last word should go to Dominique Larrey who said: 'It is necessary to begin always with the most dangerously injured without regard to rank or distinction.' Not an easy principle to follow in his day, yet one that still defines medical ethics.

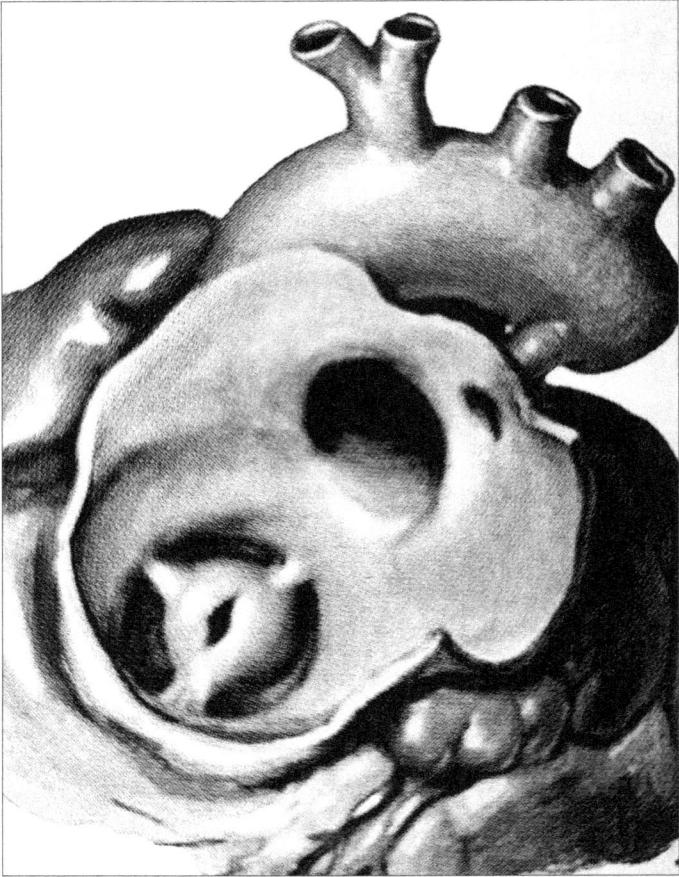

Fig 2.1 Pulmonary valve stenosis with patent ductus arteriosis
between the pulmonary artery and aorta.

Save the Children

Do what you feel in your heart to be right – for
you'll be criticised anyway. You'll be damned if
you do, and damned if you don't.
—Eleanor Roosevelt

Prospective parents are understandably desperate for their child to be born normal, that nothing should shorten their lives nor render them miserable. Sadly destiny does not lie in the stars, it is determined by the genes in every cell. And one in a hundred or thereabouts will be born with a congenital heart defect; likely to preclude a happy life. Or life at all for that matter.

The scope of congenital heart defects is considerable. The simplest includes a persistent ductus arteriosus, the tubular connection between aorta and pulmonary artery. Then a narrowing of the aorta called coarctation, an isolated narrowing of the valve to the lungs called pulmonary stenosis, and a hole between the heart's collecting chambers, atrial septal defect.

Infants may survive into adult life with few symptoms with these simpler defects, though problems will eventually emerge. In contrast more complex deformities such as tetralogy of Fallot, double outlet right ventricle transposition of the great arteries, pulmonary atresia or hypoplastic left heart syndrome may cause death within hours of birth when the ductus arteriosus closes naturally. All told around half of all children with congenital heart disease die within two years if left untreated. I know the misery these deformities cause because I have operated on all of them.

Congenital heart disease is perhaps the only domain of cardiac surgical heritage that wasn't dominated exclusively by the alpha male. The first expert in the field was a fine Canadian lady who was declined a medical school place at McGill University because the institution didn't accept women. Maude Abbott subsequently graduated from Montreal's Bishop's College then spent three years in Europe studying pathology. On return to Canada she was offered the post of assistant curator of the McGill University Medical Museum which she soon found unsatisfying. In an attempt to improve matters, she set out for Baltimore and the Johns Hopkins Hospital to consult with William Osler, the most respected physician of his time. Osler encouraged Abbott to make a comprehensive study of inherited cardiac defects resulting in her *Atlas of Congenital Heart Disease* based on one thousand autopsy specimens she sought out in mortuaries and museums. He praised her efforts as 'the very best thing ever written on the subject' and asked her to contribute the congenital heart disease chapter for his next textbook. Undoubtedly her work did much to improve the understanding of the range and complexity of inherited cardiac deformities.

One of Osler's principal contributions was the recognition of the platelet as the third blood cell together with its role in clotting and blood vessel thrombosis. He had several notable aphorisms used in his teaching including 'Medicine is learned at the bedside not in the classroom', then 'a physician who treats himself has a fool for a patient'. Yet perhaps his most telling quote was that 'In science credit goes to the man who convinces the world, not the man to whom the idea first occurred', best exemplified in the giants of cardiac surgery and particularly pertinent in the emergence of the 'blue baby' operations. The widely-employed term 'ward round' emanated from the bedside teaching of Osler with his surgical colleague William Halsted around the famous circular building at Johns Hopkins.

Osler relocated to Oxford in 1905 having been officially invited to do so by Prime Minister Balfour. That surprised and dismayed his colleagues at Hopkins with whom he had previously joked: 'Do you think I am sufficiently senile to become Regius Professor in Oxford?' Meanwhile Abbott had a friend and soulmate in the cardiologist Helen Taussig at McGill.

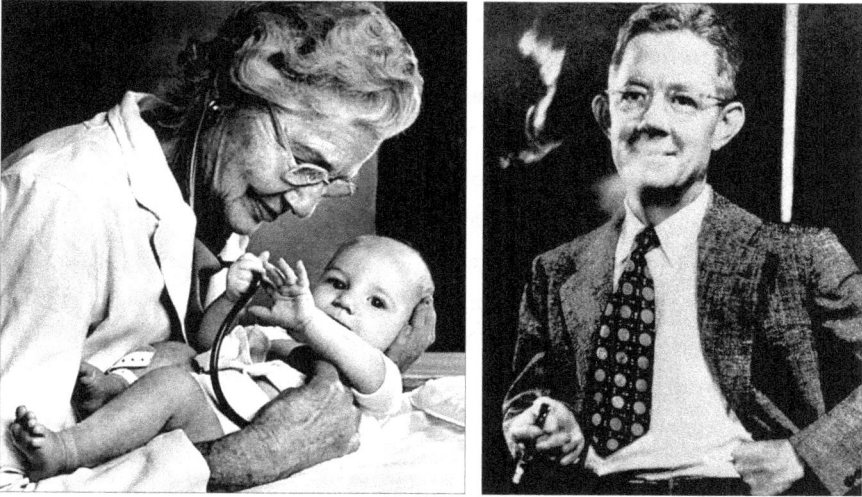

Fig 2.2 A. Dr Helen Taussig caring for one of her young patients with congenital heart disease. B. Alfred Blalock.

As a woman Taussig had similarly been refused admission to read medicine at Harvard, registering instead at Boston University. Here the Professor of Anatomy handed her a cow's heart to study advising that it would do 'no harm to be interested in one of the larger organs of the body'. After graduation he encouraged his bright female student to apply for a post at Johns Hopkins where she was eventually put in charge of the Harriet Lane Children's clinic. There she committed to taking an ECG and fluoroscopy of every young patient born with a heart defect.

The surgeon Richard Bing wrote of Taussig: 'She really understood the anatomy of congenital cardiac malformations. Her hearing was seriously impaired from an early age so the stethoscope was not her forte. Under the fluoroscope however she could see the anatomy very clearly and could correlate it with her profound knowledge of pathology.' Seeing many blue babies and infants for whom there was no treatment, she gradually defined the clinical, radiologic and electrocardiographic profile for tetralogy of Fallot, the most common category of cyanotic children. She noticed that among this group, those who had continuous heart murmurs through a ductus arteriosus that failed to close, were significantly less blue than the others. So what is the significance of the ductus arteriosus?

In the womb the lungs of the foetus are airless with oxygen delivered from the mother by the placenta. Within the baby itself bloodflow bypasses the developing lungs through two temporary channels, a hole or 'foramen ovale', between the right and left atrium, and the ductus arteriosus between the pulmonary artery and the aorta which then distributes the blood around the body. The existence of the ductus arteriosus was known to the Roman physician Galen in the first century AD. In his book of human anatomy he states 'the ductus joining the aorta to the pulmonary artery not only ceases to grow after birth when all other parts of the animal are growing, but it can be seen to become thinner and thinner until as time progresses it dries up and completely wears away'. Should it not close the lungs may be flooded and the pressure in the pulmonary circulation is too high. That is why surgeons need to close it.

In March 1937 a sick febrile 22-year-old woman was admitted to Johns Hopkins with a virulent bacterial infection on a patent ductus arteriosus. At the time, thanks to Osler, it was widely believed that congenital heart defects were more susceptible to endocarditis than normal hearts. What's more, in pre-penicillin times such infection within the heart or blood vessels could never be cured and would invariably prove fatal. With little to lose, the surgeon, John Streider, reasoned that if the ductus could be closed surgically the infection would have the chance to resolve through the body's own defences.

Positive pressure ventilation of the lungs had not been introduced as yet but the bold Streider opened the young woman's left chest widely and closed the ductus with a series of plicating stitches. Great operation – but the poor woman died five days later! The cause of death was said to be acute dilatation of the stomach which probably occurred through damage to the vagus nerve which supplies the abdominal organs and passes close to the ductus in the chest. Unlucky, but the principle was sound.

The next attempt occurred the following year at the Boston Children's Hospital. Robert Gross was an ambitious young surgical resident who spent many hours in the autopsy room and worked out a method to simply ligate the tube with a braided silk ligature. The patient, a 7-year-old girl had been referred to his distinguished boss William Ladd by the Rheumatic Fever clinic, but the man himself refused to consider surgery. Ladd's precise instructions to his chief resident as he left for the summer vacation were: 'Don't try to operate on that little girl's patent ductus. She will die.'

Gross was one of eight children born in Baltimore and mechanically gifted. So much so that he dismantled the engine of the family car at the age of twelve. When his father found the pieces strewn around the garage floor he ordered Robert to restore the working engine before the following morning – which he did. Later in life Gross kept a tool chest of his own in his operating theatre which was painted gold by his nurses. He used it to fix the lights, the autoclave and the squeaking door. His interest in the cardio-vascular system stemmed from reading the brain surgeon Harvey Cushing's biography of Sir William Osler given to him as a Christmas present at medical school. Cushing had operated on Osler's son Edward after he was seriously wounded in Flanders during World War I. The lad did not survive and Osler never recovered from the loss. Seemingly it was a small world at the medical coal-face, and Gross was keen to join the club.

Irrespective of the warning not to interfere with the child, Gross went ahead and operated on 26th August, successfully closing the ductus with a ligature. The girl recovered uneventfully, and Gross and his junior resident colleagues were out celebrating when they by chance encountered Ladd in the city. Ladd asked Gross 'anything new Bob?' The laconic chief resident replied, 'nothing much'. When visited by the patient decades later in his retirement home in New York State Gross laughed with her and said 'you know Lorraine, if you hadn't made it, I would have ended up here in Vermont as a farmer'. I know just how he felt. The first successful surgical cure of bacterial endocarditis on a ductus arteriosus was then achieved by one of my old bosses Oswald Tubbs at the Brompton Hospital in December 1939.

Helen Taussig was energised to hear about the operations on the ductus for one good reason. She already visualised the creation of an artificial ductus to boost blood flow to the lungs in cyanosed infants. Accordingly she set out for Boston to ask Gross whether he might consider this. Surprisingly given the significance of the procedure he declined outright. Taussig subsequently wrote: 'It was extremely fortunate for me when Alfred Blalock was appointed Professor of Surgery as he was a known vascular surgeon.'

Blalock had spent his internship at Johns Hopkins in the early 1920s but when he was not appointed chief resident, he moved to Vanderbilt University. In the laboratory there he experimentally reproduced the condition pulmonary hypertension (high blood pressure in the lungs) by relocating the artery to the left arm to provide high pressure and flow in the pulmonary artery. When his research eventually led to the Professorship at Hopkins, Blalock discussed this shunt procedure as an option to bypass the aortic narrowing known as coarctation. But Taussig immediately suggested the artificial ductus approach to boost lung blood flow in tetralogy of Fallot. Whilst watching Blalock ligate a patent ductus in the operating theatre one morning she remarked: 'The truly great day will be when you create a ductus for a baby dying of hypoxia, not when you close one for a child with too much blood going to the lungs.'

Blalock saw merit in the proposal but was cautious. He wanted to test the concept first and perfect the approach in the laboratory. Did he have time to do that himself as head of the department? Not really, but he knew a man who could.

Vivien Thomas was the Afro-American grandson of a slave in Louisiana. In an era when institutional racism was the norm in the Deep South, Thomas attended the local high school in Nashville, graduating with honours in 1930. He really wanted to study medicine but given his ethnicity and background he understood that there was no chance for an appropriate university place. Instead he secured a post as laboratory assistant in Blalock's laboratory at Vanderbilt University, where he worked on shock and learned anatomy and physiology on the job.

Though he rapidly mastered the vascular surgical techniques needed for Blalock's animal work he could only be paid as a janitor.

Frankly, Thomas was a much better technical surgeon than Blalock who insisted that he move with him to Baltimore. Within weeks the young man was charged with the task of creating a dog model of pulmonary stenosis and then correcting the condition with a man-made ductus arteriosus as Taussig had suggested. This required meticulous surgical dissection then faultless vascular stitching but after two years and two hundred dogs there was sufficient confidence in the group that the procedure was safe and effective. That said, it was difficult to perform in the dog and would prove even more taxing in a small child.

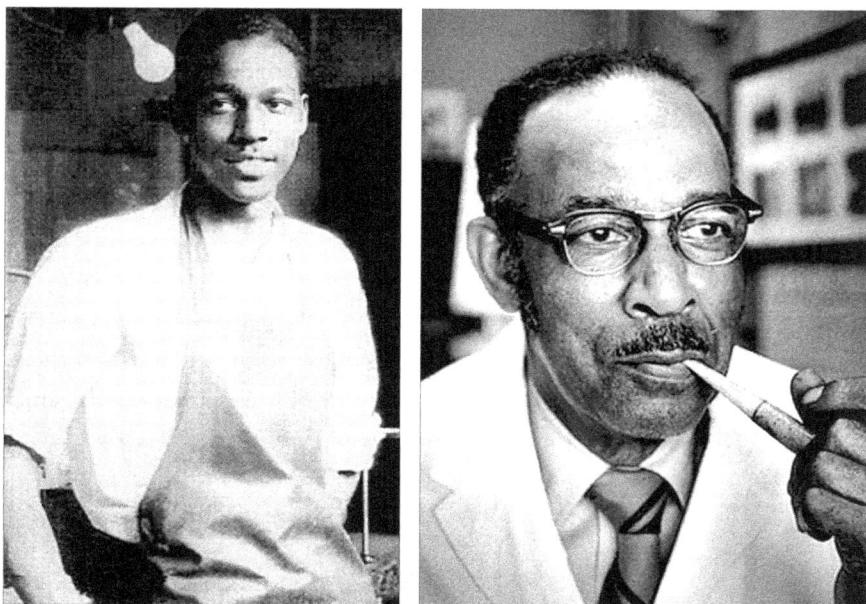

Fig 2.3 A. The young Vivien Thomas in Blalock's laboratory at Vanderbilt University before the move to Johns Hopkins. B. Thomas in his vintage.

It was a grey November day in 1944 when the disconsolate Blalock summoned his chief resident William Longmire to the office. He was sitting behind a desk in his pinstripe suit smoking a cigarette as he did forty times each day. 'I want to show you a patient Dr Taussig wants us to operate on,' said the boss. 'She's on the third floor in the children's ward.' But why so downcast? Over the past months he had attempted a number of innovative abdominal operations on sick adults but many of them had died. He was now being pushed to attempt another complex procedure but was already encountering opposition. Moreover he wasn't very confident with microvascular surgery himself.

Little Eileen Saxon lay in an oxygen tent panting for breath. At fifteen months she had been born with tetralogy of Fallot at Hopkins but her life was coming to an end. Her face was grey with blue lips, her fingers and toes a deep shade of purple. This was the natural history of tetralogy and other conditions with obstructed blood flow to the lungs where a hole in the heart shunts blue deoxygenated blood into the left ventricle and around the body. Half of these children would not live to see their third birthday.

Longmire's instinct told him the child would not survive the anaesthetic never mind an operation on the chest where the left lung would collapse. The senior anaesthetist Austin Lamont had already suggested as much and declined to participate. That was why Blalock had concerns about attempting his new operation on such a desperate case. But the parents wanted him to try and Taussig was pressing him. What was there to lose? The little girl was on a steep downward trajectory anyway.

The evening before the fateful operation even Thomas was fretting. 'I don't think I'll go,' he told a technician colleague. 'I might make Dr Blalock nervous – or even worse, he might make me nervous.' But Blalock would have none of it. He knew he needed Thomas to be there looking over his shoulder.

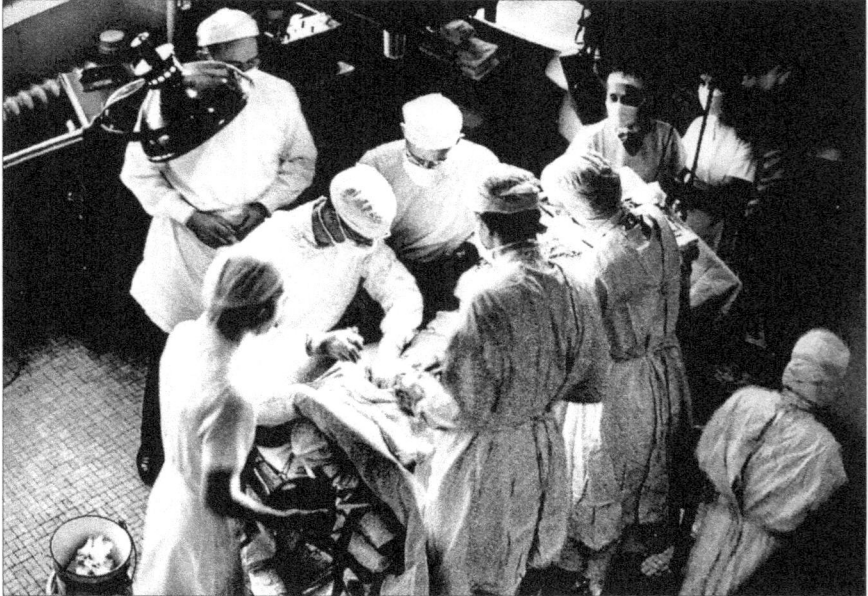

Fig 2.4 A. The first Blalock shunt procedure.
Thomas is standing directly behind Blalock.

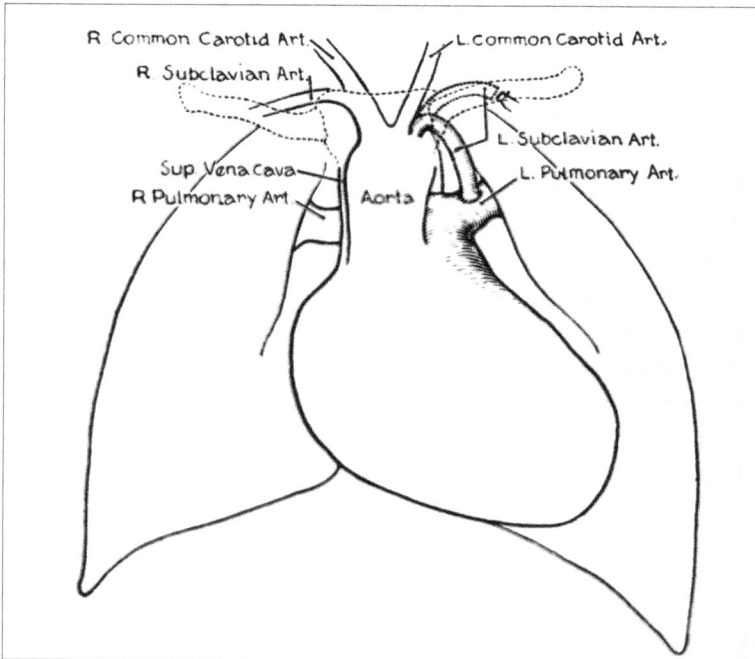

**Fig. 2.4 B. Diagram from the published paper
depicting the Blalock Taussig shunt.**

Indeed at one point he turned to him and said: 'Will the subclavian reach the pulmonary artery once it's divided?' Then 'is the incision (in the subclavian) long enough?' 'Yes, if not too long' came Thomas's reply. The atmosphere in the operating theatre that day was graphically recorded through the words of Harry Minetree, a surgical resident.

'On November 29th students and professors, including Dr Taussig, crowded into the double-deck observation gallery above the eighth floor operation room of the Halsted Clinic. Because there was a danger of losing the child before the operation began, Dr Merel Harmel decided not to use a strong anaesthetic and put her slowly to sleep with a diluted mixture of ether and oxygen. Dr William Longmire the chief resident was first assistant. Charlotte Mitchell was scrub nurse. After inserting an arterial needle for blood oxygen tests, Vivien Thomas, who in the dog lab had proved himself a master at vascular suturing, stood by in the event that his advice might be needed. Dr Denton Cooley administered fluids.

The tiny pliable ribs were retracted and the pleural cavity containing the child's atrophied lungs and small twisted heart was opened. The heart and lungs seemed infinitely more complex in miniature. With the advice of Thomas, Dr Blalock found the subclavian artery, clamped it at its origin and began dissecting away the tissue that clung to it. The instruments were clearly too large and awkward. Using bulldog clamps fitted with rubber tubing so as not to crush the vessels, Blalock, again with Thomas's help, carefully prepared a site for attaching the subclavian to the pulmonary artery. A small transverse incision was made between two clamps on the pulmonary artery, then using china-beaded silk on fine needles Dr Blalock completed the juncture that re-routed the baby's blood from the left arm to the lungs. She immediately went from waxen blue to pink. Dr Helen Taussig had watched the operation from the head of the table.' For her it was a dream come true.

At one point Blalock was heard to say 'Is this all right, Vivien?' Then a moment later 'Are those bites (of the stitches) close enough together?' It was clear to all which of them was the master surgeon. Would the left arm survive and grow having lost its blood supply? Thomas said it would. The dogs never complained.

As anticipated the initial post-operative course was stormy and they almost lost the child with a collapsed lung. Yet once recovered her blue tinge had gone. She was pink, energetic and two months after the surgery she was allowed home. Taussig's outpatient clinic follow-up charted her progress with weight gain and fewer bouts of cyanosis and fainting on exercise. Finally she learned to walk and could play with other children. Happy parents, but of course it wasn't a cure.

On February 3rd 1946 the team operated again, this time on a debilitated 9-year-old girl who could only walk a few feet without the characteristic squatting and panting of cyanosed children. Blalock wasn't a paediatric surgeon so the operation was easier on a larger subject and the recovery more expedite. Then four days later with increasing confidence the team operated on perhaps the sickest of the first three patients. This time, having had difficulty in manipulating fine needles and silk with adult instruments,

Blalock changed his approach. The innominate artery is the large first major branch of the aorta supplying blood to the head and right arm. At Thomas's suggestion Blalock cut through it just before the separation into arm and head branches (the subclavian and carotid arteries) then joined it directly to the (pulmonary) artery to the right lung. On removing the clamps he encountered brisk bleeding between the stitches needing to re-clamp and insert more. On releasing the clamp for the second time Dr Harmel immediately announced 'He's a lovely colour now. Come and look.' And so he was. With the larger artery the change was dramatic and convincing. It raised the spirits and expectations of the whole department, yet before long the relationship between surgeon and cardiologist soured. So much so that Dr Cooley became their go-between.

Blalock rapidly wrote a paper describing the operation and optimistic outcome with the first three patients which he sent to the *Journal of the American Medical Association*. As the story goes the document was leaked to a journalist and soon became headline news. Whilst Blalock gave Taussig credit for her participation in his report, Taussig went as far as to suggest that she alone had devised the procedure. She published several articles on follow-up studies without acknowledging Blalock, and of course no one acknowledged Thomas's contribution at any stage.

In a letter to a friend Blalock wrote: 'I must say that if I make a statement to you that you could improve the condition of patients with aortic stenosis should you be able to find a means to allow more blood to reach the body, I would be far from solving the practical problem.' In other words, to suggest a solution is some distance from making it happen though Taussig didn't see it that way. And without Thomas it couldn't have been done.

Aside from internal discord the response to the news was overwhelming. Within weeks the paediatric wards at Johns Hopkins were full of children not just with tetralogy but with all congenital anomalies where blood flow to the lungs was restricted. But a bed and operation at the clinic didn't come cheap. For less affluent families local newspapers ran public appeals so dying children had their chance. And reporters would arrive with them. Blalock was inundated with work but had the remarkable surgical talent of both Longmire and Cooley to help. Until Cooley was dispatched to Italy on war service that is.

Russell Brock studied at Christ's College Cambridge, then at Guy's Hospital Medical School in the 1920s.

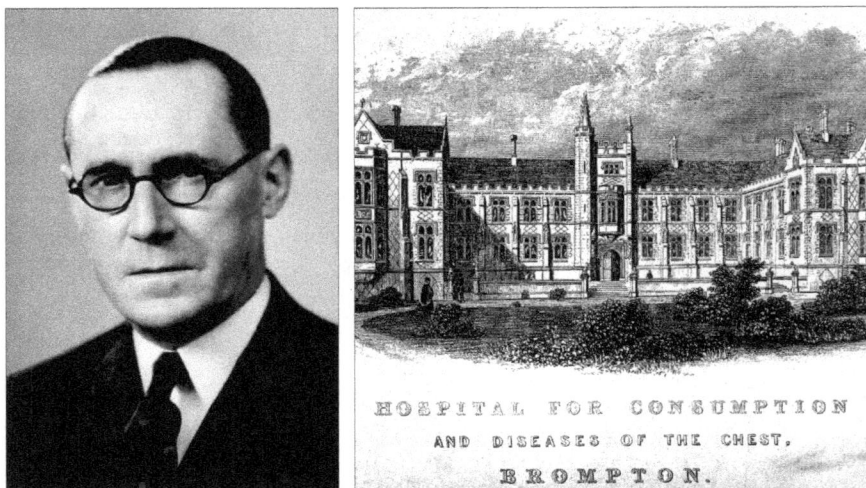

Fig 2.5 A. Russell Brock. B. The old Brompton Hospital.

Nevertheless it was his year as a surgical fellow with the thoracic surgeon Evarts Graham in St Louis that defined his future. Writing to Graham on return to London, Brock was effusive in his praise for the American experience. 'The impressions and inspiration I gained as a young surgeon visiting Barnes Hospital and numerous other great centres in your country was such a powerful influence on my thoughts and career.' In 1936 Brock was appointed consultant thoracic surgeon back at Guy's and the Brompton Hospital and was one of the surgeons who watched Harken operate on the heart in the Cotswolds. Surprisingly he remained sceptical as to where it would lead. 'I really don't see what useful purpose we can put this (intracardiac surgery) to after the war,' Brock told Harken. 'We won't see such fragments in hearts then.'

Harken emphatically disagreed. 'Russell if you'd read the manuscript of your own marvellous Laurence O'Shaughnessy you'd know he already had the idea of doing something very like what I'm doing. With the same technique I could probably open a congenital pulmonic valve stenosis. If he hadn't died at Dunkirk, O'Shaughnessy would have come back and done it. I'll show you.'

We know Brock went back to search for O'Shaughnessy's paper which remained unfinished when the war intervened. It included a drawing of an obstructed pulmonary valve and a description of a suggested operation to open the orifice using a cutting instrument passed through the wall of the right ventricle. After all, Blalock's shunt didn't cure a patient. It was only palliative.

On learning of the Blalock-Taussing procedure, Brock invited them both to spend a month in London to operate at Guy's. It was the late summer of 1947 when Blalock set sail for Southampton with his wife Mary on the Mauretania having spent the previous day acquiring a month's supply of Viceroy cigarettes which were not sold in Britain. Brock sourced ten debilitated children with tetralogy of Fallot for Blalock to operate on, and every one survived – perhaps more a testament to the anaesthetic team than the shunt operation itself. Again the press latched onto the show resulting in desperate parents rushing their babies to London hoping for a cure before the circus moved on.

At the end of the visit both the surgeon and paediatric cardiologist presented their experience at the British Medical Association, a venue that was packed to capacity. At the conclusion of Blalock's lecture the room remained dark after the projection of lantern slides, when suddenly a long wartime searchlight beam traversed the Great Hall in dramatic fashion. The light fell on a Guy's nursing sister in dark blue uniform holding a small blonde, curly haired two-year-old with tetralogy, now pink after her shunt the week before. The heart-warming effect provoked tumultuous applause from the audience. Blalock's tour proved a great stimulus towards cardiac surgery in Britain and Europe following as it did Harken's heroics with missile wounds to the heart.

Brock proceeded to undertake autopsy studies of children's hearts with right ventricular outflow obstruction bearing in mind what Harken had told him about O'Shaughnessy's concept. Observing the pinhole orifice of the congenitally narrowed pulmonary valve with extreme thickening of the muscle beneath he came to the conclusion that a direct attack on the valve was warranted. With this in mind he designed an instrument named the valvulotome with which to open the valve through an incision in the thin-walled pulmonary artery above. Though unreported we know that initial approach to have caused the tragic death of a 17-year-old girl from bleeding, after which he elected to pass the valvulotome through the muscle of the right ventricle instead.

On February 16th 1948 Brock operated on an 18-year-old girl with critical pulmonary valve stenosis. On this occasion the purposefully curved valvulotome was introduced through the body of the right ventricle, reached the valve easily, and was pushed through without incident. When opened forcefully the narrowing, followed by her symptoms, were instantly relieved. Brock repeated the procedure twice more with survival before publishing the three successful cases in the *British Medical Journal* in 1948. Then two weeks later another pulmonary valvotomy was reported in the *Lancet* by Brock's great rival Thomas Holmes Sellors at the Middlesex Hospital. That operation had actually been performed earlier on 4th December 1947. The 20-year-old male patient with tetralogy was found to have advanced tuberculosis of both lungs which mitigated against the Blalock shunt originally planned. Why? Because dense inflammatory adhesions had obscured the vessels by sticking the lung to the chest wall. Holmes Sellors therefore proceeded to open the pericardial sac near the midline instead. He then advanced a long tenotomy knife through the cavity of the right ventricle to incise the valve directly. This relieved the obstruction so that the patient lived for another nine years before succumbing to tuberculosis. Although their hospitals were just three miles apart in central London it appears that neither was aware of the others efforts.

Before the advent of cardiac catheterisation, then echocardiography, it was impossible to differentiate between isolated valvular pulmonary stenosis and the long muscular sub-valvular narrowing characteristic of tetralogy of Fallot. In the event of encountering muscular obstruction Brock designed a blunt-nosed punch with which to core out a channel through to the valve itself. Having tried it on a single patient with a modicum of success he introduced it to the USA when invited by Blalock for a reciprocal visit.

Brock's impact in Baltimore was no less impressive than Blalock's in London. He arrived at the Johns Hopkins Hospital as the cardiologists were presenting patients to surgeons at a meeting in the Medical School.

Brock wandered into the rear of the auditorium wearing a grey top coat, Homburg hat and carrying his suitcase. Distracted by the unannounced entrance, Blalock made an introduction of the esteemed guest to his colleagues then invited him to examine the patient under review. Brock set down his suitcase and without removing hat or coat, stepped onto the stage, took a stethoscope from his pocket and examined the child and his x-ray. 'Coarctation of the aorta, surgical correction advised', was all he said to the amusement and delight of the audience. It was on this visit that Brock met Cooley, learned of his great dexterity and persuaded him to spend time as chief resident at the Brompton Hospital.

Some 75 years later when I knew Dr Cooley well, I asked him what he recalled about those epic times at Johns Hopkins. Needless to say he was far more frank and illuminating than the accepted historical accounts. He had arrived at Hopkins as junior resident in 1940, the same year as Thomas and had high regard for him. 'Blalock could never have done it without Vivien,' Cooley said. 'Vivien had practised the operation so many times and taught it to his boss.' In an interview with the *Washingtonian* magazine, Cooley explained that: 'Even if you'd never seen surgery before you could do it because Vivien made it look so simple. He became a teacher to surgeons without even being a doctor. There wasn't a false move, not a wasted motion.'

Apparently in the laboratory Thomas developed an operation for babies born with the aorta arising abnormally from the right ventricle and the pulmonary artery from the left. 'Transposition of the great arteries' is the medical term for that and of course with the veins connected normally the blood just circulates round and round in two separate circuits proving rapidly fatal unless a connection between the two is created. Thomas approached that by excising the interatrial septum, the wall between right and left atrium, allowing oxygenated blood from the lungs to cross to the circulation of the body. 'Atrial septectomy' became the surgical term when introduced into patients. As legend has it when Blalock was shown the meticulously executed suture line he was prompted to remark: 'Vivien, this looks like something the Lord made.' *Something the Lord Made* was the name of a wonderful movie made about the pair years later.

Blalock's relationship with Thomas was made complex by the race issues. And it wasn't always harmonious. In his own biography published after Blalock's death Thomas describes an early altercation.

'Something went wrong. I no longer recall what but I made an error. Dr Blalock sounded off like a child throwing a temper tantrum. The profanity he used would have made the proverbial sailor proud of him. I told him he could just pay me off, that I had not been brought up to take that kind of language. He apologised, saying he had lost his temper, that he would watch his language and he asked me to go back to work. In retrospect I think that incident set the stage for what I consider our mutual respect throughout the years.'

All Thomas's ambitions to attend medical school disintegrated during the great depression. As Blalock's technician he was paid $12 a week with no overtime pay for a sixteen-hour day. But he continued to read anatomy, physiology and chemistry textbooks as he sat monitoring the animal experiments at night quietly hoping that one day things might be different. It was the Prohibition era and Blalock kept a ten-gallon keg of whisky hidden under a blanket in the laboratory. He would share this with Thomas in the evening when everyone else had gone. Thomas would act as bartender at Blalock's parties at home to boost his meagre earnings. He had a family to support but when Blalock celebrated his sixtieth birthday in a hotel in Baltimore they were not invited. The racial divide between them was never crossed in public. Yet such was Blalock's reliance upon Thomas, even before moving to Baltimore, that in 1937 he declined the chairmanship of surgery at Detroit's Henry Ford Hospital through their policy not to hire coloured people.

At Hopkins Blalock's relationship with his technician would mystify the visiting surgeons who came to learn the shunt technique. The coloured man on the stool behind was not a doctor, nor an assistant, yet Blalock would continuously turn to him for reassurance. As Dr Cooley explained: 'Dr Blalock was a great scientist, a great thinker, a leader, but by no stretch of the imagination could be he considered a great cutting surgeon.' So skilled was Thomas at operating on animals that he became the unqualified veterinary surgeon for the pets of Hopkins faculty members, and in time further afield. The first dog to become a long-term survivor of the shunt,

Anna as she was called, took up permanent residence in the Old Hunterian laboratory as Thomas's pet. In turn, Thomas hired a further twenty black laboratory technicians over the years, two of whom subsequently went to medical school. Others became formal physician's assistants within the surgical service.

Taussig went on to write *Congenital Malformations of the Heart* published in 1947. She followed the thousands of children under her care through generations which gave her an unrivalled view of both the natural and surgically modified history of the many children's heart defects. It soon became clear that the shunt was a temporary procedure at best. She and the professor never did get on.

Blalock retired in 1964 when he was deteriorating with a malignant tumour and could barely stand. Thomas would push the white-haired professor down the hallway of the Alfred Blalock Clinical Sciences building in a wheelchair and at one stage Blalock confessed to a colleague, 'I really should have found a way to send Vivien to medical school.' But he didn't.

Blalock died from cancer in 1965 after which Thomas stayed on as Director of the Laboratory he spent his life in. He was eventually awarded an honorary doctorate in 1976 with an official appointment to the Hopkins medical school faculty. There was a thunderous ovation when he stood in his gold and sable academic robe causing him to remark: 'The applause was so great that I felt very small.' His portrait now hangs opposite that of his mentor in the Blalock building. Many other distinguished surgeons went on to carry the torch for children with congenital heart disease but blind efforts to improve complex deformities could never be the answer. Some radical and as yet unforeseen development was needed but where would that come from?

In retirement Helen Taussig continued to work on congenitally defective bird hearts sent to her by friends. She was fatally injured on 20th May 1986 whilst backing her car out of the driveway at home. She had already donated her body to the medical school.

Denton Cooley became chief resident at Hopkins before taking up Brock's offer to become senior registrar at the Brompton. By then Sir Russell's heart and lung service was arguably the most innovative in the world. Later in life Brock wrote this about Cooley's arrival.

'Denton Cooley came to the Brompton Hospital as a young man, I recall, with the great advantage of physique. A very good-looking young man with charming manners and a nice way of expressing himself, all of which were undeniable attributes. It was immediately apparent that his practical performance as a surgeon was in keeping with the high standards suggested by his physical attributes. He was an extremely active worker operating all the time. A very rapid and able operator with lung as well as heart surgery. I was struck by his extreme restlessness, his pronounced eagerness to do more and better things than anyone else.' As it happened, that was an accurate prediction.

Two months after Cooley arrived on the Fulham Road, Oswald Tubbs developed pulmonary tuberculosis and required part of his right lung removed.

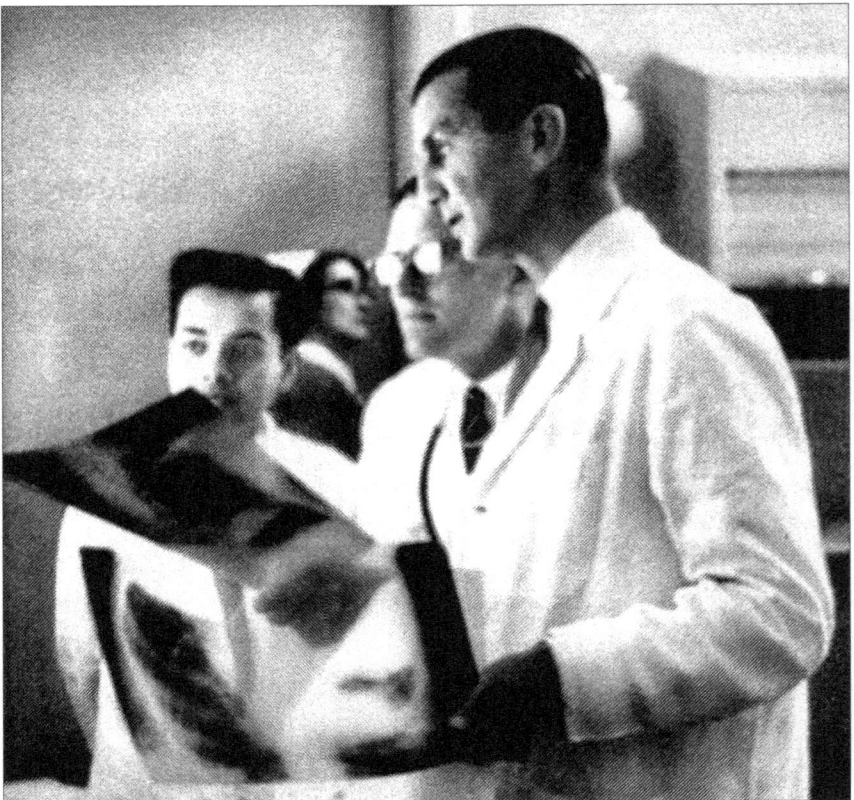

Fig 2.6 Oswald Tubbs conducting a ward round.

The nervous Tubbs requested for good reason that Cooley should be Brock's first assistant at the operation. Two hours before moving to the operating theatre Tubbs called the young American to his bedside and explained the way he wished the procedure to be performed. In particular he wanted the nerve to the diaphragm to be crushed allowing the paralysed muscle to rise and fill the space vacated by the excised lobe. In turn he would hand over his practice to the senior registrar until he was fit. Brock removed the diseased part then wandered off leaving Cooley to close the chest. So Cooley dealt with the nerve himself.

The notoriously skilled operator was summoned one day to help one of the Brompton senior surgeons Norman 'Pasty' Barrett who had ripped the wall of the left atrium whilst attempting to dilate a mitral valve. As Cooley entered the operating theatre there was an air of panic with blood all over the floor. His agitated senior exclaimed: 'Cooley, this operation should be awfully simple, but I've made it simply awful.' That was cardiac surgery in those days. The young Texan certainly left his mark on the Brompton though he left London earlier than expected to take up a post in Houston.

Brock became President of the Royal College of Surgeons and then Lord Brock. I found his operating boots discarded in a dusty old cupboard at the Brompton in 1974 and inherited them. I would wear them whilst assisting Tubbs as his last resident surgical officer. Memorable times, never to be repeated.

Blind Faith

Every surgeon carries within himself
a small cemetery where from time
to time he goes to pray.
—Rene Leriche

My own cemetery was not so small.

What Pasty Barrett intended to do was to dilate the orifice of a mitral valve that had been narrowed by the ravages of rheumatic fever. I encountered many of those valves and was occasionally confronted with the necessity to perform a 'closed mitral valvotomy' myself. The first was early in my career and the young woman was pregnant. In those days a foetus would die if the mother was placed on the heart-lung machine so I decided to resort to a traditional instrument given to me by Oswald Tubbs on his retirement. 'Blind' surgery was nerve-wracking. That's when I realised how brave if not reckless the pioneers had been.

A normal mitral valve is a thing of beauty. With thin and pliable leaflets it is anchored to the wall of the left ventricle by muscular pillars, the papillary muscles. These in turn are attached to the edges of the anterior and posterior leaflets by fine strong struts, chordae tendinae. The leaflets flash open and shut as the heart beats anything from 50 to 150 times each minute producing a characteristic sound audible with the stethoscope. When the valve performs normally there is no turbulence or murmur as the ventricle fills from the left atrium. It's the same for the tricuspid valve which sits at the orifice to the right ventricle.

In the pre-antibiotic era rheumatic fever was a curse, occurring as it does in healthy young people after a simple Group A streptococcus throat infection. In the early part of the twentieth century it was the leading cause of death in individuals younger than twenty years, and second only to tuberculosis in those between twenty and forty. Untreated, a vicious autoimmune process triggered by the body's own reaction to the streptococcus may attack the heart, the joints and the central nervous system. And many patients particularly in deprived areas suffered multiple attacks. Once in the chronic phase of the illness the mitral valve is affected in half of the cases and there is combined involvement of the aortic and mitral valves in a fifth. Involvement of the tricuspid valve is limited to one in ten cases and the pulmonary valve is rarely affected. That said I operated on all four valves at once on a number of occasions in less privileged countries.

What rheumatic fever does to the mitral valve is hideous. The leaflets become thickened, retracted and immobile sticking together through the inflammatory process. The chordae stiffen and shorten, dragging the orifice open. Over the years the once delicate structures change into a rigid obstructive mass gnarled with calcification. Only a small orifice remains so the blood flow is compromised and the pressure within the left atrium rises. The chamber distends markedly with a stretched wall that will burst on touch. That's what Barrett encountered that day before Cooley managed to sort it out.

Rene Laennec the French physician who invented the stethoscope described the characteristic murmurs of the narrowed or leaking mitral valve in 1818. Then surprisingly it was the surgeon Theodore Billroth who gave a name to the streptococcus bacterium responsible for such diverse illnesses as scarlet fever, impetigo, and cellulitis. In 1898 the London physician Daniel Samways suggested that the obstructed mitral valve might be amenable to surgical enlargement. In the *Lancet* he wrote: 'I anticipate that with the progress of cardiac surgery some of the severest cases will be relieved by slightly notching the mitral orifice.' It was an optimistic prophecy at a time when only a handful of penetrating wounds had been repaired with surgery. And indeed there was no response until Sir Thomas Lauder Brunton suggested the same thing after cutting into rheumatic mitral valves in the autopsy room.

Brunton was an eminent physician at St Bartholomew's Hospital, a Fellow of the Royal Society and had a career-long interest in the effect of drugs on the heart. In his *Preliminary note on the possibility of treating mitral stenosis by surgical methods* in the *Lancet* he emphasised the hopelessness of medical treatment and 'felt it reasonable to suggest that a suitable instrument might be introduced blindly through the left ventricular muscle to engage with the valve by sense of touch.' Interestingly he had reason to suggest the transventricular route over an atrial approach. Whilst engaged in a commission to investigate the effects of chloroform on the heart he had found ventricular wounds to bleed less than atrial perforation. He had experimented with drugs on animal hearts for thirty-five years and found that they tolerated manipulation, so his opinions were expressed in the light of considerable experience.

Provoked for a second time, the *Lancet* published an editorial rebuking Brunton who in their words had 'proceeded no further than the table of the dead house in making his investigation'. They regarded the difficulties as 'underestimated, requiring a technique that in itself would prove fatal'. Samways wrote a letter in support but Ludwig Rehn having succeeded with a cardiac stab wound came out firmly against the prospect stating that heart valves were *noli me tangere*. Not to be interfered with. Brunton made an indignant reply to Rehn stating that 'he had no intention of abandoning the idea', and that the wimpish surgeons should get on and find a solution. But it took time and a great deal of experimental work before the efforts reached an operating theatre.

Elliot Cutler studied medicine at Harvard then interned with Harvey Cushing at the Peter Bent Brigham Hospital in Boston.

Perhaps unusually for a brain surgeon, Cushing's main interest seemed to be the creation of heart valve lesions in dogs so that he could study the damaging effects. From these studies came the notion that a leaking mitral valve was better tolerated than a narrowed one. Cutler spent two years in the Surgical Research Laboratories at Harvard learning to deal with an open chest and endotracheal anaesthesia in preparation for an approach to the heart but was instead dispatched to Europe in World War I. In charge of the Harvard American Ambulance Unit, then the Fifth General Hospital in Paris, he was regarded as a determined and courageous young man who went on to receive the Distinguished Service Medal.

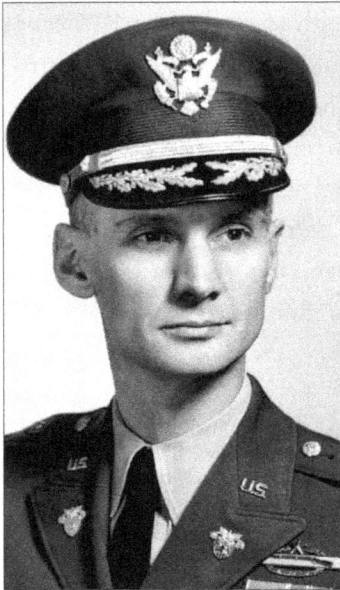

Fig 3.1 A. Elliot Cutler.
B. The Cutler Valvulotome.

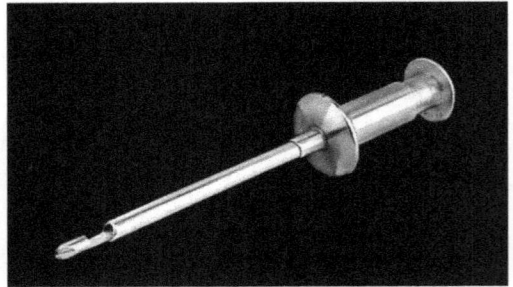

Events behind the scenes in war-torn France provided some encouragement for Cutler. The accomplished surgeon Alexis Carrel had worked on techniques for joining blood vessels together in preparation for his prospective venture into organ transplantation. Taking advantage of the newly-introduced positive pressure airway ventilation in his experimental efforts, he published papers on surgery of the aorta and even used a tube of the vessel to the join the apex of the heart to the aorta as it descended on the back wall of the chest cavity. Carrel correctly reasoned that this technique could be used to bypass a narrowed aortic valve, a coarctation or indeed an aneurysm of the aortic arch.

By 1912 Carrel and his colleague Theodore Tuffier decided they should apply their laboratory experience to help a patient. The opportunity came when a 26-year-old man with rheumatic heart disease and a severely narrowed aortic valve was admitted to the clinic. Their plan, perhaps naively, was to expose the heart using Milton's new sternum splitting approach, make an incision into the ascending aorta then pass a finger down into the valve to separate the fused commissures. On 13th July they took the patient to the operating theatre, exposed the heart but then hesitated through anxiety. It was a misguided concept and seeing the aorta bounding away at high pressure, Tuffier wisely decided not to cut into it.

After conferring with Carrel, Tuffier decided to invaginate the aortic wall a short distance above the valve using his index finger then try to disrupt the severely narrowed orifice. Afterwards he described feeling 'extremely lively vibrations' and at the Fifth Congress of the International Surgical Society they claimed that the patient had improved after the procedure. Historical accounts report the pioneering effort but frankly it was nonsense. It was never going to be possible to reach an aortic valve in that way. Nevertheless spurred on by Tuffier's account, a flamboyant and skilled surgeon Eugenie Doyen decided to have a go at opening a congenitally narrowed pulmonary valve by passing a bladed metal instrument through the right ventricle. In essence this was a forerunner of Brock's operation but was spectacularly unsuccessful. The 20-year-old woman had no benefit, remained cyanosed throughout and died a few hours later. Autopsy showed severe muscular obstruction below the valve with no evidence that the instrument had engaged the valve itself. Undeterred, Doyen next prepared to attempt mitral valvotomy with the same instrument but he himself died prematurely at the age of 57 before he had the chance.

When Cutler returned to Boston after the war he found that others had been working on a 'cardioscope' intending to directly inspect the inside of the heart along the lines of the cystoscope for the bladder. This ingenious device had an electric bulb with a lens and small knife at the tip but proved completely useless when deployed within dark red flowing blood. The stage was nevertheless set for the war hero to take the next step. When presented with a breathless bedridden 12-year-old girl who was coughing up blood there was little to lose. Her parents had been told that she would die very soon from mitral stenosis and were desperate for the authoritative and confident Cutler to try to help. He did so on the morning of 20th May 1923 at Peter Bent Brigham Hospital.

The emaciated girl's sternum was cut down the middle, continuing the incision to within two inches of her umbilicus. Spreading the bone edges widely with a retractor he opened the pericardium to expose the struggling heart with a tensely dilated right ventricle. In contrast the left ventricle was underfilled given the obstructed valve which Cutler planned to cut open. To do so he had to displace the organ towards himself to access the apex, but in doing so it objected by throwing off a run of rapid rhythm with a precipitous fall in blood pressure. Worrying, but the lower the pressure the less the bleeding. Cutler responded by dripping adrenaline solution onto the muscle before plunging his scalpel through into the left ventricle. Introducing the curved instrument with a blade on the end he cautiously advanced it towards the mitral valve until it encountered resistance. His only option then was to cut blindly hoping it was the thickened valve leaflets not the chordae tendinae that he was chopping through. Twisting the blade he made two purposeful incisions into the tissue then withdrew rapidly and closed the entry incision. The whole procedure took little more than an hour and the girl survived unscathed.

Cutler's blind effort undertaken a full quarter of a century before Brock's pulmonary valvotomy, was the very first planned cardiac operation to succeed. Unfortunately the physical signs of mitral stenosis were unchanged and she remained restricted but at least the coughing of blood abated. She eventually died at the age of sixteen after which post-mortem examination showed little evidence that the valve had been touched. This was not curative surgery. Big operation of little help but a lasting legacy.

News spread fast and many more unfortunate individuals were referred to the hospital. Cutler repeated the operation just twice in the following months but both patients died in the immediate post-operative period. Again there was little autopsy evidence that anything had been achieved, so he tried again with a new spring-loaded punch. The next two patients lived for seven and three days respectively but on the second occasion he was unable to reach the mitral valve. Though well intentioned 'blind' surgery was just that. Defending the approach Cutler claimed that all four fatalities were inevitable through advanced disease and fibrosis in the heart muscle. He didn't make further attempts.

At the Middlesex Hospital in London the cardiologist Strickland Goodall examined many post-mortem cases of mitral stenosis drawing the conclusion that the recently inflamed valve leaflets were amenable to separation in many cases. Despite having designed a double-edged knife for the purpose it was never used due to profound negativity amongst the surgical community. Nonetheless the effort was not wasted. Sir Henry Souttar was aware of Goodall's efforts and encouraged by them. Souttar, a general surgeon had gained a double first in engineering and mathematics at Queen's College, Oxford before studying medicine.

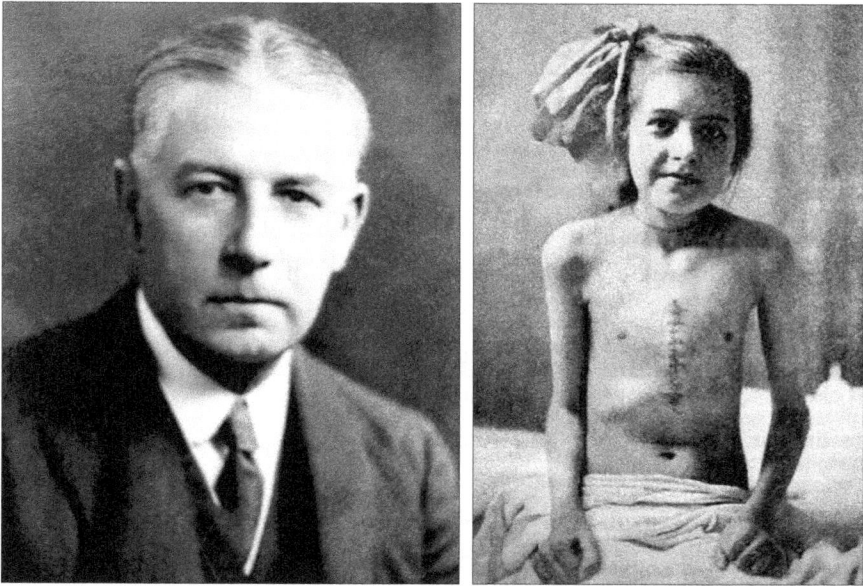

Fig 3.2 A. Henry Souttar. B. His patient Lilly Hine.

He had an engineering workshop over his Harley Street house and a fine mahogany breakfront bookcase in his operating theatre at the London Hospital for his instruments.

Souttar was referred a ten-year-old girl, Lily Hine from Bethnal Green, who was one of six children of a labourer with tuberculosis. After three attacks of rheumatic fever she was admitted to the London with inflammation in both the heart and brain. Rheumatic carditis and Sydenham's chorea were the medical terms for it. Originally under the care of Lord Dawson of Penn she improved and was discharged only to be readmitted seven years later, now coughing up blood through severe mitral stenosis and heart failure.

On humanitarian grounds and much in the face of prevailing negativity, Dawson persuaded Souttar to operate on her as a last resort. Was there anything to lose? Yes there was. Surgeons were repeatedly derided for their misjudgement when the inevitable happened.

The operation on May 6th, 1925 employed an improved anaesthetic technique whereby ether vapour was blown into the windpipe and inflation pressure increased when the chest was opened to keep the left lung expanded. Souttar divided third and fourth ribs to produce a rectangular flap and a window on the left atrium. This has an appendage like a bent finger sitting in front of the two veins from the left lung as they enter the chamber. He clamped the base of the appendage, made an incision of around 1.5 centimetres then slipped his index finger into the hole to stem the bleeding. Digitally exploring the left atrium he could feel the rigid valve leaflets with their fixed opening.

Applying gentle pressure at each end of the orifice with the fingertip was sufficient to separate the adhesions until a jet of regurgitating blood was readily apparent. That was the time to withdraw.

As the finger came out his inexperienced assistant tightened the purse-string suture but the delicate atrial wall tore releasing 'a voluminous gush of blood'. I know just how he felt as the warm red fluid gushed over his gown. That 'Pasty' Barrett moment when exsanguination seems likely. But he succeeding in gripping the remnant and applying a clamp to what remained of the base. A job well done by an abdominal surgeon who hadn't handled a beating human heart before.

Lily was sent to the countryside for convalescence but then returned to the slums of Bethnal Green where she suffered another bout of rheumatic fever the following year. Even the brave Souttar was not convinced that his operation had achieved a great deal. The cardiologists, believing rheumatic heart disease to be predominantly a problem of muscle fibrosis, didn't refer him another case. In 1930 Lily was admitted to the London for the last time in terminal heart failure having suffered a blood clot to the brain and stroke with hemiplegia. That was the natural history of this miserable disease and not a single mitral valvotomy was attempted in Britain for another twenty years.

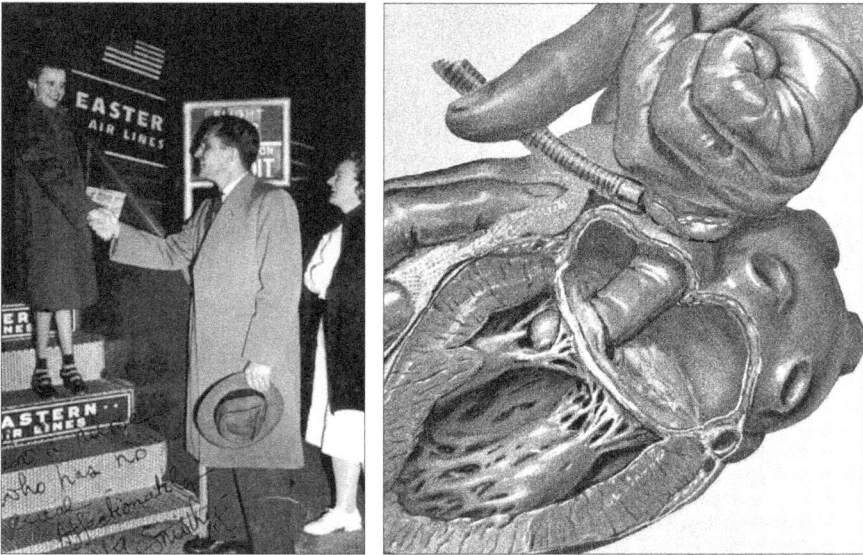

Fig 3.3 A. Horace Smithy and Nurse Agnes Bowen Kleckley bid farewell to Betty Woolridge at Charleston Airport. B. Finger dilation of the mitral valve as originally used by Souttar.

In World War II Souttar was made Surgeon-in-Chief of the field ambulance at the siege of Antwerp, then in Furnes on the Flanders coast for which he was awarded the Order of the Crown of Belgium. Having met the physicist Marie Curie in Belgium he cooperated with her on the medical applications of radium, particularly for abdominal cancer. But he never operated on another heart.

Horace Smithy was born into a wealthy family in Virginia. Troubled by frequent colds and sore throats attributed to the east coast climate, he was sent down South to the Miami Military Academy for his college education.

There the handsome and athletic young cadet excelled at baseball, American football and boxing, so there was little to indicate that his own chosen career would be blighted by rheumatic heart disease.

It was at the University of Virginia Medical School when Smithy purchased a stethoscope and listened to his own heart sounds. He was shocked by what he heard. A harsh pansystolic murmur over the upper sternum best describes the finding in medical terms, but life goes on. He married a classmate and moved on to Charleston, South Carolina for his residency with the surgeon father of an old school friend. But his performance on the football field was increasingly restricted. Breathlessness on exertion was how the doctors described it. He was subsequently diagnosed with rheumatic aortic stenosis at the age of 28, the same year that he began his surgical practice. From then on Smithy was obsessed with finding a solution to his ailment because he knew just what to expect. The inexorable decline from exertional breathlessness to heart failure with breathlessness at rest. The prospect of his wife and children having to watching the dismal helplessness of it all, so he tried to do something about it. It became a deeply personal battle for the rest of his life.

Working in the laboratory and with autopsy specimens from the hospital, Smithy developed a thin-barbed valvulotome which he introduced into the aorta above the valve hoping to open the deformed cusps. Of course that might cause the valve to become regurgitant but at the time a leaking valve was considered much less of a problem than a narrowed one. With Souttar's efforts largely unknown in the USA, Smithy presented his experimental findings at the 1947 American College of Surgeons meeting in New York. Though he was unaware of the fact, there was a science editor for Associated Press in the audience, so the innovative work made big news at a time when many thousands of patients were incapacitated by heart disease.

Spurred on by the publicity Smithy developed a different instrument for the more complex mitral valve. To help he enlisted the head of the hospital's machine shop and together they produced a plunger inside a hollow tube which in combination formed a set of sharp jaws. Smithy visualised introducing this through a purse-string stitch at the apex of the left ventricle then advancing it into the narrowed orifice of the scarred valve. When the plunger was pushed the jaws would close to bite out a portion of the scarred tissue. The instrument, still on display at the Waring Historical Library in South Carolina, would then be withdrawn and the purse string tied down. Simple, or was it?

On reading the newspaper articles one desperate soul, Betty Woolridge from Canton, Ohio, wrote to Smithy on 29th November. 'I am twenty-one years of age and have had mitral stenosis following scarlet fever since the age of ten. For the past two years I have been in cardiac failure with extreme congestion of the lungs and liver and all the accompanying symptoms. Just now the condition is worsening and the usual procedures – diuretics, diet and bed rest have lost their effect. My doctor mentioned an operation some time ago and on reading your report I have felt I should be very much interested in any information or help you can give me. I shall appreciate hearing from you at your earliest convenience.'

Apparently there was a discouraging response from Smithy but the disconsolate and emaciated Betty was unwilling to abandon what little hope she had left. On 6th December she followed up with: 'Couldn't you find some way to help me? You won't be losing anything. It will be me. I am taking, and asking for, the chance. Please reconsider my offer. Experiment on me and I will do my part or even more.'

This pleading letter from 1947 is an important document providing real insight into the need for a surgical solution for valvular heart disease. Both rheumatic heart disease and congenital deformities decimated young lives and filled hospital wards with patients for which there were no solutions. The physicians with few expectations still seemed to have their heads in the sand. This left a handful of surgeons to risk their reputations and livelihood trying to operate blindly on critically important anatomy they could not see. Many patients' lives were terminated by cardiac arrest or exsanguination in vain efforts that were never recorded.

Betty did come to Charleston having travelled hundreds of miles in an aeroplane. Smithy noted: 'When I met her, I immediately had second thoughts. Her abdomen was distended with fluid and a congested liver. She was unable to lie flat for me to examine her and had to be propped up on three pillows just to breathe with comfort.' All physical findings confirmed that she was dying from severe congestive heart failure and it is likely that Smithy recognised this as his own destiny should he decline to help.

Betty's operation was scheduled for 30th January 1948 and, on the evening before, six litres of fluid were withdrawn from her swollen belly to help her breathing. There was no intensive care unit in that era. No prospect of being kept alive on a ventilator after the procedure. Just an oxygen tent. Smithy opened the left chest and approached the obstructed mitral valve through the apex of the left ventricle just as he had done in the dogs. His novel instrument engaged the rigidly fibrotic valve leaflets and punched out a segment around one centimetre long.

From Smithy's own account: 'The p.m. procedure was without incident and no change occurred in the character of the atrial fibrillation which was present during the operation. Post-operative convalescence was uneventful. Orthopneoa (breathlessness on lying flat) disappeared entirely and the liver became impalpable. Of interest was the reversion of atrial fibrillation on the third post-operative day to normal sinus rhythm.'

Though crude and beset by risk, the operation had made a difference. Betty recovered surprisingly quickly, thanks to a modest improvement in the valve orifice and the helpful return of normal heart rhythm whereby contraction of the left atrium improves filling of the ventricle. A heart-warming archive photograph shows Smithy and Betty's nurse Agnes Bowen bidding the frail young woman goodbye as she climbs the steps of the plane back to Ohio.

Reports appeared in newspapers throughout the USA, some more explicit than they should have been. The *Atlanta Journal* revealed that 'like many research men Smithy is pioneering in a field where he himself is a sufferer'. *Time* magazine included this quote: 'So far only Dr Smithy has tried the operation. Someday some other surgeon who will need long laboratory training might operate on Dr Smithy himself, whose own heart was damaged in childhood by rheumatic fever.'

This was the first occasion when cardiac surgery and the media interacted to any great extent, and whilst projected into celebrity, the man himself was not comfortable with it. One national radio show declared: 'We had hoped and anticipated that Dr Smithy would participate in this broadcast, but he considers that his personal involvement would be in danger of being misunderstood and misinterpreted. Personal public appearances by physicians and surgeons regarding their professional work is not ordinarily done. Dr Smithy feels that while the public should be informed the procedure itself has limitations some of which may not yet be apparent.'

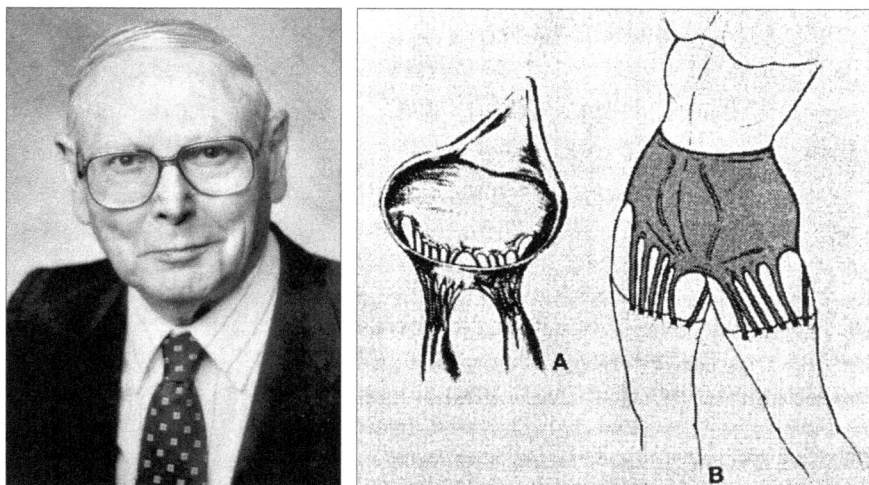

Fig 3.4 A. Charles Bailey. B. Cartoon drawing the analogy between mitral valve morphology and ladies' girdle. The artist was Walt Disney in his early days as a medical illustrator. Bailey sent the author his cartoon the year before he died.

Smithy was aware of Blalock's 'blue baby' surgery at Johns Hopkins and wrote to tell him about Betty's operation. Blalock replied immediately stating that he would keep and value the letter as a record of a very important landmark in surgery. But there was another aspect of the correspondence. Smithy sent Blalock a duplicate of his valvulotome prompting the response: 'Thank you ever so much for being good enough to have the instrument made for me.' I wonder if Blalock already knew where this was heading.

Smithy went on to operate on just six more patients, all young women. The second procedure on 1st March 1948 was unsuccessful because the instrument simply couldn't cut into the calcified valve and the unfortunate 25-year-old died ten hours afterwards. The next patient the following week also succumbed to pneumonia within days of the surgery. However the following four patients all survived including one 36-year-old who had an aborted left atrial approach followed by a successful attempt from the apex of left ventricle. Those where a segment of valve was removed with the instrument showed some degree of improvement. Others went through the operation without gaining benefit.

During the spring of 1948 Smithy himself experienced worsening heart failure from his narrowed aortic valve. On 20th May 1948 Dr John Boone, Chief of Medicine at the Medical College of South Carolina sent an urgent letter to Blalock at Johns Hopkins. 'I am writing to you at the request of Horace Smithy. He is very anxious to come to Baltimore soon and consider with you the possibility of having an aortic valvotomy done on himself.' Obviously Blalock was sympathetic. Four days later Smithy received a letter stating: 'The ideal thing would be to have you come to Baltimore and for the two of us to try to round up a couple of patients on which you could operate with my assistance.' He went on kindly, 'Nothing would give me greater pleasure than being able to help you by the use of your own method.'

Within days an optimistic Smithy travelled to Hopkins where he worked in the laboratory with Denton Cooley and Vivien Thomas, trying to perfect his vision of aortic valvotomy. He also had a test case in mind whom he brought from South Carolina. It was a crucial mistake. The man was in his late thirties, overweight and fluid overloaded, so much so that the chief nurse anaesthetist Miss Berger was pessimistic about his chances. Sure enough during induction of anaesthesia whilst Smithy and Blalock were at the scrub sink the patient developed an arrhythmia then cardiac arrest. In desperation the surgeons opened his chest to perform internal cardiac massage but he could not be revived. What's more Blalock was alarmed by the thickness of the left ventricle having never approached the heart with aortic stenosis before. It seemed that poor Smithy had destroyed his own chances by poor judgement.

Dr Cooley, who was to be first assistant had the surgery gone to plan, wrote his recollections of the atmosphere in the operating theatre. 'Anaesthesia was started and I began the incision over the fifth intercostal space. Just as I opened the pericardium the patient developed ventricular fibrillation. Despite all our efforts to defibrillate and resuscitate, that heart was not going to start.' Cooley was desperately disappointed for Smithy. 'I looked over at him and saw his face fall. He believed that this was his only chance at having an operation himself.' Sadly that was correct. Blalock was too anxious to proceed with an attempt on a colleague. Cooley would have done it but was not in the driving seat at that stage of his career.

Fate having dealt its lethal blow, poor Smithy returned to his family in despair. Predictably his health soon deteriorated. Betty Woolridge learned of the decline and wrote to nurse Bowen. 'I learned Dr Smithy was quite sick. I sure feel bad about it. I hope he will soon get well.' In fact it was Betty's aunt who penned the letter. The girl herself was too ill, and the very next day, 28th October 1948 Smithy passed away in an oxygen tent at Roper Hospital. Nurse Bowen was holding his hand. Ten days later Betty died in Canton, Ohio. She had been a great success story but not for long. Autopsy even revealed a contained leak from the site where the valvulotome was introduced into the ventricle and her valve was dismally deformed.

When the *Journal of the American Medical Association* published Smithy's obituary it contained a single non-committal phrase about cardiac surgery: '…is said to have performed the first successful heart valve operation'. An insulting remark that wasn't even true.

Long before Smithy's demise others were entering the cardiac arena. As a young boy Charles Bailey had watched his father die miserably from mitral stenosis and was motivated to find a solution. Ironically he may have been helped in that quest through selling ladies' girdles door to door in his school holidays. He saw the suspender belt as a skirt-like structure with numerous garters arising from its lower margin, attaching front and back to the tops of the stockings. It reminded him of the multiple strings, or chordae tendinae, which attach the anterior and posterior mitral valve leaflets to their papillary muscles on the ventricular wall. So taken was Bailey with the analogy that he had an aspiring young medical artist draw the valve and girdle side by side for him. He sent me an early reproduction of the illustration. Who was the artist? It was a certain Walter Disney, soon to be known for other cartoons.

Bailey was confident that mobility could be restored to deformed mitral valve leaflets by splitting the fused commissures stuck together by inflammation. And he was correct in that as long as the assault was made soon enough. He considered an approach through the left atrium to be safest and was aware that sudden severe mitral regurgitation was poorly tolerated. Against the background of numerous animal studies Bailey began to operate on patients in 1945. The first died through exsanguination from the tense atrium before the valve could be reached. The second left the operating theatre alive, but was dead from heart failure within forty-eight hours. Autopsy showed barely no widening of the valve orifice and the trauma had caused blood clot formation on the leaflets which further occluded the narrowing. Bailey then designed what he called a commisurotomy knife which he fixed to the palmar surface of his right index finger. The sharp edge together with ability to 'feel' his way into the valve orifice was a significant advance which almost succeeded in a 38-year-old man. Whilst the initial result seemed encouraging Bailey on the basis of his previous thrombosis death decided to use an anticoagulant post-operatively. This time the patient died from internal bleeding but at least that allowed an autopsy which showed the valve splitting to be encouraging.

By 1948 three of five hospitals in Philadelphia had banned Bailey from operating causing him to reflect on his state of mind. 'Finally you have to face the moment of truth, and the poignancy is so great that I can't really express it. You know that almost the whole world is against it; you know that you have a great personal stake and might even lose your medical licence or hospital privileges if you persist. In fact, the thought crosses your mind that maybe you really are crazy. And that you feel that is has to be done and that is has to be right.'

In what he regarded as the last chance saloon, Bailey scheduled one case at the Philadelphia General Hospital where he still had a morning operating slot, then another at Episcopal Hospital where he had afternoon privileges. He planned the day so that if the first patient died he would have one last opportunity before he could be stopped for good.

On the appointed morning, 38-year-old Bailey had measles with a rash and had to put off both procedures. One month later on 10th June 1948 he tried again. The first patient, an elderly man who had pulmonary complications, suffered a cardiac arrest before he even reached the mitral valve and could not be revived. So Bailey left the hospital quickly. He and his team drove directly to Episcopal Hospital where a 24-year-old woman Constance Warner was waiting irrespective of the fact that her family had begged her not to go ahead with surgery. With extreme trepidation he used the commissurotomy knife attached to his finger like a sharp claw and forcibly split open the valve. He then removed the instrument to digitally explore the final result. Sure enough the rigid leaflets were moving again with a whiff of mitral regurgitation, but Claire tolerated the procedure well and recovered. Just a couple of days later, bullish Bailey took her a thousand miles on a train to Chicago where he triumphantly presented the case at the conference of the American College of Chest Surgeons. This should be regarded as the world's first effective mitral valvotomy as Constance survived for another thirty-eight years without further surgery. Moreover her cause of death was viral pneumonia, not heart failure.

On 16th June, after two previous failures, Dwight Harken in Boston operated on a third patient using a modified Cutler valvulotome passed through the left atrium. This time the 28-year-old man survived claiming marked symptomatic improvement. However six of his next ten patients died leaving Harken devastated. So much so that following that tenth and fatal case he left the operating theatre and went home to bed, telling his wife that he had killed yet another patient and would never do another heart operation. Fortunately his cardiologist dissuaded him from that decision stating: 'Dwight you have never killed anyone. I have never sent you a patient who wasn't dying.' Downtime helped and eventually the program resumed with some adjustments in surgical technique. Like Bailey, Harken went on to dilate the valve with his index finger and lost only one of the next fifteen cases. Brock used the same technique successfully in London on 16th September 1948, generating a wave of optimism on both sides of the Atlantic. I was just three weeks old at the time.

The mitral valve procedures of Smithy, Bailey, Harken then Brock made 1948, the *annus mirabilis* of cardiac surgery as predicted by Cutler some twenty years before. Unfortunately Cutler did not live long enough to witness the progress he initiated. He died the previous year at the age of fifty-seven. But what about the aortic stenosis that ended Horace Smithy's life?

Was that amenable to the same approach. It seemed not. It was soon apparent that to punch out a segment of the aortic valve resulted in severe and potentially fatal valve leakage. Bailey tried various methods to alleviate aortic regurgitation in the laboratory. One concept was to remove the jugular vein from the dog's neck in an attempt to create an artificial valve. He did this by pushing a hollow cork bore through the aortic wall from one side to the other stretching out the opened vein patch above the leaking valve. Innovative but frankly useless. He tried using patches of aorta and pulmonary artery containing a single valve cusp but this was similarly abortive. It was difficult to control bleeding and too risky to experiment with patients.

With real ingenuity Bailey then decided to bypass the valve altogether using a tube from the apex of the ventricle to the aorta in the back of the chest. For this he used a long tube of preserved donor aorta with the valve in situ. Having obtained an appropriate length he divided it and reconstituted the conduit with the valve in the middle. Wizard in principle but there were far more failures than successes in the laboratory, so back to square one. He returned to simply punching out a piece of valve and hoping that the leak would be tolerated. On 9th March 1950 Bailey operated on a 26-year-old woman. Through a stab incision in the left ventricle he first introduced a knife but was unable to engage with the aortic valve. Undeterred, he then used a longer Heath-Robinson dilating instrument with which he managed to traverse the critically narrowed valve orifice – but it became stuck. Catastrophically so. Manoeuvres to remove it proved fruitless and the poor woman died through exsanguination on the operating table during the attempts. A brutal end to a tragically short life.

Next the intrepid surgeon devised an instrument with an umbrella-like tip which could be expanded by a screw at the end of the handle. On 6th April, less than a month after his previous disaster he tried again, this time introducing the instrument retrogradely through the right carotid artery in the neck. After railroading it through the narrow orifice he avulsed it forcibly, breaking the valve and causing severe aortic regurgitation. The poor patient survived the procedure but didn't do well. This caused Bailey to resort to the transventricular route again and over the following months he operated upon a further eleven patients. At least one third of these were known to have died as a result, but those who survived were said to be improved symptomatically.

Ever the determined optimist, on 8th April 1952 Bailey performed the first planned double valve operation, attempting to dilate both mitral and aortic valves. But by this time the intense rivalry, and indeed, acrimony between Philadelphia and Boston spilled over into clinical meetings. Bailey and Harken couldn't abide each other so their discussions at conferences always descended into undignified rows. Bailey is known to have commented: 'My mother was a redhead, my daughter is a redhead, I never was, but Harken was. We just tore at each other with the classic vigour of red-headed people!' And by that point each had filled a small cemetery.

By the autumn of 1952 Brock was able to report a series of ten mitral volvotomies undertaken through the left atrium with promising results. Declaring that 'heart surgery is now a reality' he commented that 'the finger alone splits the valve with an accuracy and speed that no instrument could rival'. Certainly these were brave, daring and in some cases reckless psychopaths who were not deterred by the body count. But the blind tearing of valves on a hit or miss basis could never be the answer in the long term. Heart surgery still needed a miracle to make it a reality. In the words of Arthur C Clarke: 'The limits of the possible can only be defined by going beyond them into the impossible.' It was coming.

Cooling Off

Start by doing what's necessary;
then do what's possible, and suddenly
you are doing the impossible.
—Francis of Assisi

The vascular surgeon Henry Swan summed it up eloquently in 1951: 'Finger vision is capable of limited success but bears the same relation to real vision that it does in life – one can read Braille with moderate facility but the chromatic values of the Mona Lisa escape one. And to shoot a winging mallard or fly an aeroplane is impossible. That the blind but educated finger is capable of accomplishing much within the heart is to be admitted and admired; that it should be considered the best method in the long run is absurd.'

Of course, Swan was correct, though 'closed mitral valvotomy' was used for many years to come. In an era when there was no reliable x-ray or ultrasound technique to demonstrate details of the pathology there had to be a way to directly visualise the defects under repair. The prospective but naive cardioscope might have helped if blood was transparent but in a bright red world it was useless. So was there anything else that might help? Could it ever prove feasible to interrupt the circulation altogether, given that nerve cells are damaged within minutes when deprived of oxygen? Damaged brain, life down the drain!

The first experiments in cooling the whole body for medical purposes emerged in 1940 when the American neurosurgeon Temple Faye attempted to slow the growth of cerebral tumours. He speculatively treated more than a thousand patients by cooling them down to 31°C for as long as several days using cold blankets. There was a justifiable fear of hypothermia at the time and sure enough the method had a high mortality rate. Metabolic studies on whole body cooling produced equivocal results with a surprising increase in oxygen consumption when it was expected to fall. The finding was confirmed by a German research programme initiated after the deaths of Luftwaffe pilots who ejected into the North Sea. Immersion experiments on dogs simulating the experience showed an average increase in metabolism of around 200% and sudden death from ventricular fibrillation at temperatures below 20°C. They found that the shivering in response to cold was responsible by dramatically increasing the basal metabolic rate by up to 400% in some animals.

Cold weather generated particular interest in hypothermia in Canada. In the winter of 1941 the young surgical resident William Bigelow encountered a number of patients at the Toronto General Hospital where frostbite had progressed to gangrene. Bigelow was surprised at the lack of information on the subject, so after carefully documenting the progress of individual patients he published his own medical review entitled *The Modern Concept and Treatment of Frostbite*. This explained that tissue death with gangrene followed shutdown of the peripheral circulation and was not caused by direct damage from cold temperatures on the tissues and cells themselves.

During World War II Bigelow was sent to England with the Canadian Army in preparation for the Normandy landings. As an army surgeon he also had an interest in injuries to the major blood vessels which more often than not required amputation of the affected limb. It was predictable therefore, that he explored cooling as a method to preserve tissue viability for longer until complex vascular repair could be undertaken.

Bigelow succeeded in persuading the British War Office to build him a purpose-built cooling cabinet. At the same time he requested a supply of the new anticoagulant heparin from the Toronto General Hospital, who had introduced it in 1935. Together with fine arterial sutures, and newly-designed vitallium tubes to aid vascular reconstruction, he embarked with the Sixth Casualty Clearing Station for the Normandy landings, anticipating many wounded blood vessels to repair. But he didn't encounter one. Amputations were still needed for shattered limbs should the soldier survive. Frustrating.

On his return to Canada Bigelow was sent south to train with Blalock at Johns Hopkins having been promised a vascular surgery post at Toronto General. Cooley was chief resident by then and Hopkins was a magnet for would-be thoracic surgeons worldwide. Nonetheless Bigelow made one key observation. Whilst the prolific shunt procedure was inspired it was far from curative. With growth, children who had improved initially were returning to Dr Taussig's clinic with further symptoms. Meaningful surgery could only be achieved under direct vision within the heart, and from his work with hypothermia Bigelow felt that the simplest option would be to cool the body, reduce the brain's oxygen consumption, then completely stop the circulation. For a few minutes the heart could then be opened. The concept simply shifted his strategy of local limb cooling towards reducing the temperature of the whole body.

When Bigelow began his studies it was still anticipated that the brain, heart, liver and kidneys would require more rather than less oxygen during hypothermia through the shivering effect. At the Banting Institute in Toronto Bigelow experimented by reducing the temperature of anaesthetised dogs with a cooling blanket. And, as anticipated, this reproducibly caused an increase in muscle tone followed by tremor and a concomitant increase in metabolism. Oxygen requirement went up not down which was a problem.

Then by chance came the solution. The introduction of muscle relaxants. Overnight a more sophisticated cocktail of anaesthetic drugs eliminated the increase in muscle tone and stopped the shivering. It was a Eureka moment. From then onwards surface cooling produced a consistent linear fall in oxygen consumption by the tissues. And cooling protected the brain against low oxygen levels. Bigelow's painstaking investigations included the effects of low body temperature on blood pressure, heart rate, and blood chemistry. They showed that the lower limit of safe cooling in an adult animal was between 20°C to 23°C but new-born puppies tolerated cooling to much lower temperatures. And importantly no brain damage was detected after rewarming.

Bigelow went on to experiment with basic heart operations on the cold animals. He found that a body temperature of 30°C decreased oxygen requirements to 50% of normal. Then profound hypothermia at 20°C would allow complete interruption of blood flow to the brain for at least 45 minutes thereby allowing the heart to be opened for more complex direct vision repair. Of course with a couple of minutes needed to cut into the cardiac chamber then at least five minutes to close, the safe duration to operate within the heart was still limited. But some deformities could be repaired.

By tightening snares around the superior and inferior vena cava, the main veins draining into the right atrium, the cold slowly-beating heart would eject its contents and empty. In the dog, the right atrium could be opened to inspect the interatrial septum then by looking through the tricuspid valve a clear view of the interventricular septum was possible. Thus holes in the heart should be accessible in children. After fifteen minutes the right atrium was stitched closed, the snares released to fill the heart with blood again and the animal rewarmed in a warm water bath. Bigelow was excited and motivated by his findings.

This is an appropriate point to declare that I am an animal lover and very much disliked vivisection. But what was the alternative. No one would breed children for research purposes and it was generally deemed unacceptable to experiment on sick patients.

Of the first three dozen dogs whose hearts were operated upon by Bigelow, half survived and the ground breaking observations were presented at the 1950 meeting of the American Surgical Association. In November of that year the corresponding scientific paper was published in the *Annals of Surgery* where Bigelow wrote: 'The use of hypothermia as a form of anaesthetic could conceivably extend the scope of surgery in many new directions. A state in which the body temperature is lowered and the oxygen requirements of tissues are reduced to a small fraction of normal would allow exclusion of organs from the circulation for prolonged periods. Such a technique might permit surgeons to operate upon the 'bloodless heart' without recourse to extracorporeal pumps and perhaps allow transplantation of organs.' And then the crucial point: 'A bloodless heart excluded from the circulation is necessary before further progress can be made in the field of cardiac surgery.'

For the next two years Bigelow's team worked cautiously to increase the safety of hypothermia, in particular to reduce the risk of ventricular fibrillation and a fatal complication known as rewarming shock which was ill understood. Monkeys were found to tolerate cooling to lower temperatures than dogs and could be safely rewarmed in a water bath seemingly without suffering shock. Remarkably hibernating mammals such as groundhogs could be cooled to 5°C, and then tolerate an open heart procedure for two hours with recovery. So finally Bigelow felt ready to attempt a human operation. Indeed the Toronto cardiologists had already identified a number of straightforward congenital heart patients with atrial septal defect or pulmonary stenosis for him to begin with. But unknown to the group others had been working towards the same goal.

In Minnesota Floyd Lewis and Mansur Taufic employed surface cooling to create atrial septal defects in dogs, but with high attrition rate through fatal arrhythmias. They even re-operated on surviving dogs to close the hole, recording survival in 17 of 26 animals. Of more importance they observed that after opening the heart residual air bubbles entering the coronary arteries were responsible for most fatalities. Clearly coronary air embolism was a complication to avoid in prospective patients.

After following the research efforts at conferences and in the literature it was Charles Bailey who made the first attempt to use hypothermia in a patient. The 32-year-old woman with an atrial septal defect underwent surgery on August 29th 1952, but died afterwards from coronary air embolism and intractable ventricular fibrillation. Little is known about the exact circumstances, other than the procedure followed a number of 'Atrio-septo-pexy' operations where he had attempted to close the defect blindly by invaginating the wall of the right atrium. The unfortunate hypothermia patient had already been subject to this technique but unsuccessfully. And on this occasion Bailey did not rush off to a conference to present the case.

Four days after Bailey's fatality Lewis and his colleagues entered the clinical arena, in the knowledge that if they didn't press ahead Bailey might try again and be the first to succeed.

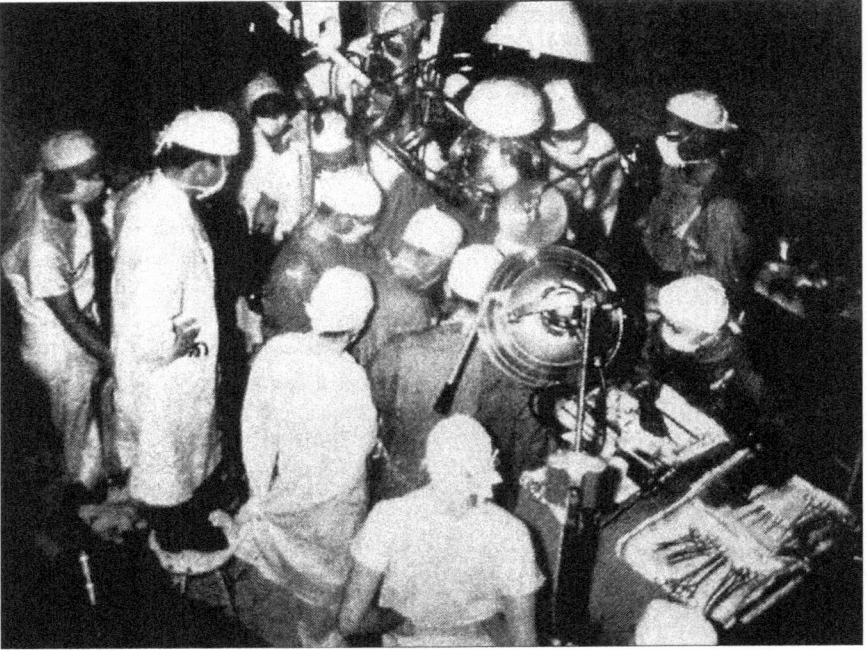

Fig 4.1 A. The first direct vision closure of an atrial septal defect by
Floyd Lewis and Mansur Taufic using moderate hypothermia
at the University of Minnesota on September 2nd 1952.

On 2nd September they took a child to the operating theatre and subsequently reported the case as follows alongside their animal experiments.
'The patient was an underdeveloped, sickly 29 pound 5-year-old girl in
whom the diagnosis of an atrial septal defect had been established by cardiac catheterisation. She was anaesthetised with Pentothal sodium and the
muscle relaxant curare and the trachea intubated. She was then wrapped
in refrigerated blankets until after a period of two hours and ten minutes
her rectal temperature had fallen to 28°C (82°F). At this point the blankets
were removed and the chest was entered through the bed of the right fifth
rib. The cardiac inflow (superior and inferior vena cavae) was occluded for
a total of five and one-half minutes and during that time a septal defect
measuring approximately 2cm in diameter was closed under direct vision,
in the manner described in the section on experimental method. In one
respect the procedure was easier than it had been in dogs, for the right

atrium was dilated and hence roomier to work in. When the Satinsky clamp and ligatures had been removed the pulse promptly regained its strength. At the conclusion of the operation which lasted fifty-eight minutes, the patient's rectal temperature was 26°C (79°F). To rewarm her she was placed in hot water kept at 45°C (113°F) and after thirty-five minutes her rectal temperature had risen to 36°C (96.8°F) at which time she was removed from the bath. Recovery from anaesthesia was prompt and her subsequent post-operative convalescence has been uneventful. She left hospital on the eleventh post-operative day. Her cardiac murmur has gone.'

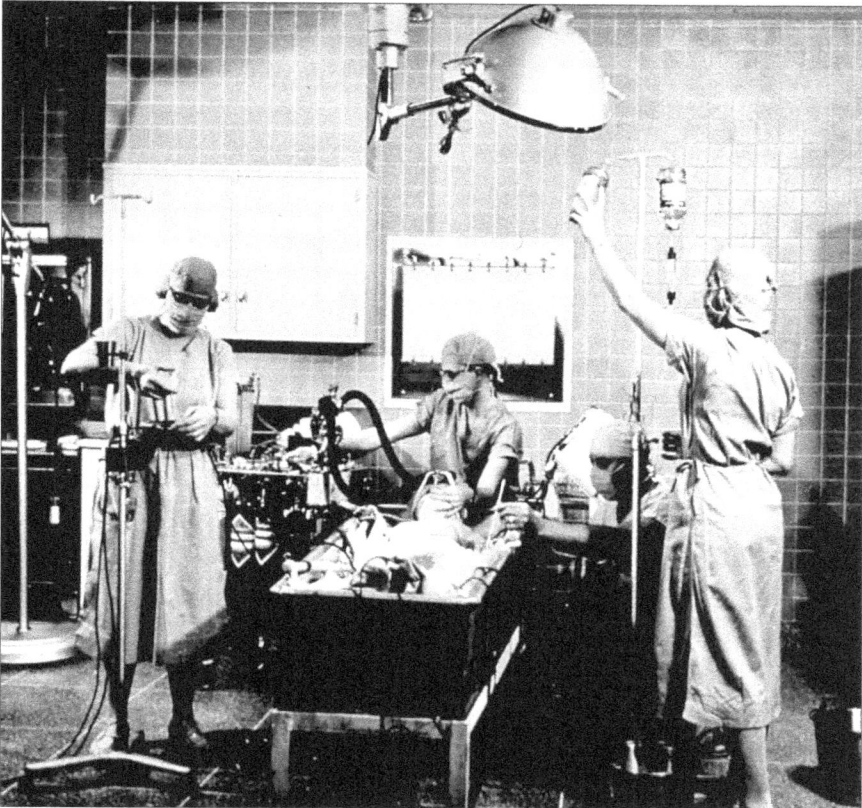

Fig 4.1 B. Water bath cooling under general anaesthetic.

Lewis had used the Satinsky clamp to occlude the aorta and origins of both coronary arteries to prevent the lethal air embolism problem. Coronary arteries are very small in children so tiny bubbles of air can easily aggregate and completely occlude them. Lewis assiduously worked to expel air from within the chambers by inserting a polythene catheter through the stitches in the atrial wall and infusing salt solution. That worked well particularly when combined with use of the aortic clamp.

By the early 1950s other innovative solutions were being considered to close holes in the heart. Robert Gross the first surgeon to close a ductus arteriosus, developed an ingenious method himself at the Boston Children's Hospital. Curiously he found that it was possible to open the right atrium whilst the heart continued to beat and support the circulation. In the landmark paper *A Method for Surgical Closure of Interauricular Septal Defects'*, he wrote: 'It seemed to us that it might be possible to attach temporarily to the heart some sort of hollow cylinder, into the base of which the atrium could be opened. Blood would rise up into the receptacle for a distance equal to the intra-atrial pressure, which ought not be more than a few centimetres. If it were possible to couple such an appliance to the heart it might be feasible to work through this pool of blood in a blind manner, but deliberately with the guidance of exploring fingers, so that an atrial septal defect could be approached and closed by appropriate means.'

Gross was sceptical about hypothermia and the interruption of blood draining back into the heart with snares on the venae cavae. He predicted fatalities through allowing air into the chambers and stated dismissively: 'This drastic manoeuvre cannot be continued for more than a few minutes and would certainly seem impractical for the closure of large defects. Furthermore in the presence of a septal defect it would be impossible to prevent embolization of air into the major arteries.' He was correct about that, given the many deaths from coronary air embolism, and disabling strokes from bubbles to the brain.

Gross's invention was a rubber cylinder, or 'well' which he sewed to the side of the right atrium of dogs and used heparin to stop blood clotting on the surface.

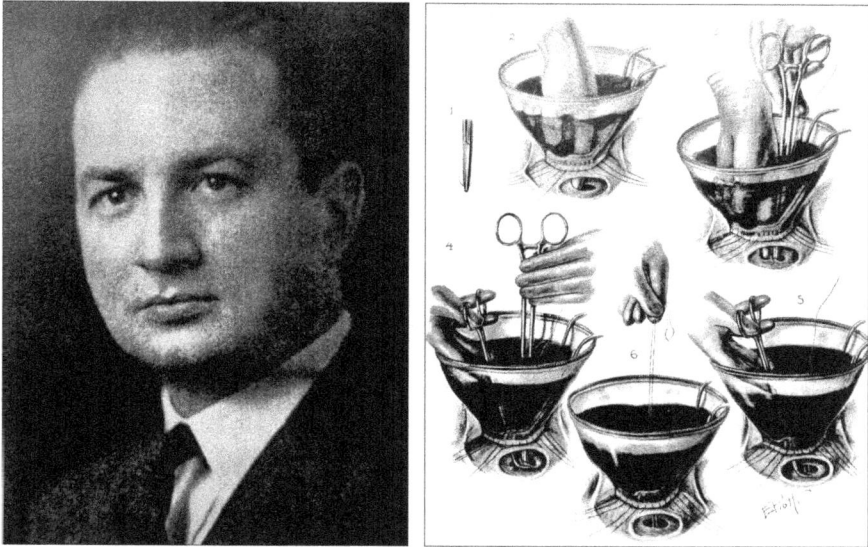

Fig 4.2 A. Robert Gross who performed the first repair of coarctation of the aorta. B. The ingenious Gross atrial well technique for closure of atrial septal defects introduced in 1953. Blood rises for several centimetres in the rubber well to the level of the intra atrial pressure. This allows the surgeon to work by finger palpation through an incision in the right atrial wall.

Numerous designs were tested before settling upon the most suitable. This was then used in 114 dogs to perfect the best approach for attachment to the heart and give access to the interatrial septum. Two special instruments were designed to help the process, the first being a clamp to pinch off and isolate a segment of right atrial wall. The second was a self-retaining retractor to hold the base of the well open. This provided access for the surgeon's fingers and a needle holder with which to sew the defect closed. And predicting a fall in the patient's blood pressure when the well filled, blood for transfusion was always kept on standby.

Despite the detailed preparations things did not go as planned when the technique was used for patients. The first application was in an 8-year-old girl who had suffered worsening heart failure since the age of four. The heart was hugely dilated, her liver grossly enlarged with abdominal distension and the poor child was breathless on the slightest exertion. She was a typical end stage case which characterised most first attempts in that era. That is why the preliminary laboratory work was so important.

On April 3rd 1952 Gross operated on her through the right chest, cutting the fifth and sixth ribs front and back. On retracting the lung and opening the pericardium he confirmed that the right atrium was hugely enlarged as expected. A large rubber well was sewn to the wall with silk stitches and naturally caused bleeding. When the incision was made blood rose within the cylinder to a level of 6cm. At that point Gross could feel the edges of the interatrial defect but the heart rhythm became irritable. Not knowing how much manipulation the heart would tolerate, Gross decided to close the septum with a purpose-made lucite button which gripped the edges of the defect with steel prongs. As he then noted: 'The size of the heart diminished greatly and the thrill in the pulmonary artery disappeared.' The well had been open for just twelve minutes before the atrium could be closed again.

For the first few hours things the child recovered satisfactorily with stable pulse and blood pressure. But then everything changed. She gradually turned blue with distended neck veins and became breathless again. Inhaled oxygen didn't help so Gross concluded that the button had displaced and was obstructing the tricuspid valve. Fluoroscopic x-ray examination confirmed that suspicion so on April 28th she was taken back to the operating theatre. Again there was no difficulty in attaching the atrial well, making the incision and confirming the diagnosis. The main portion of the septal defect was indeed open and the button displaced. Gross removed it and on this occasion closed the hole with silk stitches. But sadly as the chest incision was being closed the heart rhythm slowed then stopped entirely. There was an air of desperation in the room. After a period of manual internal cardiac massage Gross injected adrenalin then calcium which caused ventricular fibrillation. A single electric shock restored regular rhythm with ejections that gradually increased in vigour for several minutes but in Gross's words, 'skin colour was poor and peripheral pulsations were unobtainable'. A seizure followed after which no heart sounds could be heard and the electrocardiogram again showed ventricular fibrillation. Shortly afterwards the poor girl flat-lined and was declared dead.

Autopsy showed extensive bleeding into the lungs and brain. Whilst the atrial well technique worked as planned, surgical error had caused her death.

Two further attempts that same week were on fragile, wasted girls of 4 years and 8 years respectively. The first was shunting seven litres of blood per minute from left to right atrium whilst the second had twice that amount with huge dilatation of the right ventricle. Inexplicably both received a 'Hufnagel' lucite button again for expediency. It failed in both and they each died on the third post-operative day. Three young girls, three successful approaches to the atrial septum, then three device failures precipitating tragic post-operative death. A miserable experience with three bereaved and distraught families all in one week.

Did Gross throw in the towel after these disasters? Not at all. The next attempt on April 15th was on a 9-year-old boy whose defect he closed successfully with a stitched nylon patch. The lad survived and his debilitating symptoms resolved constituting the first success with the atrial well technique. Patient five, a 14-year-old girl similarly recovered causing Gross to state: 'Four months after the operation this child appears to be in excellent health. She is most exuberant. She likes to play tennis and other strenuous sports, all of which are entirely new experiences for her.'

Inexplicably, the next patient, a 16-year-old boy also died from surgical error. A sheet of polyethylene was used to close the septal defect but the size was ill judged. In his operation note Gross wrote: 'Digital palpitation of the anchored sheet disclosed that the hole was completely closed over but that the piece of plastic was too long, and therefore projected down over the annulus of the tricuspid valve. We were loath to remove it as the well had already been kept open for two hours and five minutes.' Autopsy following death on the third post-operative day showed that blood clot had formed on the kinked patch and obstructed the tricuspid valve. Misery. Yet Gross deemed the collective experience a great success and others adopted the method. Ironically I doubt that occluders nor patches were needed to close these atrial septal defects as edge to edge closure with stitches is simpler, safe and more expedite.

John Kirklin was the son of a radiologist in Muncie, Indiana. During World War II the Harvard graduate spent two years as a trainee neurosurgeon with the US army treating head trauma patients evacuated from Europe and the Pacific. Notwithstanding that experience it was a six-month residency with Gross at the Boston Children's Hospital that switched his focus to the chest. In Kirklin's own words: 'Gross looked like a surgeon sent from central casting – handsome, quiet and very stimulating. He was such a magnetic personality and his work was so fascinating to me that I switched to the idea of being a cardiac surgeon.' He continued, 'My fellow residents and I would fill pages of notebooks with drawings of how we might close ventricular septal defects, and repair tetralogy of Fallot once science gave us a method to get into the heart.'

In 1950 Kirklin completed general surgical residency at the Mayo Clinic and began putting into practice what was learned from working with Gross. He started by using the well technique for atrial septal defects and then for a more complex deformity called a partial atrioventricular canal. His results were excellent in several hundred cases yet it was still not direct vision surgery. Something new was definitely required, because time limited hypothermia did not allow correction of more complex congenital defects or valvular heart disease in adults.

Perhaps the last word on hypothermia should go to Henry Swan who like Bigelow had worked with casualties in France during the war. Swan was a skilled technician who employed hypothermia on more than a hundred patients with a range of conditions experiencing comparatively low mortality. Yet operating with one eye on the clock didn't suit him. He confessed: 'I have always been scared to death of it because I do not know what is going on. I have some definite reasons to use it, but I like to get the job done, then get the patient back up to normal temperature as quickly as possible where I believe I can understand him better.' Brock was more forthright on the matter. 'I cannot bring myself to believe that such a procedure can have a permanent role in surgery', concluding that 'The mere presence of the iced water bath in an operating theatre is both aesthetically and surgically unattractive.'

Sure enough the prolonged ice bath cooling then rewarming process with rushed operations in the interim soon became obsolete. Nonetheless hypothermia would always have its place as an adjunct to more sophisticated surgical techniques.

Double Jeopardy

As a surgeon you have to have a controlled
arrogance. If it is uncontrolled you kill people,
but you have to be pretty arrogant to saw
through a person's chest, take out their heart,
and believe that you can fix it.

—Mehmet Oz

If asked to name the true legends of my specialty I would undoubtedly begin with three: they are Drs John Kirklin, Denton Cooley and the enigmatic Walton Lillehei. I was privileged to know them all and without doubt the label 'crazy man' could only applied to the last one. The man who was also named 'the father of open heart surgery', a label that nobody challenged in his lifetime or indeed since because of the huge number of innovations and concepts he was responsible for.

Culzean Castle is perched high on a cliff on the Ayrshire coast and was a fitting place for me to meet Lillehei. Walt was staying in the splendid top floor apartment which had been gifted to General Dwight D Eisenhower after the war. A hideaway which he secretly used during his Presidency of the United States. I'd been asked to dinner there that evening during a St Jude Valve Company conference at Turnberry golf course of which Walt was Chairman. I assumed there would be others there but there weren't. He'd invited me to share recollections for my textbook *Landmarks in Cardiac Surgery*, and given that he now had prostate cancer, he wanted his legacy to be as accurate as possible. I was keen to listen. It was a privilege to spend time with him away from the formal meeting.

He greeted me at the foot of the grand oval staircase wearing a red velvet smoking jacket with a crystal whisky glass in his left hand. A gentle slightly built figure by now, he still had that fixed tilt of his neck to the right shoulder and a broad welcoming grin which suggested that he was happy to see me. In the circular saloon directly overlooking the ocean we were met by the butler with more glasses of scotch and a plate of smoked salmon. Two well-worn armchairs beckoned in front of a log fire. I could imagine Eisenhower slumped in the larger one so I sat in it myself. This was not an evening I would easily forget as the waves battered the rocks below.

Born in Minneapolis in 1918 Lillehei was destined to spend most of his life in that same city where his father was a dentist. A mechanically minded individual he planned to follow the family practice but discovering that the academic qualifications were the same for medicine he opted for the latter instead. Soon after graduating war service intervened and he found himself caring for the wounded in Algeria then Tunisia. As commanding officer of the 33rd Field MASH unit accompanying the army pursuing Rommel, his caravan was attacked by a group of Messerschmitts which totally destroyed their equipment. Lillehei's team moved to to join the allied invasions of Sicily then mainland Italy at Anzio where he rose to the rank of Lieutenant Colonel and earned a bronze star for courage and meritorious service. All told he spent four years in the army culminating in the award of the European Theatre ribbon with five battle stars. A courageous character, he was not easily intimidated.

In 1945 Lillehei returned to the USA and the University of Minnesota to complete his residency. There he worked under Professor Owen Wangensteen, a distinguished academic, who insisted that all his trainees should spend a period in laboratory research. Walt did this with the physiologist Maurice Visscher surgically creating an 'aterio-venous fistula' aimed at replicating a hole in the heart. What he found was that infection invariably developed at the join resulting in kidney failure. Lillehei considered this to explain why infections of the heart, known as bacterial endocarditis often caused the death of children with congenital heart defects. It therefore seemed logical that surgery should be undertaken as early as possible to prevent these complications.

In the winter of 1950 he became aware of a lump beneath his right ear. Biopsy showed it to be a highly malignant sarcoma of the parotid gland with a very poor prognosis. Wangensteen was determined to do the best for his talented trainee so the day after completing his residency Lillehei underwent radical excision of the tumour together with lymph glands from the neck and upper chest. Richard Varco, Lillehei's close friend assisted the boss. Inevitably the operation followed by a hefty course of radiotherapy left scarring and permanent deformity of the young surgeon's neck which took great effort and determination to overcome.

As the fire crackled and the whisky slipped down I probed him on his reaction to the devastating diagnosis. It was just as one might expect. Initial pessimism and despair – the why me reaction? Then an injection of positivity from his supportive environment, followed by the desire to help others as his own outlook gradually improved. A determined individual before the diagnosis, he was even more committed afterwards. There were things to be done.

During convalescence Walt attended hundreds of autopsies on patients who had died from heart disease retaining organs on which he performed mock operations. He found that with an incision through the wall of the right ventricle in tetralogy of Fallot the hole in the septum could be closed relatively easily. Two other things seemed obvious to him. First, the Blalock shunt procedure did not correct the fundamental problem. Second, that curative surgery might easily be possible with prolonged access to the inside of the heart. A few minutes with hypothermia and inflow occlusion simply didn't cut it for complex conditions.

So when Wangensteen asked his recovering patient: 'What research would you care to do now Walt?' the reply was straightforward. 'Open heart surgery'.

In the meantime Richard Varco had adopted responsibility for the Blalock shunt operations in Minneapolis and to begin with he routinely opened the pericardium to confirm the diagnosis of tetralogy. Having noted that one third of the patients had predominantly pulmonary valve stenosis he opted to use brief periods of vena caval occlusion without cooling to relieve the obstruction. And indeed, these patients seemed to fare better than those receiving the shunt alone.

By 1952 the Minnesota surgeons became aware of research work on mechanical heart lung machines by John Gibbon in Philadelphia and Viking Bjork in Stockholm. But Lillehei regarded the devices as too cumbersome and beset with complications. Soon afterwards the extraordinary idea for an alternative emerged serendipitously when a research associate announced that his wife was pregnant. Why did a pregnancy throw the switch? Because all pregnant mammals provide oxygen for their offspring in the womb through the placenta. So might an artificial placenta be created by connecting the circulation of a child to that of a suitable donor. A parent would be ideal. The donor's lungs would then oxygenate the child's blood whilst the heart pumped it around the body. This would allow the patient to be kept alive whilst his own heart was operated on. Simple. Or was it?

Back to the laboratory. Using donor dogs somewhat larger than the recipient animals, the large arteries and veins were connected using plastic piping. When the smaller recipient's heart was stopped recordings from leg arteries showed that their blood pressure depended upon the rate of flow from the donor. And better levels of oxygen could be obtained by increasing the flow. Consequently a booster pump was included in the connecting tubing.

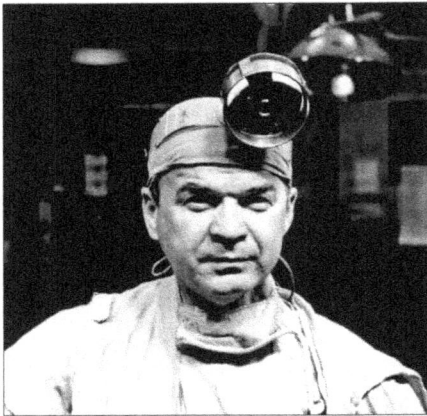

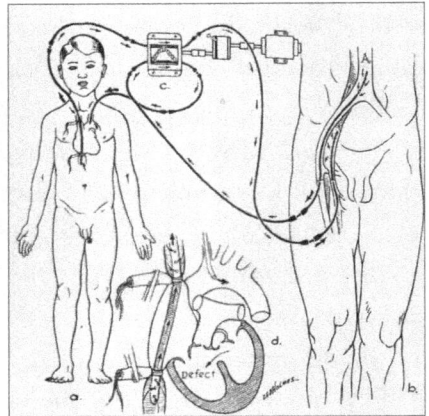

Fig 5.1 A. Walt Lillehei wearing his operating headlamp.
B. Diagram of the cross circulation technique.

At this stage all those tinkering with cardiovascular surgery at the University of Minnesota were general surgeons who were excited by the potential in the new field. Wangensteen promoted Lillehei to the rank of Assistant Professor with the remit to supervise two promising young men, Morley Cohen and Herbert Warden, in his lab. It was Morley's wife who was carrying the child and enthusiasm for the cross circulation project was gaining momentum. Refinements in the experimental procedure and improved surgical techniques meant that none of the donor dogs died even though several served in that capacity more than once. Something that wouldn't be condoned these days. By 1954 confidence in this approach to open heart surgery was such that even the laboratory technicians were asking 'when are you going to do a patient?'

Could permission ever be obtained for an operation that involved an individual who wasn't sick and inevitably risked 200% mortality? Walt took a sizeable gulp of his whisky, stared at the gilded ceiling and admitted: 'I never thought we would be allowed to do it on a patient. The stakes were too high even in those days.' He assembled a comprehensive dossier for Wangensteen including a compendium of all the experimental experience with detailed physiological analysis. A few days later there was a short handwritten response, 'Dear Walt, by all means go ahead.' Signed O.H.W. But that's not how the hospital authorities saw it, and he was told not to proceed.

This was a consistent theme throughout the pioneering years and something I encountered monotonously regularly myself. There would be no clinical advances if we listened to the administrative staff or regulatory authorities. To bring cross circulation into the operating theatre needed careful planning. There had to be two surgical teams with separate sets of instruments and anaesthetists. The extracorporeal tubing had to be modified to cover the greater distance between donor and patient, then the 'clean' techniques used in the laboratory had to be translated into sterilised protocols for the surgery.

The paediatric cardiologists were asked to select three potential candidates for the first operation, and of course their lives had to be in immediate danger to justify the controversial approach. To begin with Lillehei wanted to perform direct vision closure of a ventricular septal defect. With this in mind he took Varco and Cohen to the Mayo Clinic where they spent a day examining congenital heart deformities in Dr Jesse Edwards's laboratory. All specimens were carefully labelled in buckets of formalin, each with a medical summary. The experience alerted the surgeons to the varied size, shape and location of the holes they were likely to encounter and was time well spent.

Was it difficult to decide upon the first candidate? Of course, but there were reasons. They chose a sickly 11-month-old boy who had been hospitalised with frequent bouts of pneumonia on top of digoxin resistant heart failure. Weighing just 6.9kg he was one of 13 children in the family and one sibling had already died with a ventricular septal defect. 'Would you have chosen him if he had been an only child?' I asked Walt. Discretely he didn't answer. He just said: 'His father had compatible blood and volunteered to serve as the donor. He was a big man which helped.'

Tension grew as the date chosen for the operation approached. With opposition from the hospital authorities, Lillehei realised he could lose his job and his reputation should the child die. Worse still, if the father came to harm he had been warned of criminal charges. It was also a stressful time for the operating room nurses and anaesthetists who spent days beforehand checking and rechecking their assigned responsibilities in obsessive-compulsive fashion.

On March 26th 1954 the sedated boy and his father, were wheeled into operating theatre B of the University of Minnesota Medical Centre at 06.00 am. Most of the team had been preparing for hours without sleep, but from then on the repeatedly rehearsed steps were achieved seamlessly. Lillehei and Varco stood either side of the child whilst Cohen and Warden prepared the lightly anaesthetised father. Fine cannulas were inserted into the vessels of the patient's neck and larger ones into the main leg artery and vein in the father's groin. Cross circulation was controlled with a Sigma motor pump which massaged the blood forward within the tubing at an average of 55 ml/kg body weight per minute. Just 380 ml per minute at normal body temperature was sufficient for the boy and quite safe for his father.

With snares on the venae cavae and an empty heart, Lillehei made a scalpel incision through the beating right ventricular wall. This was gently held open by Varco using small metal retractors, and with huge relief they found themselves staring directly at the ventricular septal defect, a hole the size of a shirt button. These days we would sew in a patch, carefully avoiding the vital electrical conduction system. In 1954 they were unaware of its position and for expediency the hole was pulled closed with three individual stitches. Together with closure of the right ventricle and removal of air it was all done calmly and purposefully in 19 minutes. Photographed by a camera above, the historical record clearly shows Cohen and Warden staring intently over Varco's shoulder into the child's chest. At least the father's anaesthetist stayed with him!

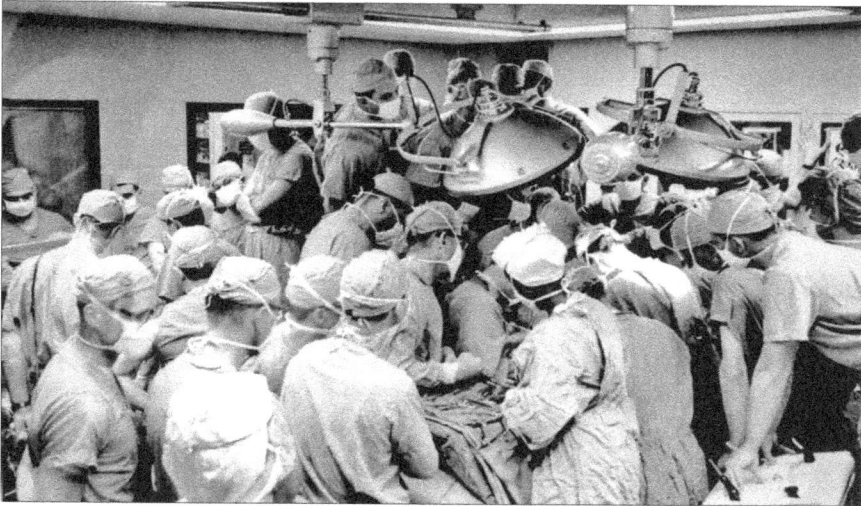

Fig 5.2 Picture taken on the occasion of the first cross circulation operation at the University of Minnesota.

As the boy's chest was being closed and the cannulas removed from his father's groin, a rapturous round of applause broke out from the observation gallery. Leading the accolade was Wangensteen himself. Warden would later confess: 'From a personal point of view, I am compelled to say that even now, the opportunity to peer into a living beating human heart for the first time was one of the most momentous, moving and humbling experiences I have ever had. I am certain that others were similarly moved.' Who could blame him? Watching blood flow from the donor vessels was not particularly exciting.

Father and son were brought out to the recovery room together where spirits were high. Both had a strong steady pulse and good blood pressure. Wakening from sedation the father asked Warden 'is Greg okay?' Thankfully he was but things did not stay that way. A week after the operation the lad contracted pneumonia, a common problem when the sore chest wound discourages coughing. But sadly it killed him on the eleventh post-operative day. Autopsy showed the boy's ventricular septal defect to be closed securely, but there were already degenerative changes in the lungs after long term shunting of blood. Fortunately the father recovered uneventfully and was discharged from hospital on day three. Obviously he was devastated when incidental infection deprived him of his son.

Three weeks later the team operated on a second ventricular septal defect, this time in a four-year-old boy using the father for cross circulation. This child survived and thrived and by the end of August a total of eight septal defects had been closed under direct vision with just two deaths.

Given the epic success, the hospital cheerfully advertised the operations to the media and the surgical world descended on the University of Minnesota. The small case series was presented at the American Association for Thoracic Surgery Meeting that year after which Sir Russell Brock, Denton Cooley and Viking Bjork headed a stream of visitors to fill the glass observation dome of Operating Room J. During discussion of the paper Alfred Blalock commented: 'I never thought I would live to see the day when this type of procedure could be performed.' He commended the Minnesota surgeons for their bravery, imagination and courage. Nevertheless Blalock predicted that it would be the emerging heart-lung machine, not cross circulation that would ultimately support open heart surgery.

Between March 19th 1954 and July 1955 Lillehei employed cross circulation for 45 patients of which 28 survived the operation and were discharged from hospital. Some mothers participated as well as fathers. Obviously the more complex the defect the greater was the risk of death but there were no serious complications in any of the parents. Notably 17 patients with repaired ventricular septal defect and two with tetralogy of Fallot were alive and well thirty years later. Eleven of the female patients collectively gave birth to 25 children, none of whom had congenital heart defects.

In the autumn of 1954 a young physician called Richard DeWall approached Lillehei with a request to join the research group. Lillehei needed someone reliable to supervise the Sigma pump during cross circulation and suggested DeWall begin with that job. The department of Surgery originally gave him the status of resident but the snooty Dean of the Graduate School of Medicine instructed that Wangensteen refuse him admission because his medical school grades were too low. When confronted with the news DeWall decided to stay on as a laboratory assistant, the difference being that his wages were doubled!

Lillehei was keen to keep DeWall when he learned of his innovative ideas about the leaking valve after closed mitral valvotomy. That pathway deviated one morning during an informal conference in the laboratory. Walt introduced the subject of dissolving oxygen in blood and whether a device could be created to do so. It was well known that when oxygen was bubbled through blue blood from the veins it would rapidly turn it red or 'arterialised' – as he put it. The problem was to get rid of bubbles and foaming which would block the tiny blood vessels. Several possibilities were discussed and at the end of the debate DeWall was assigned the task of solving the debubbling issue.

This was clear evidence that Lillehei had reservations about the sustainability of his brilliant but risk-laden cross circulation technique. It was inevitable that eventually a healthy donor would suffer a significant complication and there had already been near misses. When I queried Walt about it that evening at Culzean he was forthright about an occasion when he feared losing a father through rampant post-operative infection. That was bound to happen sooner or later, and was cause for concern when others were introducing what they called a mechanical pump oxygenator. So Walt decided to make his own heart-lung machine. And quickly.

Pumping Blood

You know what the difference between a
cardiac surgeon and God is? God doesn't
think he's a cardiac surgeon.
—Lisa Gardner

Blood is a delicate substance. The fluid component known as plasma comprises around 55% of the volume carrying with it the red and white blood cells, and the sticky platelets that initiate clotting. The objective of clotting is to seal leaks and stop bleeding from the smooth cellular lining of the arteries, veins and capillaries within our body. But what happens when blood encounters a non-biological surface such as the tubing between the parent and child in cross circulation surgery? The clotting process is triggered immediately because blood doesn't like to leave its own environment. That is what stops bleeding and keeps us alive after an accident.

In certain circumstances spontaneous clotting can occur within the circulation and thrombosis within a vessel supplying the brain, heart muscle or lungs may prove fatal through stroke, heart attack or massive pulmonary embolism. Curiously it was an embolus which ultimately gave rise to the heart-lung machine and an unfortunate young woman who had just become a mother provided the impetus.

It was February 1932 when John Gibbon, a junior resident in Philadelphia, was allocated the task of night watching the female patient. In her twenties she had been confined to bed for three weeks with high blood pressure during the last trimester of pregnancy, then shortly after giving birth she suddenly became breathless. A pulmonary embolus was diagnosed and she was placed in an oxygen tent. It didn't help. If blood doesn't reach the lung tissue it will not pick up oxygen or eliminate carbon dioxide. So she was blue, shocked and in great distress. Gibbon held her hand and tried to calm her. Intermittently the nurse read out her pulse rate and blood pressure which constantly drifted in the wrong direction. After informing his boss Edward Churchill of the deterioration they eventually decided to take her to the operating theatre and attempt to remove the clots.

Pulmonary embolectomy was both a 'smash and grab' and 'hit or miss' effort in those days. Churchill succeeded in removing a long snake-like clot that had migrated from the leg veins but, devoid of clotting factors, the poor girl bled profusely from her uterus and died. The following day Gibbon wrote: 'During the 17 hours by this patient's bedside the thought constantly occurred to me that the hazardous condition could be improved if some of the blue blood in the distended veins could be continuously withdrawn into an apparatus where it could pick up oxygen and discharge carbon dioxide then be pumped back into the patient's arteries.'

There was one huge problem with that concept in 1932. The blood would have to be thoroughly anticoagulated so as not to clot within the equipment. Though the substance heparin had been discovered in dogs' liver by the medical student Jay McLean in 1916, it was not until 1935 that Erik Jorpes in Sweden published the structure of the molecule and allowed it to be manufactured. So Gibbon was before his time.

In Toronto, Charles Best who had the distinction of discovering the hormone insulin, experimented with anticoagulation in dogs. He managed to extract much purer samples of heparin from beef liver and lungs but when the pet food industry took the bulk of these organs he switched his attention to cows' guts. Gordon Murray was the first medic to inject heparin into a patient showing that it increased the clotting time of blood from eight to thirty minutes. Clarence Crafoord, the Swedish vascular surgeon who pioneered surgery for coarctation of the aorta began to use it, and when British military surgeons requested a supply at the beginning of

World War II it was delivered across the Atlantic by destroyer rather than risking a merchant navy vessel.

Though generally understated, the production of heparin was one of the most important steps in enabling extracorporeal circulation. But something was needed to reverse its effect, otherwise the heparinised patient might bleed to death. That something was protamine, a peptide which rapidly binds to heparin to eradicate the anticoagulant effect. Isolated from fish, it is hard to believe that the whole evolution of heart surgery would depend to such an extent on cows' guts and salmon sperm.

Six months after the 'night of the pulmonary embolus', Gibbon moved to Philadelphia with his spouse Mary, who had been Churchill's research assistant. Their mornings were spent in the operating theatre and afternoons in the research laboratories. Though unable to pursue the concept that had captivated his imagination he developed a valuable working relationship with the physiologist Eugene Landis. 'It was this man,' Gibbon wrote, 'who gave me the unwavering encouragement to build an extracorporeal blood circuit capable of temporarily taking over the cardiorespiratory functions.'

Whilst Churchill remained sceptical he invited Gibbon back for another year's research at the Harvard Surgical Research Laboratories. The first apparatus designed to substitute for the lungs was a revolving glass cylinder over which a thin film of blood was spread in an atmosphere of oxygen. For the experiments the blood had to be rendered non-coagulable so supplies of heparin were obtained directly from Best in Toronto. Gibbon tested the circuit in cats, where blood was drained from the jugular vein and collected at the bottom of a stationary glass cup surrounded by a jacket through which warm water was circulated to avoid cooling. Oxygen was taken up into the blood film and carbon dioxide passed out satisfactorily before being pumped back into the animal through the main leg artery. Working with Mary he employed a simple blood transfusion pump developed by Michael DeBakey who had just been appointed Chairman of the Department of Surgery at Baylor University.

Within months it proved possible to take over from the lungs of the cat for four hours. Moreover some would recover their own heart and lung function afterwards. This was exciting and encouraging, though many still died from severe haemolysis, the disintegration of red blood cells in the machine that caused the kidneys to fail.

As Gibbon's surgical practice grew ever more time consuming Mary took charge of the laboratory work. She began by sterilising the equipment in the early morning, anaesthetising the cat, then opening the chest to expose the heart and administer the anticoagulant. When John arrived, the machine was switched on and the animal's pulmonary artery clamped to stop all blood flow to and from the lungs. The pump and mechanical oxygenator then supported the animal by taking over the function of both heart and lungs. Reminiscing about the experience much later in life he recalled 'my wife and I threw our arms around each other and danced around the laboratory'. But their nights were spent prowling the streets with pieces of tuna and a sack!

Though these extraordinary experiments were initially undertaken with the hope of sustaining life after massive pulmonary embolism, the potential for the machine to support surgery on the heart soon became apparent. When reporting his findings to the American Association for Thoracic Surgery in 1939, Gibbon stated modestly: 'It is conceivable that a diseased mitral valve might be exposed to surgical approach under direct vision and that the fields of cardiac and thoracic surgery might well be broadened.'

War service intervened as it did for so many and Gibbon was made Chief of Surgery at the Mayo General Hospital. After that came the appointment as Assistant Professor of Surgery at Pennsylvania State University, then Director of Surgical Research at the Jefferson Medical College. This was the opportunity he needed with well-equipped laboratory facilities that allowed him to work with larger animals. Then in 1946 came the real but unexpected breakthrough the programme needed. Whilst on vacation the Gibbons met Thomas Watson the Chairman of the international Business Machines Corporation, IBM as it is known. Watson was fascinated by the huge potential for extracorporeal circuits and immediately offered both technical and financial support for the project. With expert engineering input from IBM's Endicott Laboratories, a more sophisticated machine was designed to minimise haemolysis and prevent air bubbles from entering the circulation.

The smooth film oxygenator was enlarged sufficiently to support dogs and enclosed within a temperature-controlled cabinet together with the blood pump. A second cabinet housed the power system and controls. With commercial research funds behind him Gibbon selected keen young residents to work in the lab though attempts to operate on dogs hearts during cardiopulmonary bypass resulted in substantial mortality. Then a number of problems were identified in the IBM system. Oxygenation was inadequate for larger animals, controls malfunctioned frequently and blood damage remained too high. And in the meantime others began working on their own heart-lung machines, though one of them and his work remained completely unknown outside of Russia.

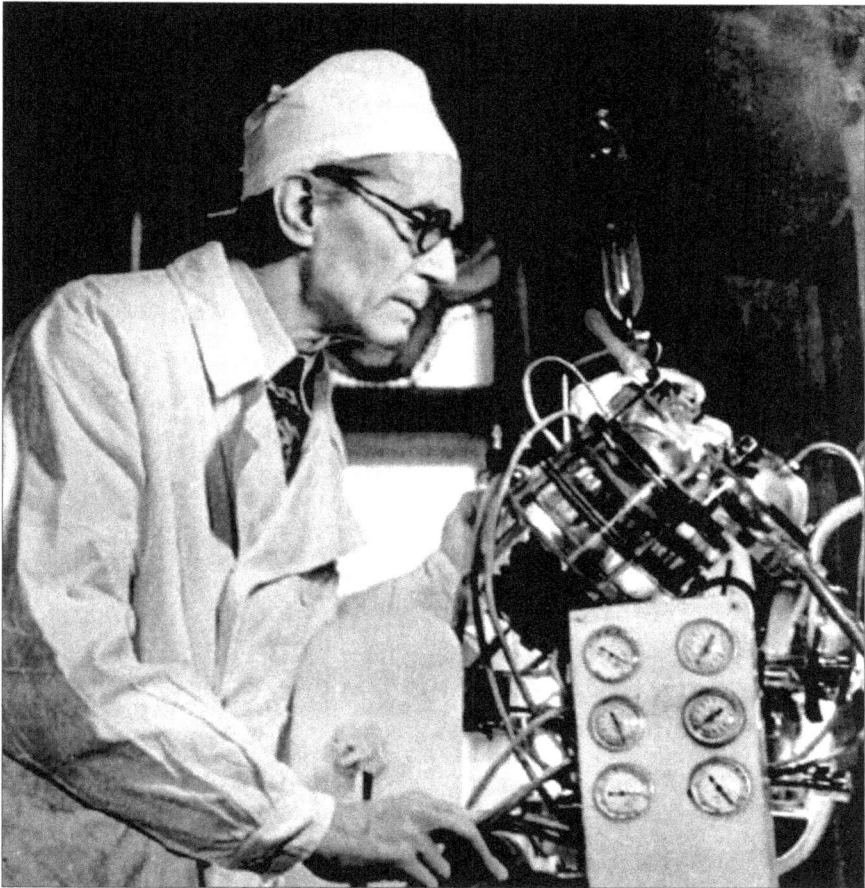

Fig 6.1 Sergei Brukhonenko and his circulatory support device.

Sergei Brukhonenko, the son of an engineer, graduated from the Medical Faculty of the University of Moscow in 1914.

He was immediately assigned to the army during World War I where he witnessed many cases of haemorrhagic shock from combat injuries to the heart and major blood vessels. With a view to rescuing the victims he began to work on an extracorporeal circuit hoping to support life whilst the life threatening wounds were repaired. His machine became known as the 'autojektor' served by two mechanically operated diaphragm pumps with a system of one-way valves in the tubing. For this work he obtained a new drug 'Suramin' from the Moscow Institute of Chemistry and Pharmacology which he employed as an anticoagulant. At this stage he did not have a mechanical oxygenator so he passed the blood through the excised lungs from a dog. As early as 1926 this extracorporeal circuit with its biological oxygenator was able to support the circulation of another animal for two hours before a brisk bleed from a chest wall blood vessel terminated the experiment. This was the world's first study of its type and after several more encouraging attempts Brukhonenko wrote: 'By conducting these experiments we wanted to clarify the possibility of surgery on the temporary arrested heart.' He concluded: 'In principle the artificial circulation may be suitable for certain operations already but improvement is necessary for its practical implementation.'

In 1931 Brukhonenko introduced a heat exchanger and profound hypothermia to the autojektor system and patented his device. The surgeon Nikolai Terebinski performed more than 250 open-heart operations on dogs with the circuit, again using a second set of dog lungs as the oxygenator. Sensibly they decided that dogs' lungs should not be used to support human patients, so Brukhonenko went on to design a bubble oxygenator. This consisted of a double-walled glass vessel with the inner unit introducing oxygen into venous blood by foaming and the outer serving as the heat exchanger. The bubbles were eradicated with alcohol before the pump returned the oxygenated blood to the animal's body.

In 1939 they achieved complete recovery in dogs cooled to 10°C and subject to ten minutes of total circulatory arrest. Seemingly none had demonstrable neurological damage. By 1941 the inventor was eager to see his ground-breaking heart-lung machine used for a patient, but World War II intervened. Although the pair resumed their experiments in 1950, Terebinski died before the system could be applied for heart surgery. Brukhonenko was appointed Head of Moscow's Laboratory of Artificial Circulation and opted to test the circuit for emergency resuscitation after sudden death. It was an original and challenging idea for its time but all the patients died. His bypass machine never was used for open-heart surgery and he died in 1960.

Besides encouraging Lillehei with the cross circulation operations, Owen Wangensteen had his own ideas about a mechanical alternative and had discussed the possibilities with Maurice Visscher, the head of the Physiology Department. Together they approached a bright young Hopkins graduate, Clarence Dennis, who had been influenced by Blalock and encouraged him to discover what others were doing in the area. Of course that was no secret. Gibbons work was well known from conferences and others had tried to keep organs alive using blood pumps and artificial lungs with the prospect of transplantation. In truth most had failed miserably so it was difficult to remain optimistic that similar efforts might support the whole body. But some persisted.

Having worked on the origins of lung cancer with Tudor Edwards at the Brompton Hospital, Viking Bjork returned to Sweden's Sabbatsberg Hospital under the mentorship of Clarence Crafoord. Crafoord was now working towards his own heart-lung machine and through his broad chest surgery experience, Bjork was asked to take over the project which employed two milking machines as pumps. After encouraging results oxygenating freshly heparinised blood on the laboratory bench, he attempted to perfuse dogs' brains. It was a disaster. All the animals died and Crafoord left his researcher to his own devices.

Undeterred Bjork devised a rotating disc oxygenator, to which he applied an artificial lining of silicone, following advice from chemical engineers in a nearby factory.

With coating of all areas exposed to blood-foreign surface interaction the blood handling of the whole system was much improved. Using a compressed air pump with the stainless steel discs rotating at 120 revolutions per minute the system provided effective oxygenation of the blood without excessive damage to the red cells. Bjork found that by simply increasing the number of discs rotating through blood he could double the oxygenation capacity.

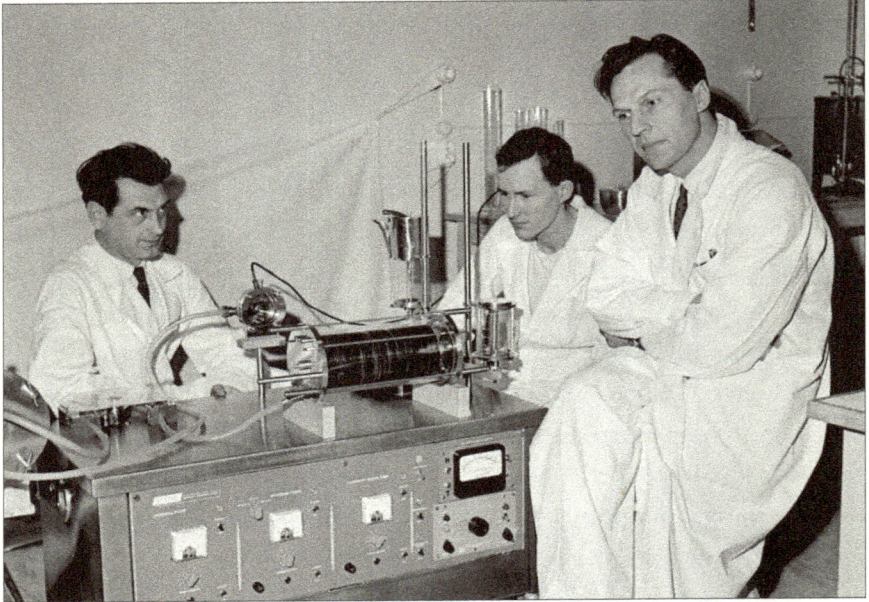

Fig 6.2 Viking Bjork (right) and his heart-lung machine.

In October 1947 the revamped machine was successful in supporting the circulation of a 20kg dog which Bjork and his chemical engineer wife then transported home to their apartment in the trunk of a borrowed car. In the morning she announced happily: 'The urine is clear without blood so haemolysis must have been low. The kidneys are fine!'

In the meantime, Gibbon's team had gone back to basics, stripping down the circuit to its bare essentials and continuously testing new modifications and components. When the second IBM model arrived at Jefferson in 1951 the laboratory outcomes were much more encouraging. But the turning point came when two residents, Thomas Stokes and John Flick discovered that introducing turbulence in the blood path substantially increased oxygen uptake. So they lined the surface of the oxygenator's revolving cylinder with an adherent fine wire screen which increased contact between red cells and oxygen by between 700% and 1000%.

This is how Gibbon described the new oxygenator himself: 'The mechanical lung performs the gas exchange by filming blood on both sides of rotating screens. The screens are made of stainless steel wire and are suspended vertically and parallel in a plastic chamber. As the blood (from the body) flows over these screens it takes up oxygen and gives off carbon dioxide. It is easy to observe that sufficient oxygen is being picked up by the apparatus as the blue blood entering the oxygenator (from the veins) becomes red as it leaves.' He also decided to persist with a DeBakey type roller pump that propelled the blood without actually touching it. A rotating wheel with three rollers at its circumference simply squeezed the blood onwards through a loop of flexible tubing, a mechanism still used in heart lung machines today.

In Minnesota Dennis and Vischer were catching up.

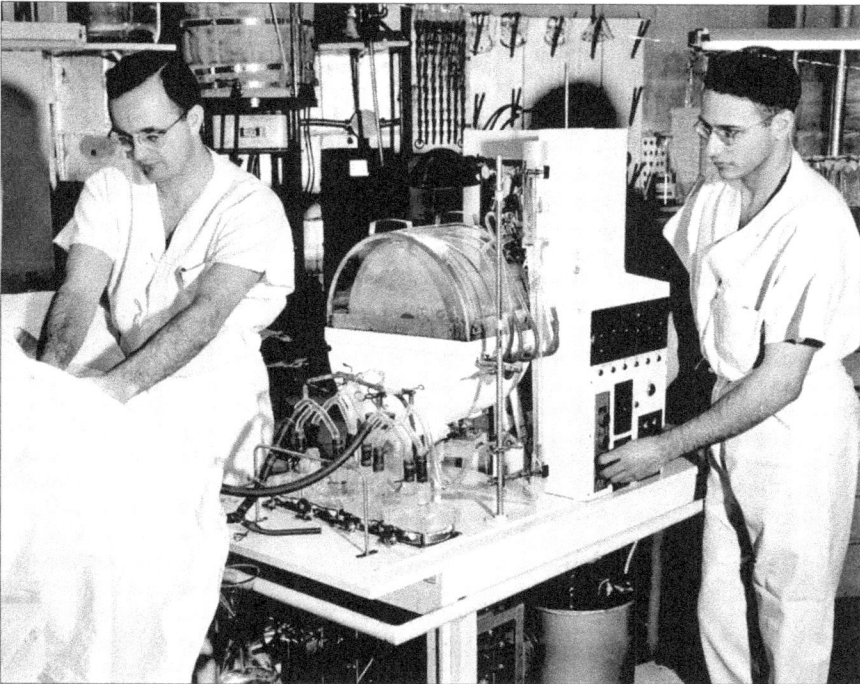

Fig 6.3 Clarence Dennis with his machine.

They had financial support from the affluent Variety Club and motion picture industry, who at the instigation of the actor Ronald Reagan, were building a new heart hospital for Minneapolis. Dennis first tried to pass blood through tubes of cellulose sausage casing in an oxygen tent. Cleverly, the casing was intended to function as a dialysing membrane. He argued that separating blood from direct contact with gas, would avoid foaming and bacteriological contamination. Good thinking but unfortunately it didn't work. The speed of diffusion of oxygen across cellulose membrane was insufficient given the rate of blood flow needed to avoid stasis and clotting. Next they resorted to direct injection of a jet of oxygen into blood flowing through a set of membranous tubes but again foaming made the approach impractical. Finally, when gas was presented to the blood in a thin film on a rotating plexiglass cylinder similar to Bjork and Gibbon's efforts, they found that foaming was eliminated and sufficient oxygen taken up to sustain the animals.

Dennis and Vischer went on to build a modified Gibbon pump consisting of a nest of stainless steel cylinders rotating through blood and oxygen. A revolving funnel collected the oxygenated blood which was then pumped back into the body. Instead of the classic DeBakey roller pump they used modified Dale-Schuster pumps which appeared to cause less haemolysis. Yet irrespective of the improvements, the apparatus proved cumbersome and difficult to clean and the majority of dogs experienced blood damage and died. It then became apparent that the equipment was frequently contaminated with bacteria, thus many of the dogs had been killed by infection.

Another year went by with more changes to the oxygenator design and more powerful antibiotic prophylaxis. Time passes and the group had to decide whether to continue the frustrating battle in the lab or progress to a patient. In April 1951, soon after the Variety Club Heart Hospital opened, the paediatric cardiologists presented a six-year-old girl with large atrial septal defect and waterlogged lungs whom they felt was on a steep downward trajectory. It was the stimulus Dennis needed and they decided to operate. But when the child was connected to the bypass circuit so much blood drained from the enlarged heart that it flooded the oxygenator. Though this was said to perform well, the child didn't. She died soon after the bypass machine was switched off, much like the dogs. This was the world's first operation with an experimental heart-lung machine and needless to say the outcome proved an enormous disappointment. But at the time there was no alternative. Neither hypothermia nor the atrial well technique had been tested in patients thus far, so it was a brave move by the Minnesota surgeons. One of many.

After twenty-three intense years of research pressure was now on Gibbon to attempt a human operation, which he did in February 1952.

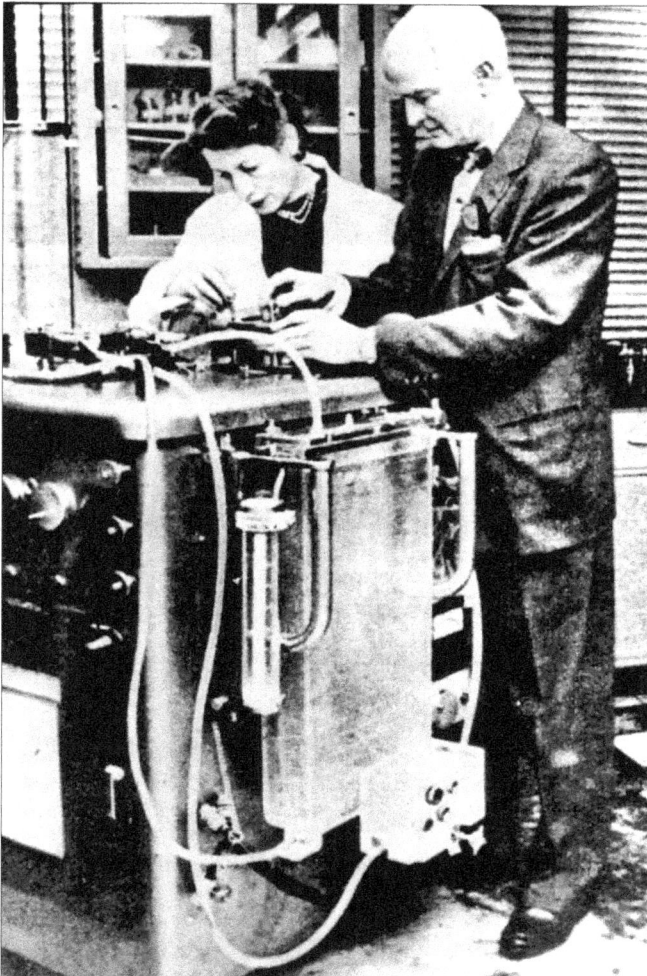

Fig 6.4 A. John Gibbon with his wife Mary working
on the first heart-lung machine to be used clinically.

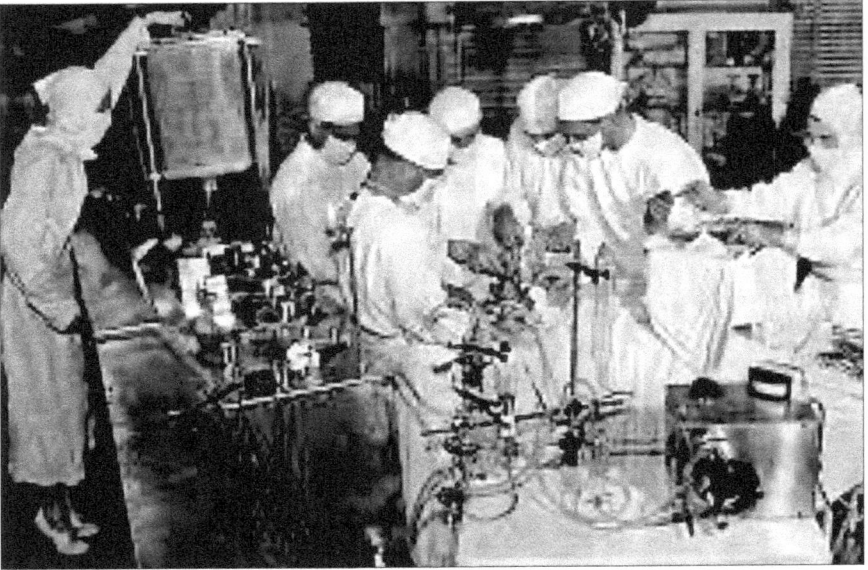

B. Picture taken in the operating theatre during Gibbon's successful operation.

This is his own description of the case which he presented at a symposium at the University of Minnesota. 'The patient was a fifteen-month-old baby that weighed eleven pounds and was in severe congestive cardiac failure. Attempts at cardiac catheterisation were unsuccessful. It was the opinion of everyone who saw the baby that her cardiac abnormality was an interatrial septal defect. We explored the right side of the heart using the apparatus and discovered that no atrial septal defect existed. The child died on the operating table and at post mortem was shown to have a huge patent ductus arteriosus which had not been recognised. This of course illustrates the importance of complete exploration of every heart which is operated upon. We might have saved this child's life it we had closed the ductus.'

Of course this was a complete disaster, which greatly disturbed a surgeon who was more introspective than most. Yet the heart-lung machine had actually functioned well so he had to try again. The next patient was Cecelia Bavolek, an eighteen-year-old student who had been fine until six months before when she developed symptoms of heart failure. In the first months of 1953 she was admitted to hospital on three occasions coughing up blood.

Cardiac catheterisation then showed that she had a large atrial septal defect with an alarming nine litres of blood passing from left atrium to right each minute. Gibbon explained this to both Cecelia and her patients concluding that her future quality of life and prognosis would be poor. Did they wish him to close the defect on the heart-lung machine? A monster of a device that took hours to prepare and which had never been used successfully. Yes they did. Either that or watch her die miserably in the next few months.

On that fateful spring morning, May 6th 1953, eager medical students queued in the corridor outside the operating theatre having volunteered to give the donor blood needed to 'prime' the machine. The whole circuit was heparinised to prevent the blood from clotting and the roller pump turned on to distribute it through the connecting pipes and suction tubes. The complexity of the circuit was awesome for those who gathered to watch, and the atmosphere in the room described as tense. The girl's chest was pre-pared with iodine solution and draped to allow the 'bucket handle' incision through the front of the chest. In a short operation note written afterwards on behalf of the emotionally drained Gibbon, the second assistant Robert Finley Jr perhaps belied the historic importance of the procedure.

'With patient under pentothal and oxygen endo-anaesthesia, the chest was opened through the fourth interspaces bilaterally. The right atrium was large but by invaginating the appendage with a finger, the large inter-auric-ular defect could be felt. The patient was then placed on the oxygenating apparatus for twenty-six minutes on total substitution of heart and lungs. The right auricle was opened and the defect closed directly with silk sutures. The patient tolerated the procedure well.'

Gibbon normally annotated his own operations. The fact that he del-egated the documentation on that day reflected the stress he was under. There had been an acrimonious exchange with the anaesthetic team when clots were seen forming on some of the rotating screens suggesting inad-equate heparinisation. There was even discussion as to whether the pro-cedure should be aborted at that stage. The first assistant Frank Allbrittan steadied the ship by suggesting direct suture closure of the hole for expedi-ency rather than using a patch of pericardium as planned. Ultimately the result was what the new specialty needed at the time. A success. As the flow from the machine was turned down Cecelia's own heart and lungs took over and she began to wake from the anaesthetic as the last skin stitches were being placed. An hour later the young woman was in an oxygen tent communicating with the nurses.

That evening a relieved and happy Gibbon telephoned Alfred Blalock at Johns Hopkins and Clarence Crafoord at the Karolinska Institute in Sweden to tell them the news. He sent a photograph of the machine and operating team to Michael DeBakey in Houston stating: 'Dear Mike, a picture of the first successful open heart operation with complete bypass of heart and lungs, May 6th 1953. Best wishes Jack.' Jack was in fact how John was always referred to. The name he preferred. Cecelia was taken home by her parents two weeks later.

In an attempt to continue the programme two five-year-old girls with atrial septal defects were operated upon in July. In the first, cardiac arrest occurred soon after opening the chest. When an hour of frantic cardiac massage failed to re-establish a heart rhythm, cannulas were placed for the bypass machine and with flow established the pulverised heart emptied turning from blue to pink. Five separate holes were closed in the septum but all attempts to wean her from the circuit resulted in distention of the heart and further cardiac arrest. In desperation the heart lung machine was kept running for four hours but when finally discontinued she died. Gibbon was inconsolable but was persuaded to go again 'because your machine works!'

Sadly on the next occasion it didn't perform well enough. The unfortunate child had both atrial and ventricular septal defects and a large patent ductus arteriosus. With the machine running the surgical field was constantly flooded with bright red blood through the connection which could not be cleared by the suckers. The procedure was abandoned and although the child left the operating theatre alive she died soon afterwards in the oxygen tent as the parents and Gibbon looked on. It was a desperately dismal tableau that Jack was not prepared to repeat. He declared a moratorium on further cardiac surgery in the department. Had Clarence Dennis not asked him to describe that one success at a symposium in Minnesota it would never have been recorded in the medical literature.

Gibbon was a sensitive family man with his own children. Did successful cardiac surgeons need psychopathic tendencies? Probably. Gibbon blamed his failures on human error, a self-effacing approach not typical of surgeons. Kirklin added his thoughts to the matter stating: 'In the deepest recesses of my heart I felt those patients died in part because of his lack of appreciation of some of the technical aspects of cardiac surgery.' That was correct. Certainly in the last child the ductus arteriosus should have been closed before going onto the bypass machine. Easily done with a ligature or clip.

Like his father, Gibbon became Professor and Chairman of the Department of Surgery at Jefferson Medical College spending the rest of his career operating on cancer of the lung and oesophagus. History accredits him with developing the heart-lung machine but he was not the man who made a success of it. That was left to those great rival surgeons Walt Lillehei and John Kirklin working a short distance from one another in Minnesota.

In Minneapolis Lillehei's team developed what was termed a 'bubble oxygenator' from first principles. Others had considered this route but had failed to overcome the lethal problem of foaming in the blood. Richard DeWall, the medically qualified research worker had the idea of coating the plastic tubing with DC antifoam used in the commercial production of mayonnaise. That certainly reduced foaming but did not completely eliminate bubbles, so the risk of air embolism persisted. The ingenious and persistent DeWall then decided that blood containing bubbles must be lighter than the bubble-free variety. Therefore should oxygenated blood be passed through a vertical tube the 'clean' proportion would sink to the bottom, whilst the bubbly bit would rise to the top. Good thinking but no cigar. That was because the hydrostatic forces which move lighter blood upwards were counteracted by the downward movement of heavier fluid through gravity. Obvious really! To overcome the viscosity factor to separation of the fractions DeWall built a spiral 'settling tube' which constantly facilitated the lighter fluid to rise upwards.

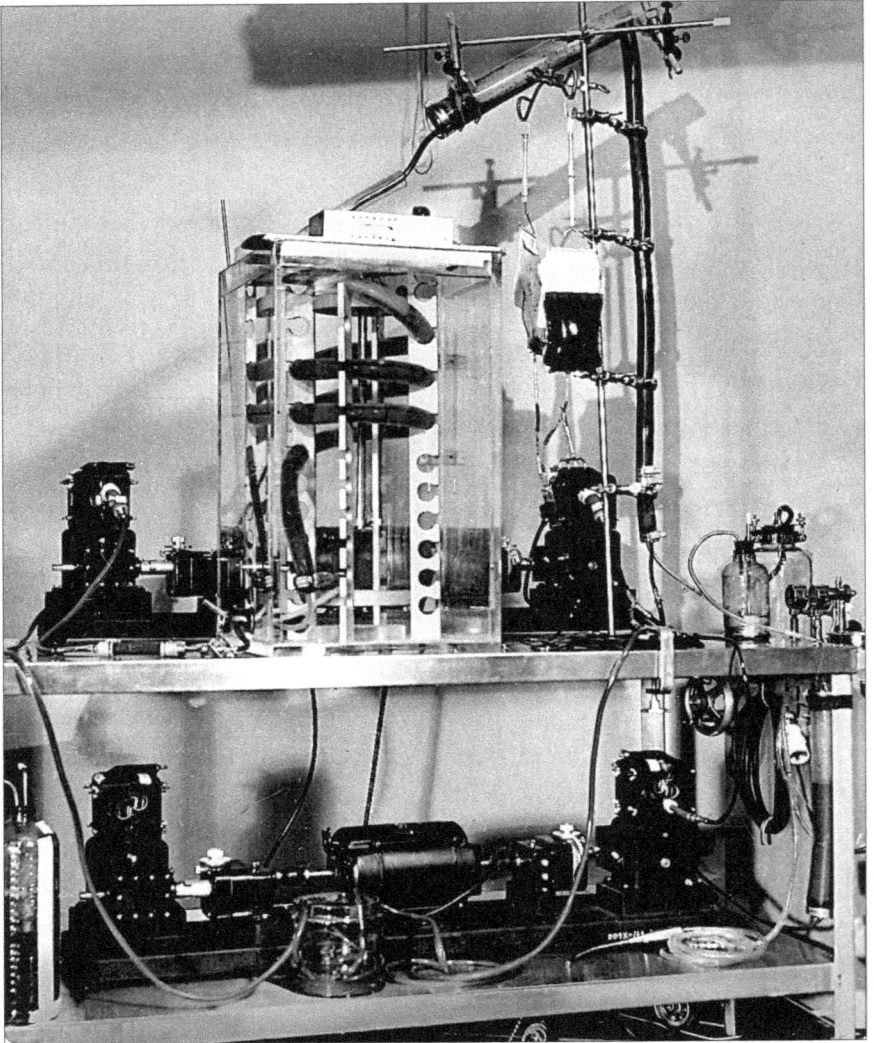

Fig 6.5 A. Lilleihei's heart-lung machine.

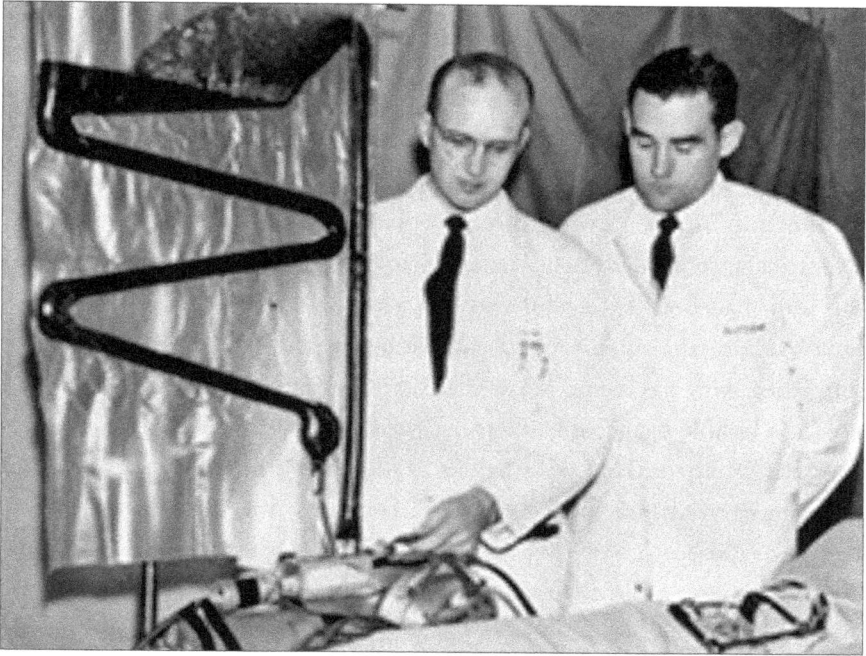

B. Richard DeWall with Vincent Gott and their oxygenator.

And Eureka, this helical system worked perfectly giving rapid, complete and dependable elimination of bubbles. The final design was a vertical plastic mixing tube with a U-shaped curve at its top. Oxygen was introduced into the bottom via multiple intravenous needles inserted through an ordinary rubber stopper. As the blood flowed upwards oxygen bubbles ascended through the rising column to the top of the mixing tube. From there it cascaded down into the U-shaped debubbling chamber containing DC antifoam A. Most of the bubbles were separated at this point whilst those remaining were removed as the oxygenated blood poured into the plastic helical coil then flowed by gravity into a reservoir. At the bottom of the helical settling tube oxygenated blood now free from bubbles passed into a reservoir followed by filters before being pumped back into the arterial system of the patient.

It was extraordinary how innovative in the engineering field these doctors could be. During the winter of 1954 DeWall thoroughly tested the bubble oxygenator in dogs. To prevent hypothermia through heat loss through the open chest he also developed a purpose-built heat exchanger utilising a water bath. Conversely this could also be used to cool the patient so that cardiopulmonary bypass with hypothermia was possible.

Finally on 13th May 1955 when Lillehei had confidence in the system he took it to the operating theatre. The patient was a three-year-old boy with a ventricular septal defect and damaged lungs, the same type of case in which the team had been successful with cross circulation. With the new heart-lung machine the surgery was a gamble but it paid off. The child survived unscathed with the defect repaired. What's more by August the group had used the bubble oxygenator for seven paediatric operations with five survivors. Relatively speaking this was a great success causing Lillehei to abandon the controversial biological equivalent. But there was a subtle difference. Patients exposed to extensive synthetic foreign surfaces during cardiopulmonary bypass suffered damage to their lungs and kidneys which became known as the 'post perfusion syndrome'. This had not happened with the biological equivalent of cross circulation and would cost many lives.

In contrast to Gibbon's elaborate blood screen oxygenators with constantly moving parts and complex controls the DeWall-Lillehei bubble oxygenator was simple, cheap and easily assembled. It could be sterilised between patients by autoclaving and the size was adaptable to the patient. Consequently the donor blood required to prime the system could be kept to a minimum. By May 1956 Lillehei had performed eighty heart operations on progressively more complex congenital defects and began to introduce protective blood cooling in longer operations. Relatively low flow rates were used to avoid turbulence and haemolysis and importantly tests performed by psychologists and neurologists could not detect significant brain damage. Many years later follow-up of 106 patients operated on for tetralogy of Fallot with the bubble oxygenator showed that 34 of them had received college or graduate degrees including two in medicine, and one in law. That was above the average for a random group from the general population.

At the Mayo Clinic John Kirklin had been prolific in his use of Gross's atrial well technique applying it to increasingly complex and ambitious operations. With his analytical mind and academic approach he carefully looked into whether the pump oxygenator and extracorporeal circuit were as dangerous as Varco had suggested in 1955. Varco was alluding to the blood damage caused by foreign surface interaction and the dangers of air being sucked into the circulation when the heart chambers were open. Whilst pressurised from within Mayo to switch to Lillehei's controlled cross circulation technique, Kirklin persisted with a modified, and even more complex, Gibbon machine to produce a remarkable series of intracardiac repairs.

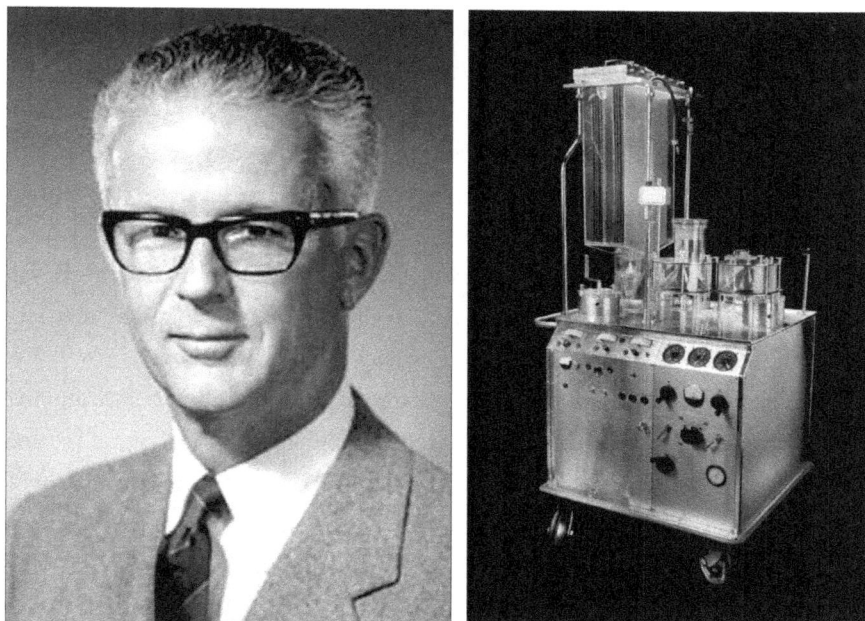

Fig 6.6 A. John Kirklin. B. The Mayo Gibbon Machine.

This included only the second but unsuccessful repair of tetralogy of Fallot months after Lillehei and Varco's first using the child's father as oxygenator.

Throughout 1955 and well into 1956, the University of Minnesota Medical Centre and the Mayo Clinic were the only hospitals in the world performing open-heart surgery. They were only ninety miles apart but fierce rivalry isolated them from one another. Visitors from all parts of the world flocked to both institutions, and whilst the surgery was superlative in each, there were substantial differences between their equipment and approach.

Denton Cooley, now at the Methodist Hospital with Michael DeBakey, was an early observer in June 1955. Later he wrote: 'The contrast between the two institutions and the two surgeons was striking. We observed Lillehei and a team composed mostly of house staff correct a ventricular septal defect using cross circulation. During the visit we also saw an oxygenator developed by Richard DeWall in the laboratory. The next day we observed John Kirklin and his impressive team in Rochester that was made up of physiologists, biochemists, cardiologists and others as they performed operations using the Mayo-Gibbon apparatus. Such a device was beyond my organizational capacity and financial reach. Thus I was deeply disappointed on our return to Houston when our cardiologist Dr MacNamara stated that he would not permit me to operate on his patients unless I used the Mayo apparatus.'

After Kirklin's first patient with tetralogy died he made four further attempts with cardiopulmonary bypass. But closing the ventricular septal defect and opening up the narrowing beneath the pulmonary valve was time consuming on the apparatus. And unfortunately all of them died afterwards. For a while the programme was paused whilst he and the team worked furtively to overcome the difficulties. One of the lethal problems was 'heart block' where the coordinated passage of electrical signals from the atria to the ventricles was interrupted. These hearts just wouldn't beat when the invisible conduction pathways were severed and there were no pacemakers at the time. Not knowing where the conduction system was located was clearly problematic.

Lillehei attempted to overcome heart block by using adrenaline but whilst this occasionally helped, all the patients eventually died. Then at a departmental pathology meeting in 1956 the physiologist Jack Johnson pointed out that a simple electrical device called the Grass Stimulator had been used to activate frogs' legs in the laboratory for years. Exclaiming 'why not try this in a human', Johnson proposed that a wire passed from the stimulator through the chest wall to the ventricles should be tested. To explore the hypothesis Lillehei's surgical residents Vincent Gott and William Weirich borrowed Johnson's Grass stimulator and tried different positions to attach the wire to the dog heart. Needless to say the right ventricle just behind the chest wall proved the most convenient and Gott succeeded in pacing the animals after surgically-induced heart block.

On 30th January 1957, Lillehei urgently summoned Gott to the operating theatre. He wanted him to help place an electrical wire on the ventricle of a 3-year-old girl with heart block who wouldn't separate from the bypass machine after a difficult tetralogy of Fallot repair. When Lillehei passed the wire through the chest wall, Gott attached it to the Grass stimulator and switched it on at ninety beats per minute. It was the first time that direct cardiac pacing had been applied in a patient and it was continued in the recovery room until the child fortunately regained normal sinus rhythm. Soon seventeen of nineteen patients with complete heart block survived with pacing whereas they would invariably have died given drugs alone.

Samuel Hunter, a junior surgical resident gave this description of the use of pacing in a 12-year-old boy with heart block after ventricular septal defect repair. 'During the closing moments of the procedure we experienced severe slowing of the heart to 30 beats per minute. Dr William Weirich was summoned and appeared shortly with a device that resembled a large table radio. Two stainless steel Teflon coated wires connected to this device were stitched to the right ventricle and subcutaneous tissues respectively by Dr Lillehei. The patient's pulse rate immediately jumped from 30 to 85 beats per minute.'

Even if temporary heart block resolved during the course of an operation the team would still leave a precautionary pacing wire attached to the right ventricle which could be withdrawn later. This is done routinely today. Sometimes heart block occurred unexpectedly in the post-operative period, and for this Lillehei would pass a hollow needle through the chest wall and feed in a pacing wire onto the right ventricle. This evolved into a method for reviving cardiac arrest patients in other parts of the hospital.

The early pacemaker power sources were large, cumbersome and potentially dangerous, yet impulses of only one or two volts were needed to cause contraction of the ventricles. Lillehei consequently believed it possible to create a compact, more user-friendly system. He sought the help of Earl Bakken, the engineer responsible for maintenance of electrical equipment in the Department of Surgery who at the time was in partnership with his brother-in-law, Herman Dsli. Together they operated an electrical business in a garage in North East Minneapolis where they repaired television sets and adapted medical equipment such as the electrocardiograph to meet particular needs.

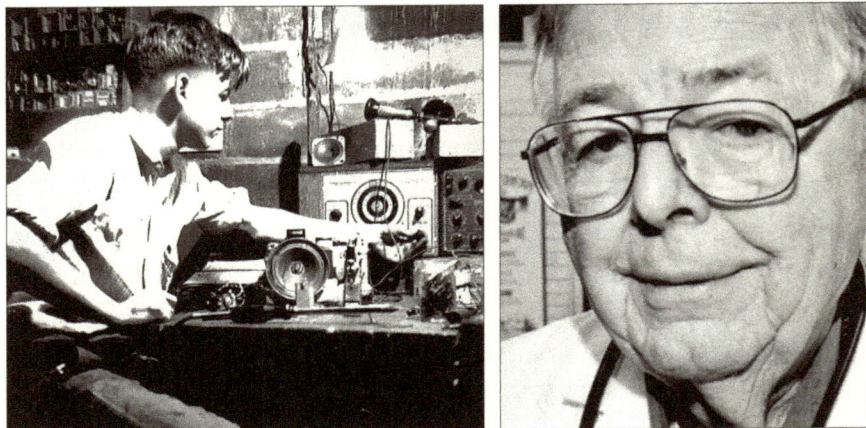

Fig 6.7 A. The young Earl Bakken working on a pacemaker in his garage. B. Later in life.

Within weeks of the Professor's request Bakken returned to the University Hospital with a small purpose-designed battery-operated pacemaker which was adjustable to provide a specified heart rate and easily portable in a small holster. This innovation was so successful that the pair soon had difficulty in servicing local demand. They formed the Medtronic Company in 1958 and within two years Lillehei and his colleagues had used their pacemaker in 66 patients. Though most regained sinus rhythm within a few weeks, one boy was safely supported by the device for fifteen months.

Sadly early recovery from heart block often didn't last. Lillehei found that two thirds suffered recurrent episodes and some died suddenly. Clearly such patients needed a long-term pacemaker in a prophylactic capacity but continuous presence of a wire through the skin often caused infection. In turn, scar tissue where the wire entered the heart muscle raised the electrical resistance and required a progressive increase in voltage. After several weeks the chest wall muscles began to twitch so prolonged use was unthinkable.

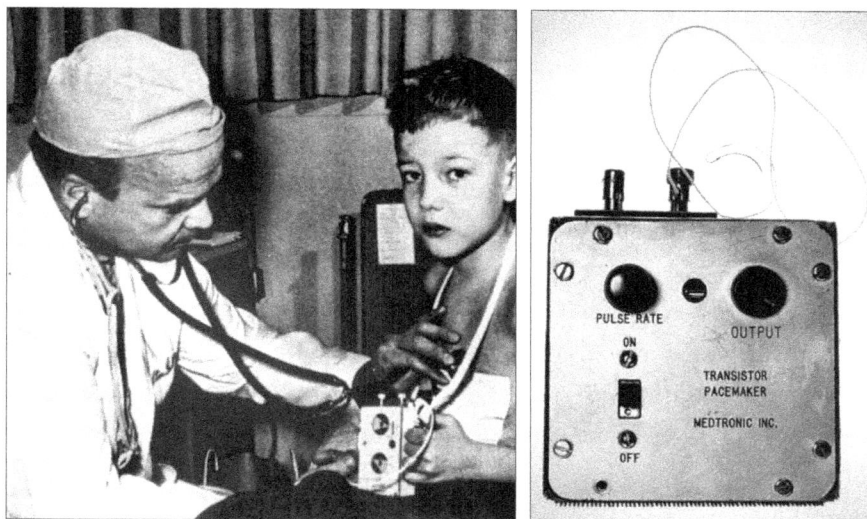

Fig 6.8 A. Lilleihei and young boy with a pacemaker after congenital heart repair
B. Metronic's first pacemaker.

In 1959 Hunter was appointed Director of Cardiac Research at St Joseph's Hospital in Minneapolis where he worked with Norman Roth, the Chief Engineer at Medtronic. Between them they developed a bipolar stainless steel electrode that required a much reduced electrical current. Hunter soon implanted his new pacemaker wire into a 72-year- old man who sustained complete heart block following acute myocardial infarction. At the same time the cardiologist Paul Zoll, who had assisted Harken with his first heart operations in the Cotswolds was working on a hand-held non-invasive system to apply high voltage transthoracic electric shocks to save patients with ventricular fibrillation.

Like William Harvey who described the circulation of the blood 350 years before, Zoll noticed that an arrested heart would respond to a flick of the finger by contracting. And sometimes it resumed its rhythm. He also realised that the closest non-invasive access to the heart was through the gullet, and began to use transoesophageal electrical stimulation to overcome heart block in patients subject to fainting attacks. By then the Medtronic transistorised external pacing system had arrived and became a standard accessory in virtually every cardiac operating theatre in the world. The survival of patients with heart block increased to 90% with use of the equipment.

The first permanent implant of a pacemaker was performed by the Swedish cardiac surgeon Ake Senning in 1959. Senning had trained with Harken in Boston and wrote to him to explain the circumstances. 'What made me make the first implantation was an energetic, beautiful woman called Else-Marie Larsson who entered my lab on 6th October 1958 and told me I had to implant a pacemaker into her husband. He had been hospitalised several times over the previous six months with heart block and fainting, suffering twenty to thirty events each day. I told her we had not completed our experiments, nor did we have a pacemaker for human use. She responded by saying: 'So make one! That day she drove several times from Elmquist's electronic lab and back and finally persuaded us. Elmquist coated two pacemaker circuits in epoxy resin using shoe polish tins as a mould. On 8th October in the evening when there was no one else in the theatre, I implanted the first, but it lasted only eight hours. Presumably I had damaged the output transistor or capacitance with the catheter and I did not have the spare which was in the lab. I implanted that one the next morning. As the early pacemakers were short lived this patient now has his 24th. He is well and has retired from an active and successful life. In the 1950s we didn't have any liability issues. The patient and relatives were happy if they survived.'

Having a pushy wife helps sometimes.

Earl Bakken and Medtronic went on to manufacture pacemakers, heart-lung machines and artificial heart valves thus establishing the cardiovascular industry. The company was recently valued at more than one hundred billion dollars and still runs the business from Minneapolis. I had the privilege of launching one of their heart valves for them in Oxford and came to know Bakken as a result. A real gentleman.

The first conference dedicated to the heart-lung machine was held in Chicago in 1957 when the following statement by Forrest Dodrill opened a session on the complications of the technique. 'One of the most serious difficulties encountered in whole body perfusion is the profound effect upon the lungs that may occur in certain patients. It is indeed discouraging to perform open cardiac corrective surgery, to have the patient remain in excellent condition throughout the procedure and for a day or two afterwards, finally succumbing to pulmonary insufficiency while the heart itself remains strong to the very end.'

This was not a problem that was easy to shake down, but the clues were there.

Lillehei's parental cross circulation didn't cause the post perfusion syndrome, because contact between blood and synthetic foreign surfaces was kept to a minimum. Blood doesn't like to leave its cellular environment so if the sickest and most vulnerable patients were to be accepted for heart surgery something had to change.

Nonetheless, thanks to those 'magnificent men and their heart-lung machines', a new surgical specialty was well on its way.

Keeping It Still

Don't be reckless with other people's hearts;
don't put up with those who are
reckless with yours.
—Mary Schmich

By the late 1950s the technical process to establish cardiopulmonary by-pass was well defined. The surgeon exposes the heart by dividing the breast bone along its whole length with an oscillating saw then opens the incision widely with a hand-cranked metal retractor. Somewhat brutal to the inci-dental observer. The fibrous sac, the pericardium is then opened by cutting with scissors, sweeping aside the remnants of the thymus gland and trying to avoid entering the chest cavity with lungs on either side. There in all its splendour is the beating heart with right atrium and ventricle at the front and left atrium and ventricle behind. The continuous rhythm and coordi-nated movement are captivating however often one watches it, and it takes less than ten minutes operating to reach this point. Bleeding in the midline is minimal and we generally stop oozing from the sternal bone marrow with electrocautery and wax smeared along the edges. The surgeon then instructs their anaesthetist to administer the heparin through a venous cannula in the neck. I would then lift and suspend the cut edges of the pericardium to the subcutaneous tissues with stay stitches. This raises the heart towards the surgeon.

The plastic cannulas to covey blood to and from the heart-lung machine are introduced through purse-string stitches with snares to secure a blood tight seal. The surgeon would usually place a plastic pipe in the high pressure pulsating aorta first to convey oxygenated blood from the circuit back into the patient and around the body. In the early days this 'arterial return' pipe was sometimes inserted into the smaller femoral artery in the groin. Two further cannulas are then introduced through the right atrial wall and fed into the superior and inferior vena cava respectively. The surgeon then instructs the perfusionist to 'go on' after which clamps are removed from the venous pipes and the heart empties. Blue deoxygenated blood drains from the veins into the mechanical oxygenator and reservoir before it is returned bright red again from the circuit into the patient.

Simple. I could teach my 'physician's assistants' to do that in half a day.

Actually not that simple. To survive a complex operation the heart still needed its blood supply through the coronary arteries, as a result of which it continued to beat vigorously. A proportion of the patients would have an undiagnosed persistent ductus arteriosus allowing the lungs to be flooded from the aorta, or indeed a leaking aortic valve so that the surgical field would be obscured by blood. Moreover when an incision allowed air to enter the cardiac chambers it could be pushed onward into the circulation and cause a stroke. As a result it became necessary to place a clamp across the aorta above the heart but then blood returning from the machine couldn't reach the heart muscle itself. Oxygen deprivation was tolerated for thirty or so minutes but prolonged periods of 'myocardial ischaemia' would cause sufficient damage to compromise the ability of the ventricles to wean from the machine at the conclusion of the repair. So, in essence, surgeons were still working against the clock when operating on more complex malformations and facing similar complications to procedures which employed moderate hypothermia alone.

On 21st June 1956 Will Sealy at Duke University, North Carolina, elected to combine the pump oxygenator with cooling to lower the oxygen requirements of the tissues in a patient. He operated to close an atrial septal defect in a seven-year-old girl but the cooling was done with external ice packs on the skin. The combination of cooling and rewarming lasted seven hours under anaesthetic whilst closure of the hole took only fifteen minutes. He repeated the process in forty more patients whilst searching for an effective heat exchanger to incorporate as part of the bypass circuit. From then on a few degrees of blood temperature manipulation took no longer than ten to fifteen minutes. Operating conditions were improved because the aorta could be clamped for longer without the oxygen-deprived heart suffering to the same extent as it did at normal body temperature. More often than not Sealy could now operate in a bloodless field, and with the introduction of a reliable defibrillator he went a step further by deliberately fibrillating the heart for up to twenty minutes. By eliminating continuous contraction and relaxation a precision repair became easier particularly in tiny children's hearts. However, fibrillation does not mean the heart is completely still since it wriggles and maintains its muscle tone. Sometimes it would spontaneously defibrillate and start to beat again in response to touch.

Ironically it was a man who had trained as an ear, nose and throat surgeon who made the next substantial contribution. Denis Melrose bemoaned the primitive operating conditions during attempted heart operations at London's Hammersmith Hospital and Royal Postgraduate Medical School in the early 1950s.

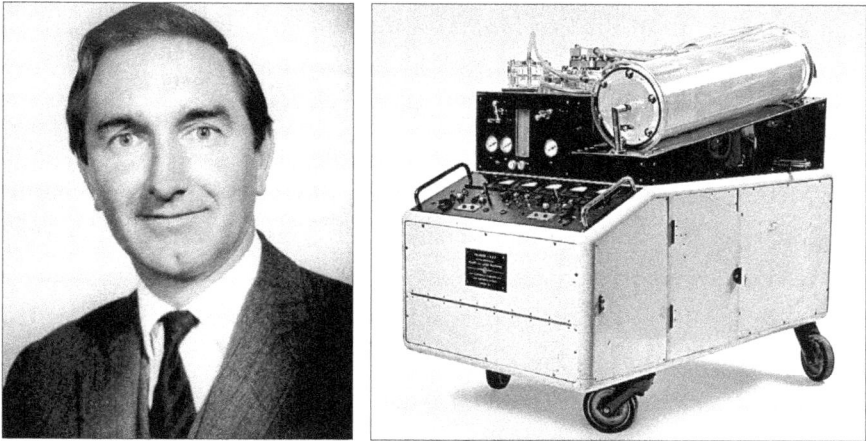

Fig 7.1 A. Denis Melrose. B. The Hammersmith Heart-Lung Machine.

'Consider a group of people practising the management of open-heart surgery in the animal laboratory. Remember the clumsy perfusion apparatus, primitive anaesthesia, little or no monitoring equipment, a host of mysteries gradually overcome. Then follows the first nightmarish attempt on a sick patient. Suddenly the rules are completely without validity, drowned in a torrent of blood streaming into the opened chambers from a patent ductus, a large bronchial anastomosis or an incompetent aortic valve above the septal defect.'

Unhappy with what was immediately available to them the Hammersmith decided to build their own heart-lung machine.

Under the guidance of the Professor of Surgery, Ian Aird, Melrose worked to improve Bjork's existing rotating disc oxygenator and succeeded in reducing the volume of donor blood needed to prime the system. In December 1953 the Hammersmith surgeons, led by Bill Cleland, used the Melrose modification for partial support of a patient undergoing blind dilatation of a narrowed aortic valve. Aird encouraged this much like Wangensteen did in Minneapolis. That year he had successfully separated Nigerian-born Siamese twins which thrust him into the public eye and, in his own mind, obfuscated his more serious research contributions. Again Melrose commented: 'As a measure of the man, it is noteworthy that in the first clinical trials of this machine Aird took on himself full responsibility, and as soon as success was ensured, relinquished it, leaving the rewards to others. He took immense pleasure in this, striving always to direct the limelight away from himself towards the staff.'

Melrose was convinced that heart surgery should and could become less intimidating. But how? As more taxing operations were being attempted on moving hearts the extended periods of aortic cross clamping, with myocardial ischaemia were causing deaths through left ventricular failure. The heart was simply not strong enough to take over again when the bypass machine was switched off. Searching the scientific literature Melrose discovered that the physiologist Sidney Ringer of University College London, just a couple of miles away, had used potassium salts dissolved in fluid to stop hearts beating. Moreover, another physiologist, Martin at Johns Hopkins, had performed numerous experiments with potassium on the isolated hearts of terrapins. Crucially the infusion of a potassium solution into the root of the aorta would stop the heart beating in a flaccid relaxed state. But when blood flow was restored in the coronary arteries after half an hour the potassium was rapidly washed out and the chambers would resume beating again normally.

These experiments had been performed at the turn of the century so no practical use had been made of the findings. Yet for Melrose the observations lit a candle in the dark. With Aird's encouragement he set up a laboratory-based research programme at the Hammersmith to explore the use of cooled potassium citrate solution at 26°C. Potassium infusion stopped the dogs' hearts rapidly in the flaccid state whilst hypothermia helped reduce the metabolic demands of the muscle. When the hearts were reperfused with warm blood the muscle tone returned within seconds and most hearts began to beat vigorously in normal rhythm. Magic. Melrose named the process 'cardioplegia' and published the findings in the *Lancet* in 1955.

The key sentence in the paper's introduction read: 'A most valuable contribution to the problems of intracardiac surgery would be the ability to arrest and restart the heart at will, suffering no damage during cessation of coronary blood flow.' The manuscript concluded that 'arrest is maintained for as long as an adequate amount of potassium citrate remains in the coronary arteries', then "normal heart beat is restored when reperfusion of the coronary circulation with blood reduces the level'. And importantly 'the oxygen consumption of the quiescent heart is very low and at normal body temperature, cessation of the coronary circulation for over fifteen minutes does not endanger the muscle'. Co-authors on the paper were Hugh Bentall, the Professor of Cardiac Surgery and John Baker, who was the Professor of Pharmacology during my own years at Charing Cross Hospital Medical School.

The heart-lung machine and cardioplegia were as 'hand in glove' and Melrose had developed both. During my own training at the Hammersmith in the late 1970s both Melrose and Bentall would take me sailing off the south coast of England in their yachts and reflect on those heady days. It was clear that they faced massive political opposition when planning to use cardioplegia in the operating theatre. No one had dared to deliberately stop a human heart before. And whilst the healthy dog heart could be resuscitated how could they be certain that the same would apply to a sick human heart? In the hospital administrators' minds the two were not necessarily aligned and sure enough there were fierce religious objections.

In 1955, well before cardiopulmonary bypass was in widespread use, the Hammersmith team audaciously employed potassium-induced cardiac arrest in the operating theatre. With the first patient established on the bypass machine Cleland and Bentall clamped the aorta well above the openings of the coronary arteries after which Melrose squeezed in potassium citrate solution through a cannula from the head of the table. As predicted the heart rapidly slowed then stopped entirely. It lay there in the pericardium both cold and floppy. Ideal conditions to carry out the repair in a flaccid bloodless organ.

This was indeed a revolution, but would it start again? Such was the angst that the regional coroner was stationed in the operating theatre with bishops of the Anglican, Catholic and Presbyterian churches standing outside in the corridor praying! Fortunately, though predictably, removal of the aortic clamp flooded the muscle with well-oxygenated blood and it reverted to beating forcibly. The cheerful heart flew off the bypass machine to the massive relief and elation of all present. For the bishops it was a miracle, for the coroner, no inquest needed.

Although Melrose didn't operate on hearts himself he rapidly became influential in the field through his major advances. He liaised closely with the renal dialysis pioneer Willem Kolff and the cardiac surgeon Donald Effler at the Cleveland clinic who built a modified Melrose heart-lung machine and began to use cardioplegia for patients in 1956. During a preliminary telephone conversation, Melrose advised Effler to limit the duration of cardiac arrest to fifteen minutes. Perhaps this was a clue that there had been problems at the Hammersmith. Nevertheless Effler persisted with 'stopped heart' operations over the following months reporting the safety and benefits of the technique, and advocating that it should be adopted on a worldwide basis. Others remained less enthusiastic and frankly frightened of the method.

In the spring of 1959 came a request from Russia to obtain a Melrose heart-lung machine alongside an invitation for the Hammersmith team to travel to Moscow and demonstrate it. Melrose was accompanied by Bill Cleland and Hugh Bentall together with the anaesthetist John Beard, perfusionist John Robson, theatre sister Phyllis Bowtle and the eminent cardiologist Arthur Hollman. They arrived at the Russian Institute of Cardiovascular Surgery on Leninsky Prospect with half a ton of equipment after which four children with congenital heart lesions were successfully operated on. Two of those cases had complex deformities which the surgeons had never previously attempted to correct. It was said to be the first occasion on which foreign doctors had been invited to teach in Russia as distinct from visitors being instructed in the wonders of Soviet medicine.

The Hammersmith team had made its mark. So successful was the trip in launching Russian cardiac surgery that the participants were congratulated by the government. The deputy prime-minister Anastas Mikoyan is said to have embraced Phyllis somewhat intimidatingly stating: 'Medicine is clean, Politics are dirty.' Who would disagree with that? As a tangible reward the glorious team were flown back to London on the inaugural flight of the Tupolev 104, the Soviet version of the Comet aircraft. It was during the Moscow visit that Melrose met Brukhonenko the year before his death and learned of the pioneering efforts during the Stalinist era. Gentleman that he was, Melrose wrote an account of Brukhonenko's research in the *British Medical Journal* so that the West might be made aware. Unfortunately some descriptions of the attempted resurrection of dead animal heads caused widespread revulsion as a consequence of which the 'autojektor' was soon forgotten.

As other groups adopted potassium cardioplegia problems began to arise. Walt Lillehei cautioned against the method particularly for patients who had sustained previous heart muscle damage like myocardial infarction. Others reported fatal intractable ventricular fibrillation after thirty minutes of cardioplegic arrest. At autopsy microscopic areas of dead muscle were found throughout the heart suggesting that the strategy was not effective. Bjork stated: 'The potassium method of Melrose seems to be a rather dangerous and doubtful one.' Then when the US National Heart Institute group reported deaths through myocardial necrosis in the *Journal of Thoracic and Cardiovascular Surgery* the technique was abandoned in America in 1960. Alternative methods such as profound surface cooling of the heart with saline, or simply clamping the aorta intermittently then re-perfusing the muscle with blood were preferred.

The rejection of the Hammersmith's flagship cardioplegia solution may have affected Aird who until then had been energetic, extroverted and a little ruthless. His first assistant for the Siamese twins' separation had described him 'as a whirlwind of a man, larger than life, who drove himself with a passion and fury that caused grave concerns to his friends'. But after the cardioplegia debacle he became depressed and was found dead in bed from barbiturate poisoning at the age of fifty-seven. Irreverently his residence on the second floor of the entrance block of the Hammersmith Hospital became the doctors' bar. Known as the Waterhole it was much frequented by future cardiac surgeons including myself.

It would be another fifteen years before chemical arrest of the heart regained popularity. In the meantime Lillehei investigated the possibility of directly cannulating the coronary arteries within the aorta and perfusing continuously with blood. I remember having to hold the two perspex perfusion cannulas in place by hand as a trainee at the Brompton. It was tedious, risked damaging the orifice of vessels and the cannulas kept slipping out and spraying the surgeon whilst he tried to replace the aortic valve. Walt eventually drew the same conclusion. He then discovered an article which explained the ability of heart muscle to take up oxygen during retrograde blood flow through the large vein called the coronary sinus which opens into the right atrium. He tried doing just that in a patient undergoing aortic valve surgery in 1956. The perfusion lasted for eleven minutes and was useful in avoiding the dreaded problem of coronary air embolism.

As senior registrar to Brock at the Brompton in the 1960s, Mark Baimbridge was alarmed by the number of patients who still died from ventricular failure through inadequate muscle protection during surgery. The condition became known as 'stone heart'. Sir Russell was now President of the Royal College of Surgeons and suggested Baimbridge consult with biochemists working in the laboratories there. From then onwards the new science of molecular biology entered the research arena combining electron microscopy of biopsies from the heart, cell biochemistry and optical biophysics to compare myocardial preservation techniques.

In 1973 Baimbridge approached Sir Ernst Chain, the Nobel Prize winner and Head of Biochemistry at nearby Imperial College to ask how he would consider protecting the heart muscle molecule myosin that was consistently found to be damaged by prolonged ischaemia. Chain referred him on to David Hearse a young researcher at the College who was studying mechanisms to prevent myocardial injury during acute coronary thrombosis and heart attack. Hearse was working with the energy molecule adenosine triphosphate, (ATP) which was depleted during lack of oxygen. He hypothesised that the stone heart phenomenon during surgery occurred through lack of ATP after which the pendulum began to swing back towards cold cardioplegia.

Baimbridge was made a consultant at St Thomas' Hospital and frankly was one of the slowest operators I ever encountered. That is an observation not a criticism but for that very reason effective muscle preservation was very important to him. He had read about the emerging myocardial protection strategies of two surgeons, Hans Bretschneider at the University of Gottingen, and Thys Sondergaard of Aarhus, Denmark, both of whom had employed the cardioplegic solution developed by Bretschneider for patients undergoing aortic valve replacement. This process involved clamping the aorta then perfusing the coronary arteries with blood containing glucose and cardioplegic chemicals. At the same time the pericardial sac around the heart was filled with cold glucose solution at 4°C. The duration of aortic clamping with no coronary blood flow had routinely exceeded an hour but the results were excellent.

Baimbridge went on to recruit Hearse to work on a new cardioplegic solution at the Rayne Institute of St Thomas'. He suggested resuming the focus on potassium, as per Melrose, together with magnesium and the local anaesthetic compound procaine as a cell membrane stabiliser. The combination was tested exhaustively on rat hearts in a solution cooled to 4°C and then introduced into patients at St Thomas' with encouraging results. Surgeons in the US were also trying to escape the tedium of Lillehei's continuous coronary perfusion with blood. Whilst trying to explain why Melrose's original solution caused injury it was suggested that the concentration of potassium was far too high. Cold cardioplegia solutions with substantially less potassium were indeed shown to be safer allowing cardiac arrest periods for as long as 200 minutes without muscle damage.

In the late 1970s coronary perfusion with blood pumped from the bypass machine was abandoned altogether. That said in 1977 Gerald Buckberg in Los Angeles showed that cold blood was a better vehicle to deliver the cardioplegic chemicals than a clear salt solution. Blood delivered more oxygen to the muscle, had more compatible osmotic pressure and conveyed a protective effect through free radical scavenging. As a result of the incremental improvements, with reliable protection for much longer periods, the possibility for even more complex operations emerged. That also meant longer time supported by the heart-lung machine, with the serious issues that generated.

My own career had started by then. From the beginning my intention was to become a cardiac surgeon and to that end I would watch operations from the rarely-used viewing gallery of my teaching hospital in London. On my very first visit in October 1966. I was alone staring down into the chest when the patient, a young woman, exsanguinated spectacularly. Her blood pressure was poorly managed and the aortic suture line simply gave way as she separated from the bypass machine. Blood sprayed the operating lights, as she died, but I was not easily put off.

In 1974 whilst still very junior, I talked my way into a resident surgical officer post at the Brompton Hospital and became Oswald Tubb's last assistant. Lord Brock, already retired, would still visit to give talks and by chance I discovered and cheerfully wore his discarded operating boots to the amusement of my bosses. Following in his footsteps you might say, and in those days the mortality was still substantial.

After a thorough general surgery training in Cambridge, where I operated day and night, I spotted an advertisement for a temporary consultant post on Hong Kong Island. Given a deep fascination for the East, I impulsively submitted an application and was hired by return.

Once in practice, word spread that I could also operate on the chest and I was solicited to help out on a philanthropic basis at a large public hospital on the mainland. Frequently there were unusual problems in Kowloon that I would never encounter in Britain. Moreover the patients had few expectations. When things went well the families were enormously grateful and I soon had a collection of jade. Contented, I would drift back across Victoria Harbour on the Star Ferry watching a blood red sun sink into the South China Sea. Romantic but lonely.

Included in the contract, I stayed in the travelling surgeon's apartment on the Peak, drove his Porsche, and was given access to the famous Hong Kong Club on the waterfront. One evening after a long days operating I found myself languishing in the sauna next to Colonel Bob Stewart, the distinguished head of the overseas intelligence agency MI6. After the predictable banter as to why I was there in the first place the conversation drifted towards the grim humanitarian situation across the border in mainland China. Did cardiac surgery exist there at all I asked? This was the autumn of 1978 not long after the death of the Chairman Mao Zedong. The Great Proletarian Cultural Revolution had reached its conclusion, but the events had proved devastating, particularly for southern China.

Mao had provoked revolution in 1966 by urging the poor, or masses being the derogatory term, to rise up and seize control of the Communist Party. Gangs of students morphed into his vicious Red Guards that were urged to 'wipe away the evil habits of the old society'. That included an all-out assault against 'monsters and demons', in other words the 'intellectual elite'. Academics, teachers, doctors and the wealthy were set upon. Many thousands were killed with sinister reports of cannibalism. Universities, schools and hospitals were shut down. Churches, shrines, shops and homes were ransacked throughout China. The British Embassy in Peking was destroyed in 1967 with the diplomats lucky to escape. As a result the borders had been closed to the West for more than a decade. No contact, no trade, no exchange of ideas.

Out of the blue, or rather through the haze of smoke in the bar, Stewart asked me whether I cared to see the consequences of the devastation of Chinese medicine for myself. Many hospitals simply didn't possess an anaesthetic machine, any investigations other than plain x-rays, antibiotics nor disposable instruments and needles. For reasons beyond my imagination he knew the chief of heart surgery in the southern port of Guangzhou some ninety-five miles away. Canton, as it was still called in Britain, had been devastated by the Revolution and their main Guangdong Provincial Hospital shut down. The surgeons had been sent to work in the fields but were now endeavouring to start over. Having been deprived of contact with Western medicine for years he predicted that I would receive a warm welcome. 'How can they possibly perform heart operations with no anaesthetic nor ventilators,' I asked. 'They use acupuncture' came the reply but I didn't believe it. That said, I was about find out for myself on a unique adventure. And sure enough, the history of cardiac surgery in China was just as compelling as in the West.

Just as in Europe, armed conflict had impacted upon progress in the specialty from the outset. In 1946 Dr Ying-Kai Wu performed China's first ligation of a patent ductus arteriosus at the Central Hospital in Chonqing.

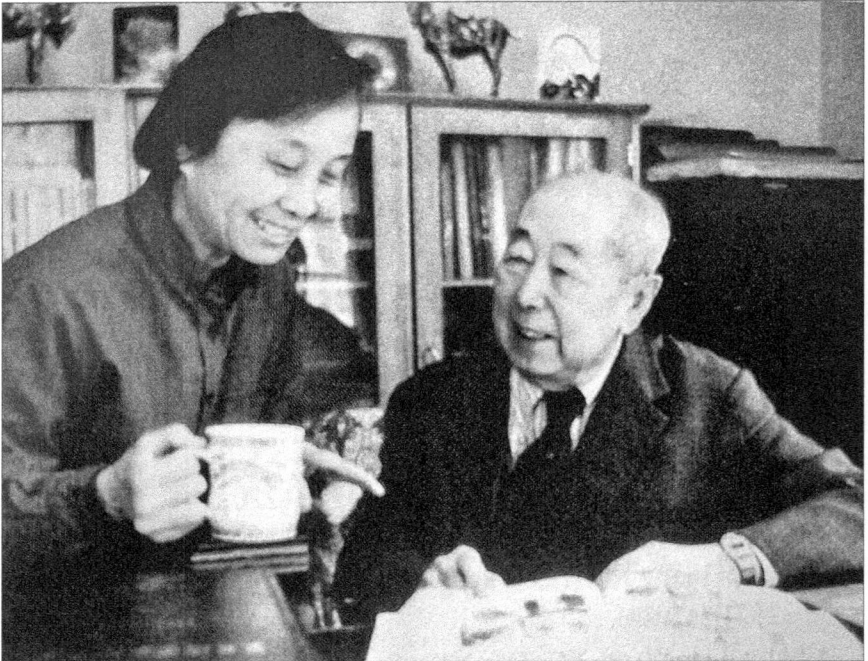

7.2 Ying Kai Wu and his wife.

This southern city had been made the wartime capital when Peking was largely evacuated during the Japanese invasion. Wu followed by performing a pericardectomy in 1947, but it wasn't until March 1953 that Mei-H Sin Shih constructed a Blalock-Taussig shunt in Shanghai.

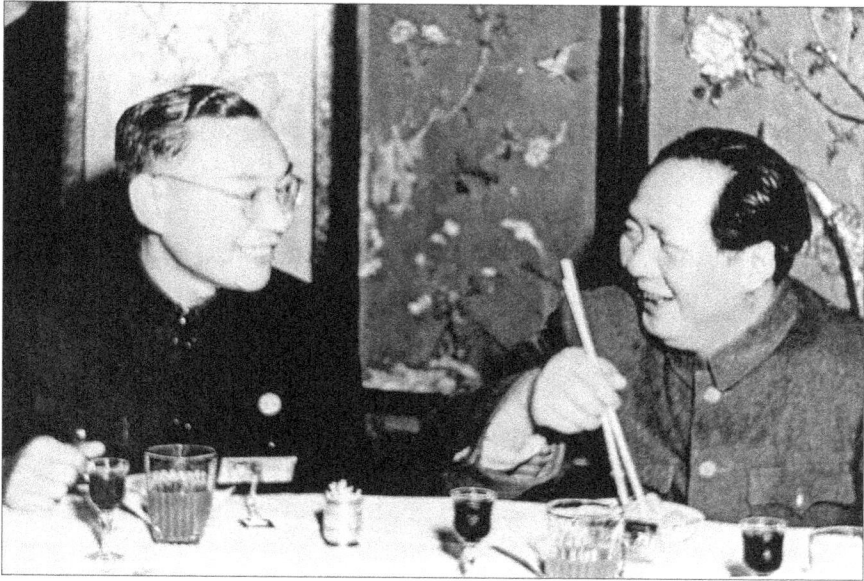

Fig 7.3 Dr Shih with Chairman Mao.

Shih had no fine needles or suture materials at his disposal so he had to fashion his own. No mean feat for microvascular surgery in new-born babies.

Influence from the outside world remained restricted after World War II, so it wasn't until 1954 that Xi-Chun Lan had attempted a closed mitral valvotomy in Shanghai. Again, he did not have the valvulotomes available in the West but achieved success using index finger exploration through the left atrial appendage. By the following year Lan reported a series of thirty-two cases with just a single death from stroke. In tandem, surgery for thoracic aneurysms began, aided by whole body cooling and using segments of human aorta from cadavers as replacement grafts. Water bath hypothermia was employed by Qi-Chen Lian at the Shanghai Second medical College to facilitate direct vision closure of atrial septal defects and open pulmonary valvotomies. Apparently it took the skilled Lian just seven minutes to open the right atrium, directly stitch the hole, and close it up again.

As in many other countries the heart-lung machine was introduced by a young surgeon who had studied in the United States. Hong-Xi Su served as an army medic in the Sino-Japanese War before being sent to train at North Western University in Chicago in 1949. Having worked on a cardio-pulmonary bypass project in the animal laboratory, Su used his own savings to purchase a DeWall-Lillehei machine and bubble oxygenator, which he shipped back home together with his new American wife, Jane McDonald.

Su was appointed head of cardiovascular surgery at the Fourth Military University, Nanjing in 1958 and soon afterwards used his heart-lung machine to close a ventricular septal defect in a 6-year-old boy. This was the first such operation in China but it wasn't straightforward. There was no air conditioning in the hospital and covered by heavy surgical drapes the lad suffered violent febrile convulsions before going onto bypass. Determined to succeed Su carried on regardless and actively cooled him with the circuit's heat exchanger before completing the operation. Newspapers throughout China heralded the advance the following day.

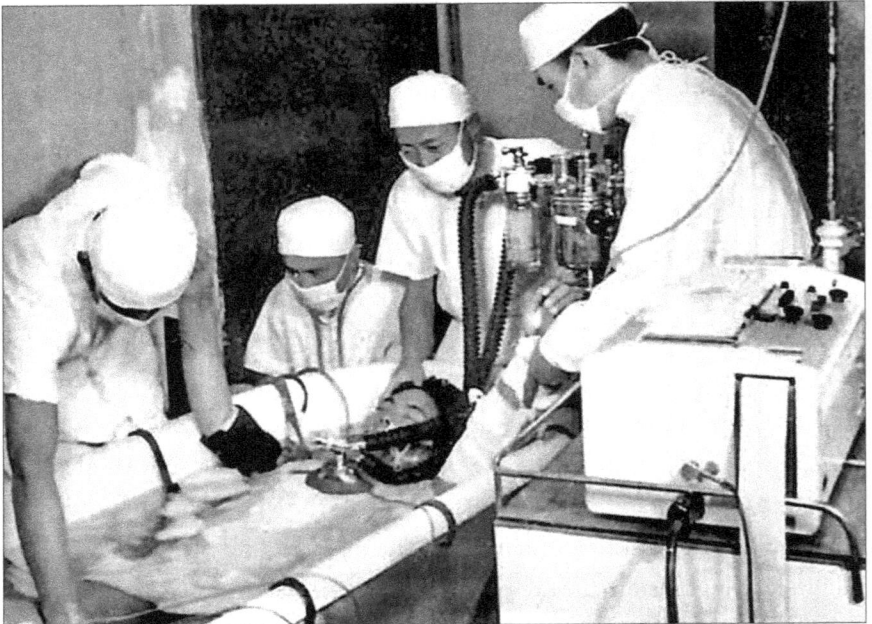

Fig 7.4 A. The Fu Wai cooling bath.

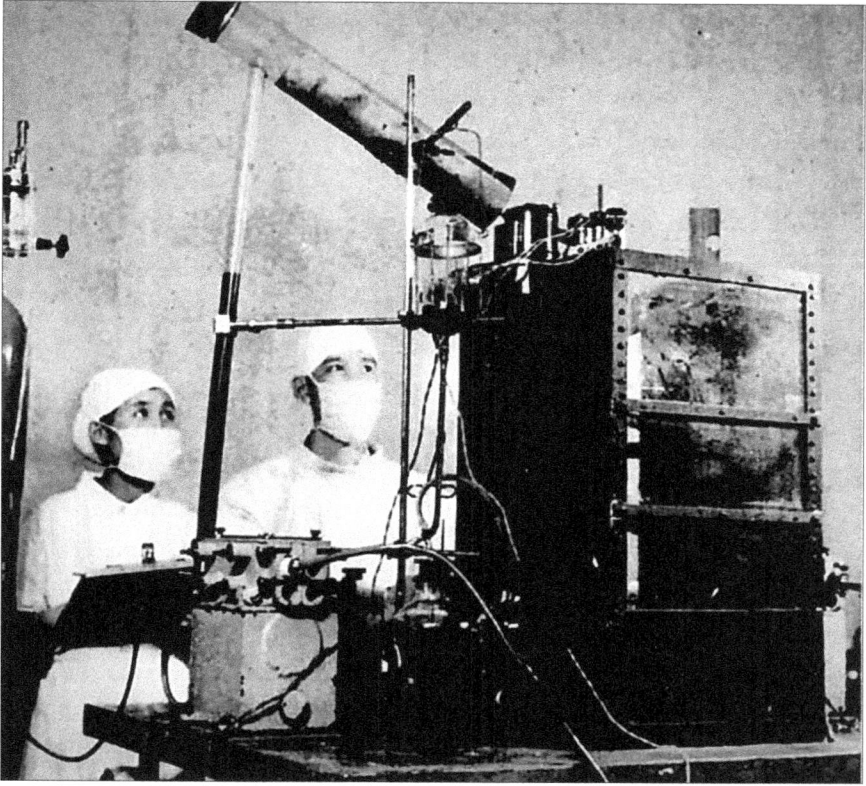

B. The Fu Wai heart-lung machine.

The very same rubber tubing and oxygenator were reused in a number of patients simply because there were no disposable replacements. But within weeks Chinese ingenuity in the form of the Shanghai Medical Equipment Factory, had copied the equipment and started to manufacture it. A vertical screen oxygenator and DeBakey type roller pump were also reproduced which Shih used to repair tetralogy of Fallot.

Beijing's newly opened Fuwai hospital then launched an ambitious programme of cardiac operations employing water bath cooling to 30°C without extracorporeal circulation.

Working against the clock You-Lin Hou and colleagues closed atrial and ventricular septal defects, repaired rheumatic mitral valves, and replaced aortic aneurysms. Then in 1959 Fuwai obtained its own bypass machine from the Chinese Academy of Medical Sciences and expanded their surgery to more complex defects.

Mao Zedong was destined to put an end to all that. The Revolution brought bloodshed, hunger and starvation after which, Maoist medicine was restricted to basic care in rural settings. Trained medical staff were replaced by the 'barefoot doctors', perhaps equivalent to paramedics yet essentially untrained. They performed first aid, moxibustion, and dispensed herbal remedies for infective illness because there were no antibiotics. Mao described his purge of the bourgeoisie as 'the great chaos under heaven'. Chaos was an appropriate term as a result of which cardiovascular surgery disappeared between 1967 and 1976. There were no imports of drugs, equipment or expertise.

Against this background, I landed in a desolate Guangzhou at the head of the Pearl River. The vast port had been China's main commercial and trading centre, the gateway to foreign goods and influence since the third century. The old Silk Road began there, but the first thing I observed was that there were no cars. Only bicycles. And I proved a novelty to the children who had never seen a Western face. As I wandered the streets dozens of kids followed me like the Pied Piper.

I was greeted at the airstrip by an English-speaking surgeon from the Guangdong Provincial Hospital, a large regional centre who were battling to resurrect a cardiac surgical service. And undoubtedly I would never learn so much in such a short time. The hospital owned one dated heart-lung machine but no disposables, so the oxygenator, cariotomy reservoir and rubber tubing were continually reused from patient to patient. Washed yes, Sterilised? Not possible. When we walked through the theatre recovery area, which couldn't justify the phrase intensive care unit, I asked 'where are your ventilators?' 'We don't have any, nor anaesthetic machines. We lost everything', came the glib response.

At that point I politely interjected. 'But Colonel Stewart said that you were doing open heart operations here.' 'We are', my escort responded. 'The patients are awake.' I was bewildered. How could anyone tolerate a saw up the sternum whilst conscious and breathing spontaneously?

According to the writings of Huangdi Neijin, the Yellow Emperor, acupuncture has been a recognised therapeutic measure for two thousand years yet only recently in the context of pain relief in surgery. Introduced into the operating theatre in 1958 it was initially used for brain and thyroid gland surgery. Yi-Shan Wang in Shanghai then introduced acupuncture pain relief during heart operations with cardiopulmonary bypass in 1972. The first patient, a 15-year-old girl with tetralogy of Fallot, was fully conscious and breathing herself throughout her procedure, then back working in the fields with her father two weeks later. An 8-cent postage stamp was released depicting the operation in celebration of the integration of Chinese with Western Medicine.

In preparation for the main event my host walked me through overhead-viewing galleries where abdominal and brain surgery were underway. In neither room was there an anaesthetic machine nor a ventilator. Both patients on the operating table were middle aged men perhaps bewildered to see a European face staring down on their exposed anatomy. We then entered the cardiac operating theatre where the immediate factor to draw my attention was the antiquity of the heart-lung machine.

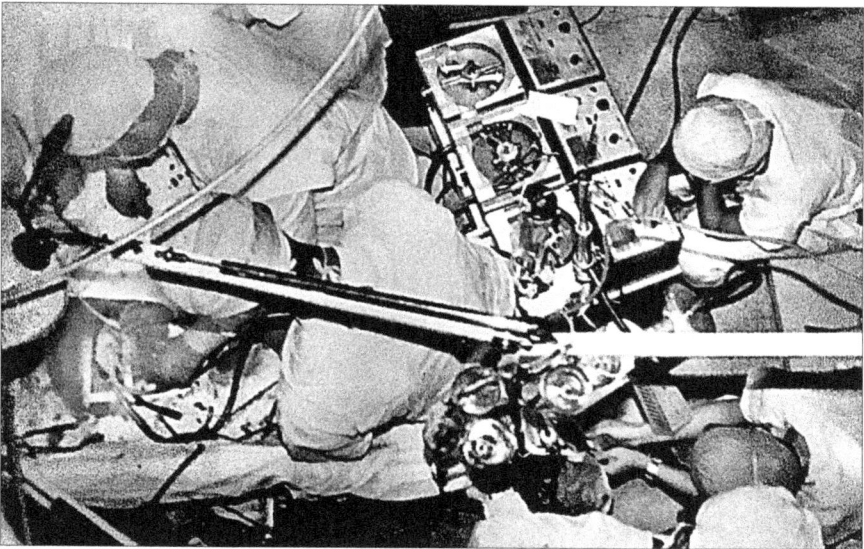

**Fig 7.5 Photograph taken by the author from a viewing gallery in Canton.
It shows heart surgery using cardiopulmonary bypass on
an awake patient with acupuncture.**

That together with the sight of worn and discoloured rubber pipes connecting it with the patient beneath the drapes. Again there was no other technology to be seen. What I then saw disbelievingly was an awake young woman with ashen white face, eyes staring intently towards the ceiling. She gave the impression of intense concentration.

So alien was the concept of cardiac surgery in a conscious patient without muscle relaxants or positive pressure ventilation, that I was curious to understand how they did it. First came the obvious retort. 'We don't have anaesthetic machines these days. They were all destroyed when the hospital was ransacked and we haven't been able to replace them. It's the same for ventilators, so we select the patients very carefully.' Indeed those chosen had to be old enough to cooperate in discomfort for long periods, have healthy lungs together with straightforward conditions amenable to repair within a relatively short time frame.

Of course I asked: 'How can a conscious person tolerate the foot long skin incision with a scalpel then burning electrocautery to stop the bleeding, followed by a saw up the length of their breast bone?' The very thought made me want to throw up. Clearly understanding what I had said, the acupuncturist took a step backwards and invited me to speak to the girl. When I put my palm on her cold forehead she shifted her gaze from the ceiling and smiled at me. I looked over the drapes and there was the beating heart with an incision in the right ventricle. The surgeon was repairing tetralogy of Fallot and in the midst of stitching a cloth patch into the ventricular septal defect. I was used to that. It was the situation on my side of the drapes that fascinated me.

I probed into the consequence if one or other of the chest cavities was opened causing pneumothorax? That was common enough. The lung then deflates suddenly due to the loss of negative pressure in the pleural space, so surely the patient would suffer breathlessness. All that was covered by the pre-operative training it seemed. At least a week to practise slow and deep abdominal breathing so chest wall movement could be kept to a minimum throughout. If a hole was made inadvertently into the pleural cavity it had to be stitched closed immediately. In the event of respiratory distress a chest drain was inserted between the ribs to evacuate air. Agonising once again so it was clear that indoctrination and compliance played a vital role in the acceptance of such intervention. Could we try it in London? Absolutely not.

The acupuncture needles themselves were inserted into the front of the chest below each clavicle and on the wrists and ankles. Needles through the cartilage of the ears had been abandoned because of the severe discomfort they caused. But how does acupuncture actually work? I was told that the sharp needles served to stimulate the central nervous system to release endorphins into the muscles, spinal cord and brain. Endorphins or 'feel good' chemicals are the body's natural pain damping agents. They can also attenuate nausea and prevent vomiting in response to the surgery.

In theory that's fine, but when I probed again how effective all that was when the burning electrocautery was generating smoke from the tissues or the oscillating saw was spattering bone marrow across the drapes, my host looked pensive or defensive even. He admitted the diathermy to be painful so they infiltrated the skin and subcutaneous tissues with adrenaline. This serves to constrict the blood vessels and helps prevent bleeding. If they had an injectable local anaesthetic they would use it, and cover the chest opening and closing phase with a sedative. They denied using morphine or heroin as the patient had to remain cooperative throughout to regulate their breathing.

Once beneath the sternum there are no pain receptors. No sensation when manipulating the heart or using ice cold fluid in the pericardium or even when electrically defibrillating. Having observed the whole procedure, I can testify to that.

But had acupuncture taken the pain away. I don't think so. Whilst watching the gentle meticulous and speedy surgery I switched to the girl's face on numerous occasions and could see that it was difficult for her. Sometimes when the perfusion pressure in the bypass machine dropped off, her conscious level drifted away in response. Pain from the large metal needles and wire stitches passing through the breast bone caused her newly-repaired heart to generate worryingly high pressures. Nonetheless the two-hour operation was successful and she drank water and smiled in the recovery room. It was disturbing to watch in many respects but a huge privilege. As taxing as those hours were for the patient she was now cured of a crippling congenital heart problem. Compliance is a cultural phenomenon. It wouldn't work in the West, but I was now better placed to tolerate the numerous deficiencies of the NHS. Of course things changed for the better in China over time and I returned many times in my career.

When I returned to the Hammersmith, Hugh Bentall and Denis Melrose were approaching retirement so as senior registrar I had the opportunity to operate for some of the country's top cardiologists. I had Attention Deficit Hyperactivity Disorder (ADHD) so paperwork didn't suit me. I was a perpetual blood and guts man, disinhibited by a head injury playing ruby and somewhat out of control. It was then whilst sailing off the cliffs of the Isle of White that Bentall suggested that I train with Kirklin in America. 'To learn some discipline' as he put it. I had no idea who Dr Kirklin was at that stage so I politely suggested that I should go to the heart transplant pioneer Norman Shumway in Stanford instead. Bentall shook his head in despair. 'If you go to California you'll be a complete write off', he snorted. Melrose smiled and nodded politely in agreement. 'Kirklin is using my cardioplegia,' he said cheerfully. So in January 1981 I went to the University of Alabama, the best move I could possibly have made at that point in my career. It was as if the phrase 'right place, right time' had been coined for me.

Kirklin had relocated from the Mayo Clinic to Birmingham, Alabama in 1966, where with unlimited resources he established the world's leading cardiac surgical unit. He was the undisputed master of surgery for congenital heart disease with a long list of operative firsts, and needless to say his carefully selected team of surgical residents were destined for positions of leadership in other centres. His opinions on the education of trainees were made clear on many occasions. As he put it: 'The most critical and important part of the cardiovascular resident's learning is in the operating room, and this is where we try to be certain that he learns well and completely the thousand and one little details of operative cardiac surgery. This means endless hours of scrubbing with them, of searching for their wasted motions and helping to get rid of them. Of increasing their perception of tissue planes and insisting that they use them in their dissection; that they keep the operation moving forward.'

One thing was for sure. If Kirklin didn't like you that was the end of a career in cardiac surgery. If he did you would make it, so I had to rein myself in – for a while that is. The boss used his operating theatre and intensive care unit as laboratories, making systematic measurements and deductions on which to construct nomograms for reliable decision-making. He believed that surgery must be conducted in a scientific and reproducible fashion, and employed rigorous statistical analysis when reporting results. Undoubtedly the strategy worked. Reflecting on the gradual improvements in outcomes he commented: 'During 1955 our mortality rate was high for the repair of tetralogy of Fallot in children. We were discouraged by our inability to make most of these patients live. Mortality in these babies started out at 50% or higher, but within five years it had fallen to 15%. By 1970 it was around 8%. In 1980 it approached zero, and is still never higher than 4% annually at the Birmingham Medical Centre.' This was all down to the discipline Bentall rightly insisted I needed, but it was certainly a culture shock.

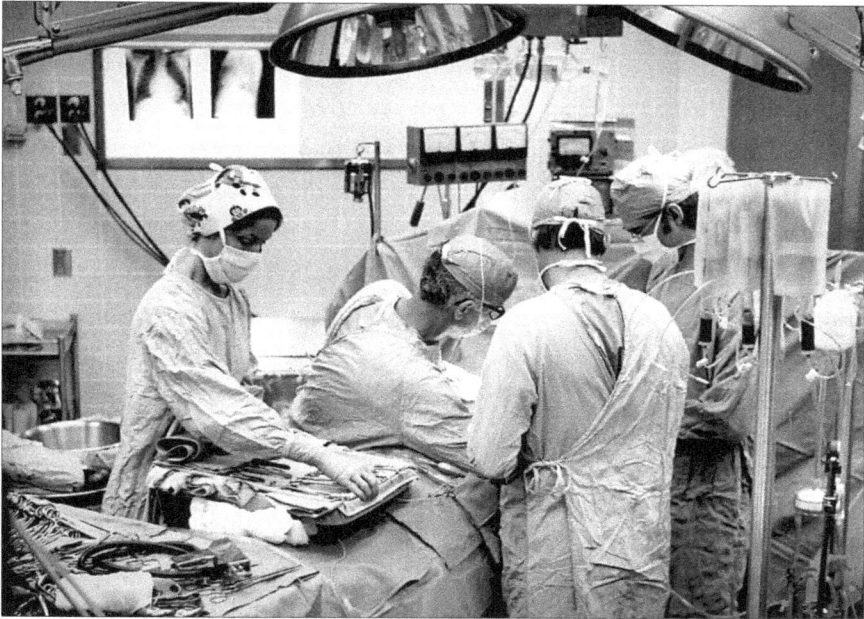

Fig 7.6 The author assisting Dr Kirklin at the University of Alabama.

The residents' morning rounds began at 4 a.m. so Kirklin could be called at 6 a.m. with a progress report on his patients or indeed anyone else's if they were not doing well. Surgery began at 7 a.m. and usually went on until the early evening. I would then go to the laboratory whilst the residents did evening intensive care rounds.

There were full departmental academic meetings on Wednesday evenings, then on Saturday mornings beginning at 8 a.m. On Sunday mornings at 7 a.m. Kirklin and his head of research Eugene Blackstone held academic business meetings to review progress in the various research projects and to finalise scientific papers for publication. This was the Alabama work ethic. Some of us thrived, others couldn't hack it and capitulated.

With Kirklin's rigorous analytic approach and well-honed operative techniques, those patients who died didn't do so through surgical mistakes. But there remained that one problem that was hard to overcome. The damage inflicted on the patient by the heart-lung machine.

At a meeting to celebrate the twenty-fifth anniversary of open heart surgery at the Mayo Clinic in 1980, Kirklin highlighted the issue as follows. 'Some of the basic problems associated with the clinical use of pump oxygenators are as real and unsolved as they were in 1953. When we repair very complex kinds of heart disease, particularly in the very young, the very sick or the very old, important risks are still imposed by the unsolved problems of cardiopulmonary bypass. These include the physio-chemical changes produced in the formed and unformed elements of the blood by exposure to non-biological surfaces which produce profound and widespread structural and functional abnormalities in the patients. Solutions to these complex problems would not only be intellectually rewarding and save lives but would considerably increase the cost effectiveness of cardiac surgery.'

The 'post-perfusion syndrome' caused damage to the lungs which became waterlogged, together with kidney dysfunction, fever, with raised white blood cell count and an increased risk of bleeding through coagulation defects. Kirklin interpreted the process as an inflammatory reaction throughout the whole body. The consequence was the need for prolonged ventilator support, often with kidney dialysis and blood transfusion during an extended stay in the intensive care unit. And of course many of the more vulnerable patients died. Then it became apparent that a similar phenomenon afflicted kidney failure patients who were placed on a dialysis machine. The common factor was the interaction of blood with the non-biological surfaces of an extracorporeal circuit which had to be triggered by disturbances in blood biochemistry.

When Kirklin and Blackstone saw that their new British fellow had a degree in biochemistry they decided to challenge me with identifying the cause. Kirklin's son James was chief resident at the time and made sure I had a wide range of patients to study. Moreover there were some original and revealing discoveries in the understanding of inflammation emerging from the Scripps Institute in San Diego. They had been sent blood to analyse from dialysis patients at the University of Minnesota and discovered activation of what is known as the 'complement system'. Toxins released during the interaction were known to activate white blood cells, and sure enough the numbers of circulating white cells were known to fall sharply during dialysis in kidney failure patients. Where had they gone to and was this a clue as to the events during cardiopulmonary bypass?

I was fortunate to be allocated an experienced laboratory technician Jack Acton to work with me. Jack was a fixer and I needed a full set of unused heart-lung machine equipment with a supply of fresh blood. My plan was to take samples of all the synthetic materials of the bypass circuit and incubate them in a test tube with blood at body temperature. We then centrifuged away the cells and sent the plasma to California for analysis. At the same time I studied 150 consecutive patients undergoing heart surgery with or without the bypass machine obtaining multiple blood samples before, during and after each operation. Their post-operative course was then monitored for days afterwards to record signs and symptoms of the post-perfusion syndrome.

What we found was fascinating and conclusive. Complement-derived toxins were immediately released during blood foreign surface interaction and were not found in patients who were operated upon without the machine. The longer the time on cardiopulmonary bypass the more toxins were released with the higher likelihood of the post-perfusion syndrome. That's what we expected but what I really wanted to know, was whether all synthetic materials were similarly involved or was there a particular culprit. When I scrutinised the results from California the answer was right there. Nylon, which was used widely in blood oxygenators and filters, avidly triggered the release of the inflammatory toxins. What's more, by taking blood samples from the pulmonary artery and from the left atrium, which receives blood returning to the heart from the lungs, we showed that virtually half of the circulating white blood cells became trapped in the capillaries when lung blood flow was restored. Why? Because cells activated by the toxins had stuck to the capillary wall where they released oxygen-free radicals to damage the delicate barrier between blood and air. As a result fluid seeped through into the air sacs effectively drowning the patient.

This was a momentous discovery for the whole department and the Scripps Institute. We had identified the cause of virtually half of the deaths after heart surgery. When I presented the findings during the Sunday morning research meeting there was a stunned silence. Kirklin and Blackstone looked at each other and smiled. But there was one thing left to do, besides publishing a paper about it. We called the manufacturers of the bypass equipment and explained carefully why they should remove nylon. When they did the severity of the post-perfusion syndrome abated. This was a simple but invaluable contribution in the quest to make heart surgery safer.

Did I appreciate the significance of the discovery at the time? Not really. As an ambitious young surgeon I was too absorbed in what went on in the operating theatres. But there was one more pivotal event for me that year.

I arrived for the early morning round on Friday 23rd July and sensed a palpable buzz amongst the residents. They were standing around the first patient's bed, but that patient was dying. So I enquired as to the source of the excitement. 'Dr Cooley implanted a total artificial heart last night', I was told. It was only the second ever. It had taken twelve years to recover from the first debacle in 1969, an operation which sparked the career-long feud between Drs Cooley and DeBakey.

The comment threw a switch in my sleep-deprived brain so that night I took the red eye to Houston, determined to meet Dr Cooley and see that artificial heart for myself.

Spare Parts

Out of difficulties grow miracles.
—Jean de la Bruyere

The extraordinary efficiency of the human heart, and indeed life itself, depends upon one crucial factor. The blood must continue to flow forward in one direction, a situation which is entirely dependent upon the integrity of our heart valves. They must not leak nor must there be obstruction to flow. Narrowed or regurgitant valves cause a rise in pressure in the cardiac chambers and the compromised organ produces very unpleasant symptoms.

When the aortic or mitral valves are deformed pressure rises in the blood vessels of the lungs causing breathlessness. In turn decreased flow to the body results in listlessness and fatigue. Similarly back pressure in the right heart from issues with the pulmonary or tricuspid valve causes resistance to blood draining back to the heart in the veins. This results in an accumulation of oedema, fluid in the tissues of the body with swollen legs and abdomen, a painful distended liver and water on the brain with confusion. This is the misery of heart failure and not just in older age groups. Rheumatic fever with heart valve involvement afflicted half a million young patients in Britain in the 1950s when medical treatment was largely ineffective.

As described the usual suspects made valiant attempts to dilate or repair heart valves without even being able to see them. Much like fixing the engine of a car in pitch darkness. But it was the only hope for the desperate or dying before our specialty evolved. Even after the introduction of the heart-lung machine there were no fail safe repair strategies for leaking valves so it was deemed unacceptable to attempt an operation before the patient became severely symptomatic. And by then heart failure had damaged the kidneys and liver, thus increasing surgical risk.

It was the unsurmountable challenge of the leaking aortic valve that spurned the development of heart valve substitutes. Early operations which utilised pieces of the patient's own pericardium or segments of vein from the leg failed miserably and led to the consideration of synthetic materials. At the Peter Bent Brigham Hospital in Boston, Charles Hufnagel was encouraged to develop an artificial heart valve by his chief Elliot Cutler, the pioneer of mitral valvotomy.

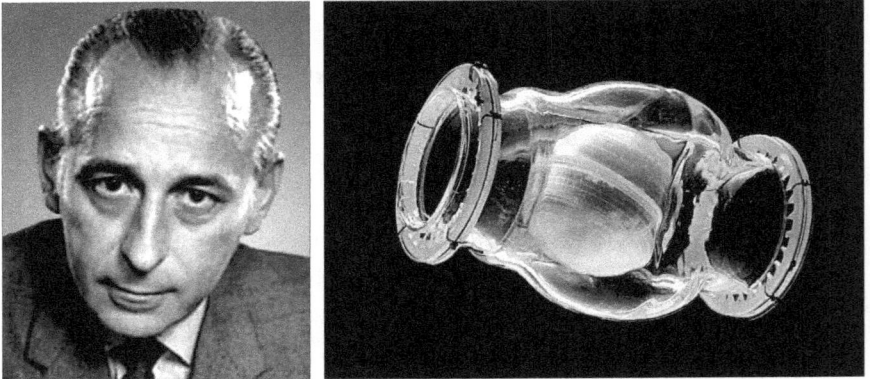

Fig 8.1 A. Charles Huffnagel. B. The Huffnagel Valve.

One of the first challenges was to determine which materials would be tolerated within the bloodstream without promoting clot formation. Thrombosis of the implant followed by an embolus to the brain with stroke would not be a reasonable outcome. So Hufnagel first tried strips of methyl methacrylate stitched into the lining of the dog's aorta and documented to his excitement that no thrombus formed on it.

On the basis of the encouraging experiment Hufnagel constructed a transparent hollow tube of methyl methacrylate with a globular 'blow out' in the middle portion into which he inserted a metal ball. At each end of the tube were fixation rings of nylon to sew to the vessel wall. By this time surgery for coarctation of the aorta, the tight narrowing high in the chest, was well established which seemingly justified the next audacious move. Supported by Cutler, Hufnagel suggested that his ball valve could be used to treat a leaking aortic valve, though not as we understand the procedure today. There was still no cardiopulmonary bypass in 1952 so Hufnagel argued that the best option would be a valve inserted into the aorta at the site of coarctation surgery. At least this should stem a proportion of the regurgitant blood flow back into the left ventricle, and further laboratory experience suggested that it did.

On the 11th September 1952 Hufnagel operated on a thirty-one-year old woman who had suffered with chronic rheumatic aortic regurgitation since the age of five. For years she had been severely restricted by chest pain and breathlessness and was more than ready to accept the potential surgical risks which included paraplegia. Her left chest was opened with a long incision between the fourth and fifth ribs, and with the inflated lung retracted towards his assistant the vigorously pulsating aorta was readily apparent. In preparation for the positioning of clamps above and below the site of implantation Hufnagel carefully tied off a number of branches which supply both the chest wall and more importantly the spinal cord. He knew that aortic clamping for periods longer than thirty minutes risked permanent spinal cord damage so was working against the clock. Subsequently he suggested that less expedite surgeons should employ a temporary bypass tube between the arteries to the left arm and left leg in order to avoid paraplegia. Either that or place the valve itself in a permanent bypass tube then occlude the intervening segment of aorta. Unnecessarily complicated when the real answer was that slow surgeons were not suited for cardiac surgery.

Hufnagel operated on a series of eighty aortic regurgitation patients with his prosthesis though in twelve the procedure had to be abandoned in the anaesthetic room when the blood pressure fell precipitously. That was a consequence of the severe valve leak and a failing left ventricle made worse by the vasodilating drugs. Indeed one in five of his patients died through spontaneous ventricular fibrillation. Nevertheless the survivors, were substantially improved with an impressive relief of breathlessness and decrease in heart size. Unfortunately a number of long-term survivors suffered clotting in the sphere and embolism to the leg arteries but at least that was better than stroke. And there was one further disturbing issue. The metal ball clicked loudly in its cage and could be heard opening and closing across the room. Or across the street in skinny patients. This caused frustration and distress leading to the metal ball being replaced by a silicone covered poppet.

Gordon Murray at the Toronto General Hospital came up with a better solution. Murray was originally a fellow of the Royal College of Surgeons in London and was an innovative and technical genius. In October 1955 he carefully dissected out the natural aortic valve from a cadaver, preserved it in salt solution at 4°C for thirty-six hours, and then implanted it into the descending aorta of a patient in a procedure similar to Hufnagel's. Of course this human valve was silent and functioned well for many years. Three more aortic regurgitation patients underwent the same operation and each was greatly improved.

Spurred on by Hufnagel's efforts and determined not to be outdone, Charles Bailey began to experiment with different plastic balls and flap valves. He suspended these within the lumen of the aorta just above the diseased valve using one or two tails, intending that they would be displaced from the flow path during contraction, then fall back to occlude the orifice during relaxation of the ventricle. For flap valve think toilet seat flipping up and down. As an adjunct for the leaking aortic valve he produced a constriction ring of nylon fabric as a sling around the outside of the aorta which he tightened to narrow the lumen. None of these methods proved satisfactory though the constriction ring provided some symptomatic improvement if the valve cusps themselves were not severely deformed.

By the late 1950s cardiopulmonary bypass gave direct access to all four valves within the heart so that meaningful valve surgery became a reality. Diagnostic techniques were improving too, so that more precise and reliable assessments could be made. In 1959 Hufnagel adopted another ingenious approach. The normal aortic valve has three thin-walled flexible cusps which open widely then coapt on closure. But one in fifty people is born with a bicuspid valve and these are more prone to degeneration and leakage. Hufnagel worked to develop a single replacement valve cusp made of

Dacron cloth which he impregnated with silicone rubber to prevent cells from growing into it. Moulded to directly replicate the human aortic cusp, it had pins on one edge to pass through the vessel wall like staples to secure it in position. Hufnagel employed these replacement cusps either singly or in groups of three but the results were less than satisfactory. That said, he implanted them in 150 patients before finally giving up with the conclusion that the whole valve needed to be replaced in a single unit. Perhaps he should have reverted to the ball valve concept he used further down in the aorta before someone else did.

The first international conference dedicated to the surgery of heart valves took place in Chicago in 1960. Here one of the key questions was 'do prosthetic valve substitutes need to mimic the natural valve?' Would that help to reduce the risk of thrombosis or infection on the foreign surfaces, both of which proved fatal? A female cardiac surgeon had opinions on that.

Nina Starr from Brooklyn had trained at the New York University College of Medicine then followed with internship at Bellevue Hospital.

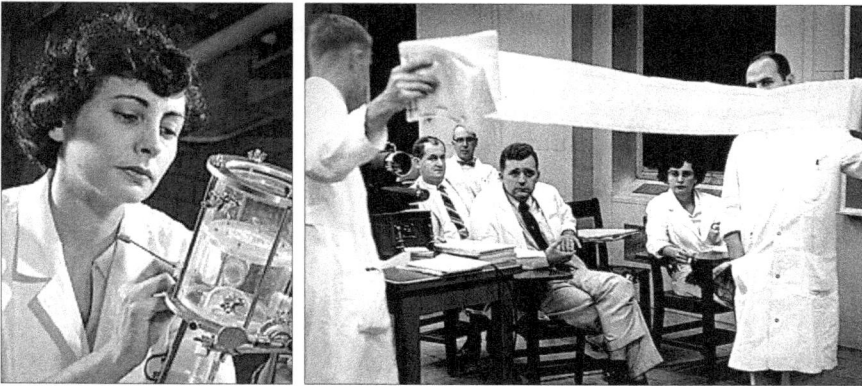

Fig 8.2 A. Nina Braunwald. B. Nina with Eugene Braunwald in a team meeting.

There she met and married Eugene Braunwald, a classmate destined to become the world's leading cardiologist. As Nina Braunwald she became Bellevue's first female general surgeon but then took a post-doctoral fellowship with Hufnagel whom she assisted with the early valve operations at Georgetown University. Fascinated by the heart she progressed to train with Andrew Morrow alongside her cardiologist husband at the National Institutes of Health, Bethesda, Maryland. It was here that she designed a mitral valve prosthesis for rheumatic heart disease patients that she modelled on plaster casts of the natural valve.

Nina's valve consisted of two flexible polyurethane flaps mounted on Dacron fabric to replace the natural valve leaflets. These were anchored to the sub-valvar papillary muscles by Teflon ribbons as substitutes for the natural chordae tendinae. This Braunwald-Morrow valve was tested in dogs with implants supported by the heart-lung machine and provided results that were thought to justify the switch to patients. That decision was made after just four animals had survived for up to forty hours together with autopsy findings that none of the valves had clotted. Not entirely convincing!

On the 10th March 1960 Nina, assisted by Morrow, performed the first replacement of the mitral valve ever attempted.

Braunwald established the patient, a sixteen-year-old girl, on the bypass machine and cut out the valve from within its annulus, removing most of the underlying papillary muscles with it. Morrow then sewed in the new valve and anchored the leaflets with the tails. Sadly it was not a success. There were technical issues with the implant and though the girl separated from the heart-lung machine she died with a leaking valve three days later. Before that case had reached its sad conclusion Morrow operated the following day on a 44-year-old woman who recovered and was well eight weeks later. Even so, the days of trying to imitate nature with plastic were numbered. Human heart valves took millions of years to evolve and are not easy to replicate.

On the same day as Braunwald's landmark mitral valve replacement Dwight Harken performed the world's first aortic valve replacement in Boston. In this case the prosthesis consisted of a Lucite ball in a stainless steel cage with a Teflon-backed sewing ring. The patient with severe aortic stenosis was supported by the heart-lung machine and cooled to 26°C. His obstructive rigidly-calcified valve was cut away and the new valve sewn into place with individual silk stitches placed through the narrow remnant or annulus as it is known. Against the odds this first patient from Jacksonville, Florida survived and the valve performed well. On June 6th Harken operated on a second patient from Massachusetts whose ball valve functioned splendidly for twenty-two years. The man then underwent a prostate operation without prophylactic antibiotics and died weeks later from infection on the prosthesis. Unfortunately Harken's next five aortic valve replacements all died causing him to suspend the programme. In the meantime the original ball valve design was modified slightly for the mitral position.

Braunwald's mitral valve replacements and Harken's two aortic valve triumphs were discussed excitedly at the Chicago meeting. Albert Starr of Portland, Oregon congratulated the solitary female surgeon on her courage and achievements and was himself preparing to implant a new prosthesis inspired by an old bottle stopper. It was the product of collaboration between surgeons and engineers that would endure for many decades.

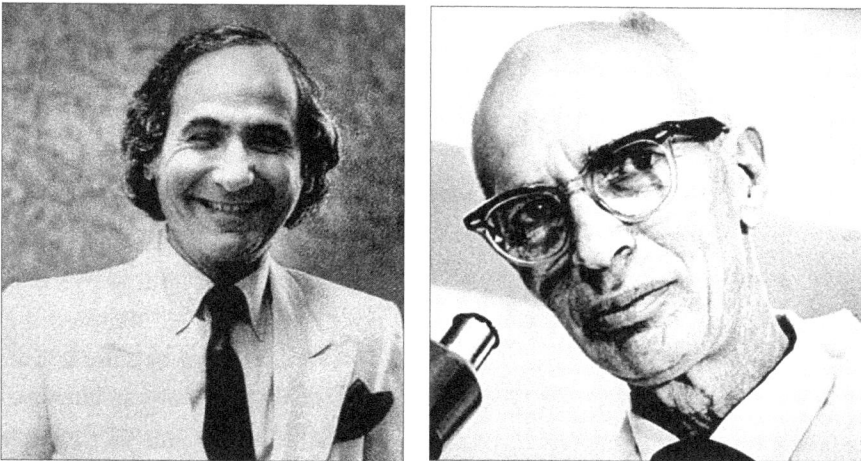

Fig 8.3 A. Albert Starr. B. Lowell Edwards.

It had been the autumn of 1958 when the retired engineer Lowell Edwards first approached Starr's office for an appointment. That morning he arrived in golf clothes and trainers and shook Starr's hand with a Parkinsonian tremor. Edwards was a successful engineer with 63 patents in an array of industries together with a number of original inventions. One was a fuel pump for aircraft that had been widely used by the military in World War II, and having come from a formidable engineering family, he was already a wealthy man. In his dotage he had the ambition to build a total artificial heart and, whilst not being explicit, it was because he had lost a close family member with heart failure.

Starr was sceptical about the blood pump issue, but recognising the potential which emanated from Edward's background he pointed out that years had been spent simply trying to produce an artificial heart valve and so wouldn't that be a good place to start? At thirty-two Starr was an experienced general surgeon who had trained with Blalock then operated prolifically on battlefield casualties in the Korean War. Seeing Edward's smart Cadillac parked outside drew him towards the eccentric engineer who was many years his senior. So together they embarked on the design of their own mechanical mitral valve.

At first they reproduced Braunwald's concept by modelling a bileaflet anatomical replica valve made from flexible plastic. Yet when tested in animals the results were uniformly poor through rapid clot deposition and device thrombosis. Starr inevitably concluded that synthetic surfaces and blood were a poor mix, much like the bypass machine without heparin. But there was no heparin tablet so patients couldn't be heparinised on a permanent basis. Irrespective of the bleeding risk, that would entail intravenous injections every few hours. Then in the mid 1950s the anticoagulant drug warfarin was introduced, a major contribution in itself with an intriguing background.

In the 1920s, cattle in Canada and the bordering states of the USA were afflicted by an unusual disease which caused spontaneous bleeding. In time mouldy silage made from sweet clover was implicated and shown to contain a substance that inactivated the blood clotting factor prothrombin. The cows were actually dying from anticoagulation, yet it was 1933 before a Wisconsin farmer drove to Madison to persuade the state veterinarian to get on and diagnose the condition. Serendipitously he found most offices closed that Saturday afternoon and by chance walked into the laboratory of the Professor of Biochemistry, Karl Link.

It wasn't until 1940 that Link managed to isolate the responsible agent, dicoumarol, and by 1948 he had synthesised warfarin, an agent which proved more potent than coumarol, and was first introduced as rat poison. The name warfarin was derived from the initials of Wisconsin Alumni Research Foundation, WARF, together with -arin, from coumarin. From 1954 onwards warfarin was used widely to prevent stroke in patients with atrial fibrillation but only after Vitamin K had been sourced as an antagonist to the potentially lethal bleeding complications.

Having abandoned God's original design for the mitral valve, Starr and Edwards took a leaf out of Hufnagel's book and pursued a ball-in-cage design.

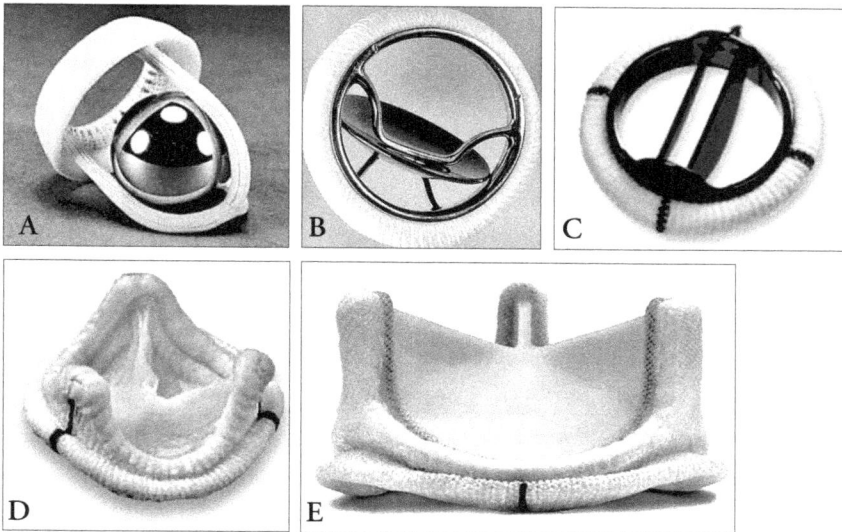

Fig 8.4 Types of valves prosthesis A. Ball-in-Cage Valve. B. Tilting disc valve. C. Bileaflet valve D. Porcine bioprosthesis. E. Pericardial bioprosthesis.

Edwards's laboratory was a shed in the garden of his summer cabin in North Oregon. The pair held frequent meetings to mull over materials and design features, finally agreeing on a plastic ball enclosed by a metal cage comprising three curved struts. The circular base of the valve, or prosthetic annulus, had a generous cloth sewing ring through which the anchoring stitches would be inserted. The concept was simple. The patient's own mitral valve would be removed including the sub-valvar chordae tendinae and papillary muscles, but leaving a cuff of tissue to sew to around the valve orifice. Stitches would then be placed through the cuff to anchor the prosthetic sewing ring and the cage slid down over them into the inlet of the left ventricle.

Once securely implanted with the heart filled with blood, the ball would slide to the end of the cage during the ventricles filling phase but be shot back to occlude the orifice when it contracted. And that is precisely what happened in the dogs. Animals implanted with the ball and cage valve survived for months rather than days. With continued refinement of the design more than forty dogs were sacrificed to the cause with one robust Labrador named Blackie surviving for more than a year.

Much then depended upon the cardiologists' willingness to refer patients for surgery since dogs don't pay bills. So Starr invited the hospital's Chief of Cardiology, Herbert Griswold, to visit the laboratory and listen to the valves ticking away in the animal's chest. Again the stethoscope wasn't really necessary as the noise was audible. It was something the patient and their spouse had to get used to. Griswold was immediately impressed that the prosthesis worked well and offered numerous patients who might benefit. But how long might the valve last? Starr and Edwards had already pondered that question. In ten years a heart would beat more than 400 million times with blood pounding the ball against the cage. Would the materials survive that stress? One of Starr's bright laboratory assistants produced an accelerometer which could mimic the valve movement as much as 6000 times per minute with pressures up to 150 mm Hg. That was equivalent to more than forty years within the heart but over three weeks of testing.

Remarkably Edwards's materials and Starr's valve design showed no significant wear under these conditions. The cage was robust enough to withstand the battering and the resilient plastic ball was virtually unchanged. Magic. In Griswold's opinion the prosthesis already merited clinical trials. The patients were desperate for help, the dogs weren't. And by 1960 no one had survived more than three months after a mitral valve replacement.

Perhaps foolishly Starr's first case was a difficult re-operation. The bedbound 33-year-old woman was confined to an oxygen tent having previously undergone two abortive valve repairs where Ivalon sponge had been inserted to support her leaking valve leaflets. As such the surgical site was an inflammatory mess and an unenviable surgical prospect.

Starr operated on 25th August eagerly watched by his engineering friend. Repeated chest re-entry with a saw ripping through the sternum is never a comfortable endeavour. With a hugely dilated heart beneath and tissues densely adherent through fibrous adhesions, the risk of slicing into the right ventricle is ever present. Fortunately it didn't happen. Soon she was established on cardiopulmonary bypass with cooling to 32°C whilst the thin-walled left atrium was separated from the adherent pericardium. The cavity was hugely dilated after months of mitral regurgitation and provided easy access to the useless valve. Starr chopped out much of it then anchored the substitute ball and cage with twenty individual silk stitches. It looked impressive with circular white sewing ring, black stitches, and the glistening ball sitting within the inlet of the left ventricle. A great result celebrated as she struggled to separate from the heart-lung machine. Or was it?

Soon after arriving fully conscious in the recovery area the poor woman could cooperate and sit up for a plain chest x-ray. But as Starr inspected it closely, what he saw generated considerable anxiety. There was a large air bubble in the left atrium which had presumably lurked in the enlarged and crooked appendage. There was no non-invasive method to remove it and tragically when she rolled over in the bed in pain hours later, the collection dislodged. The patient collapsed suddenly with massive air embolism to the carotid arteries. 'Air in the brain, life down the drain', as I used to tell my own staff. The valve through which the air passed ticked on happily until she died just ten hours after leaving the operating theatre. After a complex re-operation to implant an innovative new valve, this was a truly devastating outcome. But in this business disaster breeds resilience.

A month later Starr operated again in similarly taxing circumstances. This patient, a 52-year-old truck dispatcher Philip Amundson, had a leaking rheumatic mitral valve, subject to two separate attempts at repair. Again the surgical re-entry was prolonged, tedious and bloody but once safely on the bypass machine the valve was easily accessible and the replacement straightforward. Highly sensitised by the previous case, Starr went to great lengths to evacuate air from the heart, aspirating the chambers repeatedly with a needle and syringe and allowing the aorta to leak bubbles through a de-airing hole for a prolonged period. Amundson separated easily from the bypass machine causing Starr to wonder whether his previous patient hadn't filled her coronary arteries with air too. That was more than likely.

Amundson recovered uneventfully and Starr chose to anti-coagulate him with the new agent warfarin a week after the procedure. Though this was undoubtedly the correct decision there was debate and disagreement at first because the dogs were never anticoagulated and had not suffered embolic events. Nor did Amundson sustain any anticoagulant related bleeding over the next ten years, until tragically falling from a ladder, whilst decorating his house. He sustained a fractured skull with cerebral haemorrhage and died as a result.

Within months the Starr Edwards ball valve was in use everywhere that cardiac surgery was performed and the experience gave birth to what would become a huge heart valve industry. Recognising the opportunity, Edwards established his company, Edwards Laboratories in Santa Ana, California and in 1966 it was later acquired by the American Hospital Supply Corporation. A valve specifically for the aortic position was crafted and in November 1961 the surgeon Robert Cartwright of Pittsburgh carried out the first combined aortic and mitral valve replacements. But he did it in the most unconventional way.

Having excised the diseased mitral valve he worked through that opening into the cavity of the left ventricle to access the underside of the aortic valve. With considerable difficulty he obtained sufficient exposure to remove the calcified cusps and replace them with the Starr Edwards prosthesis. Then he inserted the second valve in the mitral position. The aorta was kept clamped to maintain a bloodless operating field and to protect against air embolism whilst the heart muscle was preserved by packing ice slush into the pericardial cavity. Though the patient limped from cardiopulmonary bypass and recovered to leave hospital, the predictable happened. The aortic prosthesis which had been implanted with excruciating difficulty became loose and leaked. Whilst the aortic regurgitation was tolerated for some time the valve eventually dehisced completely causing sudden death from heart failure.

At that point Starr himself began a series of multiple valve operations which he reported in 1964. Thirteen patients underwent aortic and mitral valve replacement, two of whom had the tricuspid valve exchanged too. The results were less than impressive with just six being completely relieved of their symptoms. The need for life-long anticoagulation with warfarin was off-putting for many patients so the search began for an alternative. Curiously it was my predecessor, an ear nose and throat surgeon in Oxford, who provided a solution.

Alf Gunning was an extraordinary character.

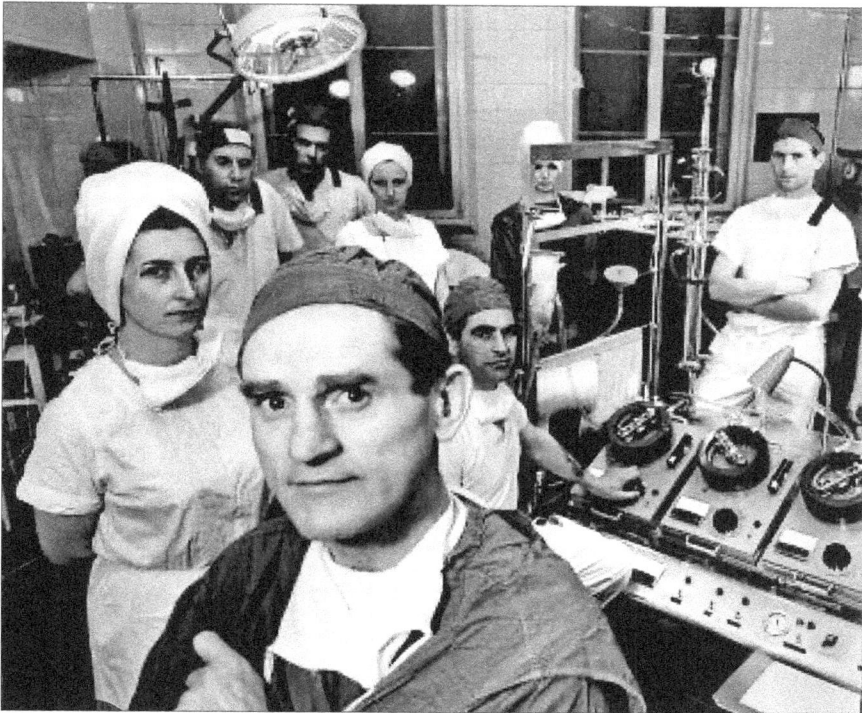

Fig 8.5 A. Alf Gunning and team.

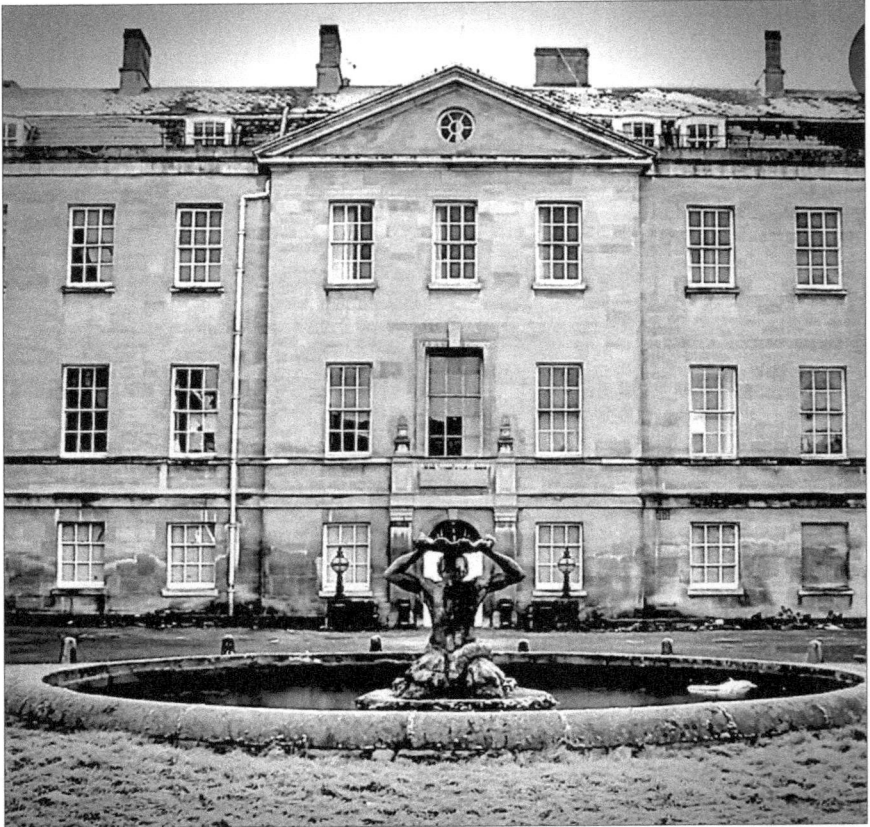

Fig 8.5 B. The Radcliffe Infirmary.

Born in South Africa he trained at Oxford's Radcliffe Infirmary, and practised general surgery. Such was the versatility of this slightly-built and mild-mannered gentleman that the hospital invited him to develop thoracic and cardiac surgery too. In that sphere he was essentially self-taught and a typical operating list would include an aortic valve replacement, a gall bladder excision and a tonsillectomy. A diverse practice that I was destined to inherit but did not continue. Thankfully.

Following on from Gordon Murray, Gunning wanted to use human aortic valves that would not need warfarin. Taking them from corpses in the mortuary he worked on various preservation techniques and a method to implant them within the patient's valve annulus so they would not obstruct the coronary arteries. It was shared access to this research that allowed fellow South African Donald Ross, at London's National Heart Hospital to perform the first human orthotopic valve implant in a patient.

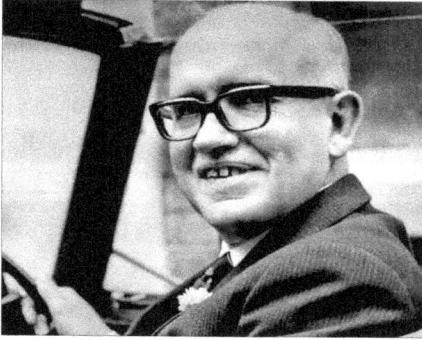

Fig 8.6 A. Donald Ross.
B. Diagram depicting
homograft aortic valve
Implantation.

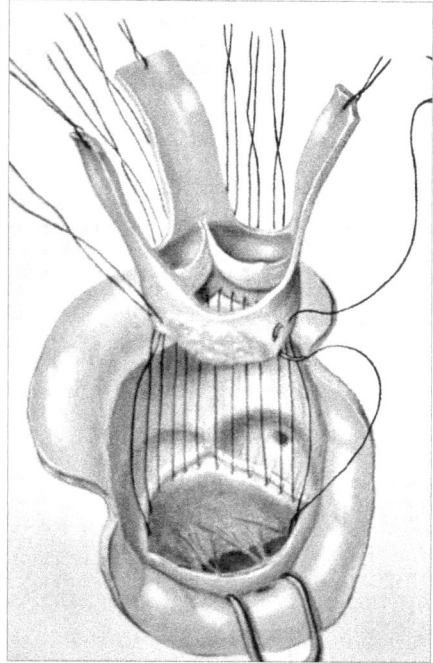

Ross had not schemed to outdo his old classmate from Cape Town. He described the circumstances of the unplanned operation as follows. 'Such was the state of unpreparedness that in June 1962, an aortic valve that I was attempting to decalcify disappeared down the sucker at a time when Starr valves were only a distant rumour. We had no alternative but to reconstitute one of our freeze-dried aortic homograft valves from the lab and sew it in with a single suture layer – a technique which fortunately had already been described to us by our colleagues, Alfred Gunning and Carlos Duran of Oxford. You can imagine our delight when the transplanted valve was not rejected and continued to function in that patient for four years. We forgot about the newly available mechanical valves – a state of amnesia which I must confess persists to this day. The homograft valve became an established surgical technique yet used only sparingly by a few persistent and courageous exponents of the method, largely in the Antipodes.'

Ross's philosophy was that the haemodynamic performance of a heart valve prosthesis should be as close as possible to the natural valve with low resistance to forward flow and only trivial backflow as the occluder closes. They should also, whenever possible, avoid the risks of anticoagulation. As such, he was very much against the Starr prosthesis with its obstructive plastic ball sitting in what should be a central flow path. The operation that bears his name, the Ross Procedure, was another bridge too far for many surgeons. He removed the patient's own pulmonary valve from the outflow of the right ventricle and used it to replace the diseased aortic valve. He then used a cadaver aortic or pulmonary valve in place of the transplanted pulmonary valve arguing that the preserved foreign tissue would degenerate at a slower pace in the low pressure environment of the right side of the heart. This was certainly a technically demanding operation that I learned from him as his senior registrar and subsequently used it on many occasions in children and young adults. It was the perfect biological substitute.

There were reasons that the cadaver homograft valve wasn't widely adopted. Firstly few surgical departments had a system to harvest them from suitable corpses in the mortuary, process them and store them in an appropriate preservative. Second, homografts were a form of transplantation and, as Ross intimated, many anticipated immunological rejection of the tissue. Lastly most found the operation taxing and time-consuming when myocardial protection was limited and prolonged surgery was likely to be followed by the post perfusion syndrome. A valve with a sewing ring needing just a few stitches was much easier but the superstars, including Kirklin, Norman Shumway at Stanford, and Brian Barratt-Boyes in New Zealand adopted the operation with excellent results. No anticoagulation required for biological tissue, and slow valve degeneration made this the perfect solution for aortic valve replacement in the young.

When Ross retired I hired his dedicated homograft technician Jill Davies from the National Heart Hospital and set up a bank of human parts in Oxford where it all began. Typically the NHS forced Alf Gunning to retire at sixty-seven so he returned to South Africa where he worked tirelessly as a chest surgeon for many more years. He died in Oxford in 2011, aged ninety-three.

To simplify homograft implantation Weldon from the Johns Hopkins Hospital began to hand mount human valves on a frame. Obviously the stented valves were much simpler to implant in patients than the freehand sewn homograft and consequently leaked less frequently. Unfortunately the stent exerted excessive stress on the tissue which in turn resulted in premature valve failure. Typically the valve would tear from the stent within four or five years whilst the freehand implanted equivalent functioned well for at least fifteen years. This dilemma spurred on the search for alternative biological tissues which proved more durable on a frame.

In Zurich Ake Senning removed strips of fibrous membrane called fascia lata from the thigh and fashioned this robust material into a trileaflet valve. Results were disappointing with almost a quarter of prosthesis failing within a year. In turn Marion Ionescu in Leeds worked with frame mounted strips of pericardium, which was more promising, and would eventually result in a commercial product with the Shiley company.

At the Radcliffe Infirmary Gunning now transferred his attention to pig valves which were easily obtained from the abattoir and preserved by freeze drying. In contrast to the term homograft, from humans, pig valves were termed heterografts and obviously their use caused alarm in some quarters and posed many questions. How would the human recipient react to a pig implant? How is tissue best sterilised and preserved? And how would the collagen and elastin molecules in the foreign valve cusps stand up to human haemodynamics over the years? The answer was 'suck it and see!'

On 23rd September 1964 Gunning performed the first clinical implant of a freeze-dried stent-mounted pig valve in a patient with aortic stenosis. Given that it was biological tissue, warfarin was considered unnecessary and follow up proved that to be correct. The introduction of tissue valve engineering then generated intense competition to produce stents with excellent haemodynamics and valve leaflets that proved immunologically inert with prolonged durability. Initially formalin was used to sterilise and fix fresh pig valves but the method was found to cause collagen breakdown with leaflet stiffening and calcium deposition in the cusps.

Some years later Alain Carpentier in Paris wrote: 'It became obvious that the future of tissue valves would depend on methods of preventing an inflammatory reaction and its penetration into the tissues.' He therefore resorted to the preservative glutaraldehyde which established cross-links in collagen molecules and rendered the valve cusps immunologically inert. In essence this single step dramatically increased the tissue durability and life span of porcine bioprostheses, allowing them to compete with the mechanical alternatives particularly in older age groups.

In 1966, the year I started medical school, the Leeds surgeons Marian Ionescu and Geoffrey Wooler produced a new type of frame for pig valves. The titanium structure had three struts and was covered inside and out with Dacron velour. The pig aortic valve was stitched within the stent and was stored with the curvature of the cusps maintained with formaldehyde soaked cotton wool. A Dacron felt ring covered with velour cloth served as the sewing ring for ease of implantation. This titanium-framed pig valve was soon marketed in the UK and US and was the precursor of the emerging Ionescu-Shiley pericardial prosthesis which proved more durable.

Why did Ionescu turn to pericardium for his valve cusps? His concept was to create a manmade prosthesis with optimised geometric configuration in order to avoid the defined anatomy of animal valves that had limitations. He mounted cow pericardium treated with gulteraldehyde on a Delrin flexible stent and demonstrated more symmetrical and wider opening than in the pig aortic valve equivalent. Yet despite initial enthusiasm the first cases of structural failure occurred in patients within five years of implantation. Examination of the valves after removal showed the pericardium to have torn away from its support. This mode of failure was often sudden causing severe and sometimes fatal aortic regurgitation. The acute failure mode was eventually avoided by introducing a thinner and more flexible frame, and sewing the pericardial tissue to its outer aspect.

Carpentier produced his own metal frame, a round rigid stent constructed from Teflon-coated stainless steel to which rings of Teflon were attached at the inlet to facilitate implantation. Human implants followed and the porcine model became the highly successful Carpentier-Edwards valve. From the haemodynamic standpoint central flow seemed preferable to the turbulent obstructive flow characteristics of the Starr Edwards prosthesis though subsequent analysis suggested an important pressure drop, or gradient, across the tissue and frame. This was due to restricted leaflet opening caused by the stent together with the geometry and stiffness of normal pig's anatomy. It was at this point that Carpentier reflected upon the potential advantages of direct vision valve repair.

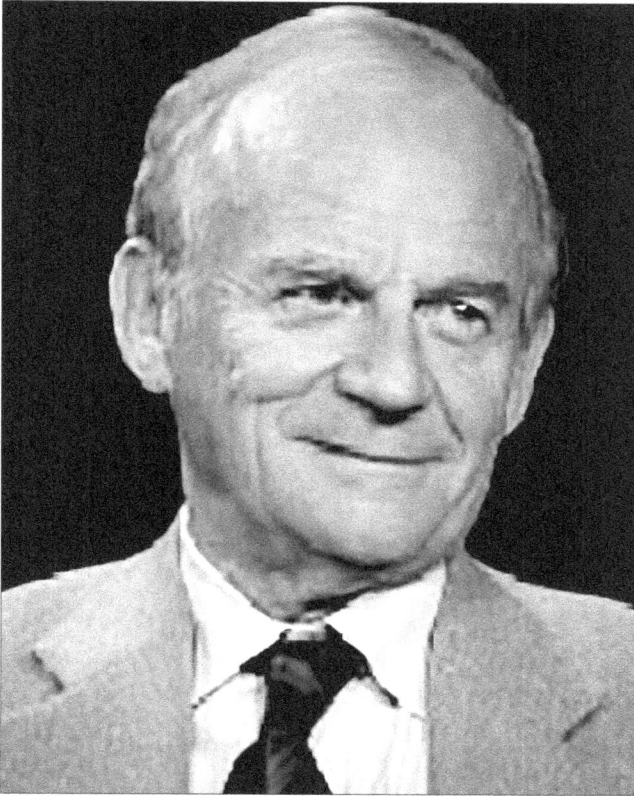

Fig 8.7 A. Alain Carpentier.

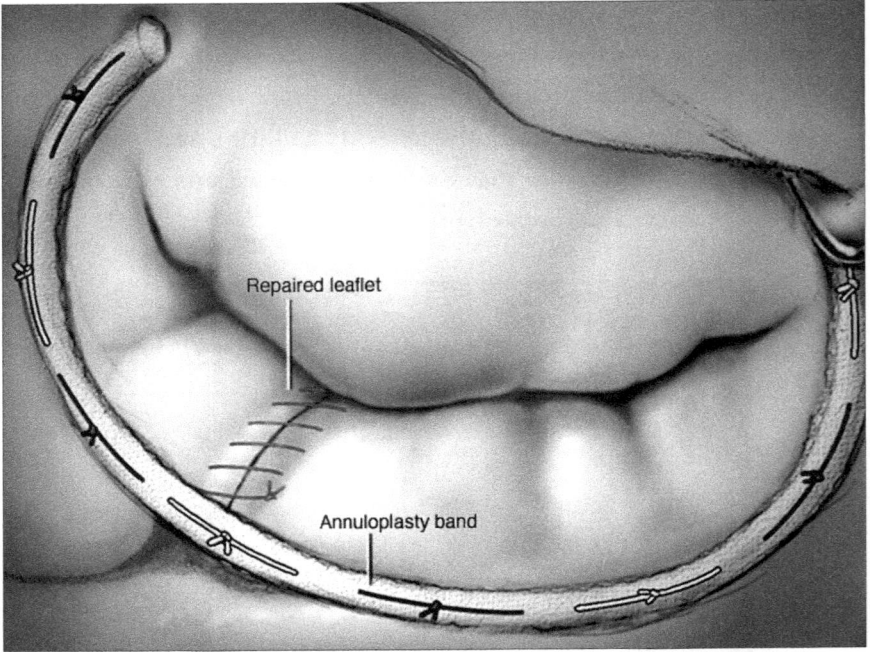

Repaired leaflet

Annuloplasty band

Fig 8.7 B Diagram illustrating the mitral valve repair technique.

Carpentier is said to have pondered the feasibility of repairing rather than replacing the mitral valve whilst walking through the ancient arched entrance of the Hopital Broussais in Paris. Observing the iron gates attached to the stone pillars as he did every day, he drew the analogy between the leaflets of the mitral valve suspended from the annulus. Should the edifice be hit by a truck and the gates damaged, workmen would rebuild it. Wouldn't that be a better option for a leaking mitral valve with a dilated annulus or prolapsed leaflets? Perhaps. But only time and experience would tell.

In contrast to the simplicity of cutting out a diseased valve and stitching in a stented replacement, valve repair required careful judgement with an important learning curve. To improve the orifice of a narrowed rheumatic valve by cutting into the areas of leaflet fusion was straightforward enough but at what point would the leaflets prove too stiff and calcified to conserve? If the annulus was dilated in degenerative disease, how much smaller did it need to be made? Or if the cusps were prolapsing and redundant how much tissue should be removed? In short these were the questions Carpentier answered in time by being determined to attempt repair in every case.

He would narrow and support an enlarged annulus by implanting a kidney-shaped ring around it, bringing the leaflet edges together. The obvious term for this was annuloplasty. Then he would remove segments of prolapsed or redundant tissue, usually from the smaller posterior leaflet and seek to adjust the length of stretched sub-valvar chordae tendinae. Carpentier coined the repair process 'the French Correction', and sure enough valve conservation soon showed advantages over replacement. In particular the pumping function of the heart was better preserved by maintaining continuity between the valve leaflets and the ventricular muscle.

Commercial competition inevitably spawns innovation with the drive to produce a better product. In 1968 Edwards Laboratories working with both Starr and Carpentier, issued their nine commandments for heart valve construction. First and foremost was embolism prevention - the avoidance of blood clots and stroke. Then, in sequence, followed long-term durability, ease of attachment within the heart, preservation of the surrounding tissues, reduced blood turbulence, elimination of blood cell damage, reduced noise, use of biocompatible materials and ease of storage and sterilisation. That was logical enough and most in the industry didn't need to be told about it.

Towards the end of the 1960s the turbulent and obstructive nature of ball-in-cage valves led to the introduction of new mechanical valve designs. The South African, Christiaan Barnard had trained with Lillehei and Varco at the University of Minnesota before being appointed both cardiothoracic surgeon at Groote Schuur Hospital and Director of Surgical Research at the University of Cape Town. Wangensteen considered Barnard an ambitious and driven young man and was motivated to help him to begin the first cardiac surgery programme in Africa. So, in a two-minute call to Washington, he asked that the US Government award Barnard $2000 for a heart-lung machine to take home followed by $2000 per year until the department was established in Cape Town. So influential was Wangensteen that Washington immediately complied. But Africa couldn't afford American heart valves so Barnard designed his own with the support of the engineer, Carl Goosen.

Constructed from stainless steel and silicone rubber these were the Barnard lenticular mitral, then the biconical aortic valves, which were implanted in patients at Groote Schuur before adoption by the Mayo Clinic. Barnard also performed the world's first tricuspid valve replacement for the congenital heart deformity, Ebstein's anomaly.

There followed a number of new mechanical heart valves from the USA the majority of which were abandoned in a relatively short period. Nina Braunwald produced a ball valve with an open-ended titanium housing covered in cloth which was manufactured by Cutter Laboratories. More than 5000 Braunwald Cutter valves were implanted in patients with excellent results, but by this time Nina was the mother of three daughters. Balancing her personal life with career demands wasn't easy, especially with a world-leading cardiologist for a husband. She would awaken very early each morning to manage the household chores and prepare the kids for school. During her pregnancies she continued to perform surgery up until each birth, stopping only when her distended belly kept her too far away from the operating table. That said, unless an emergency arose, she would always be back home for dinner. But then she would return to check on the patients after putting the girls to bed.

Sadly Nina's brilliant surgical career was cut short when she developed breast cancer and died on 5th August 1992. She was just 64 years old. In tribute, Eugene established a foundation to support women who wished to join the male-dominated world of cardiac surgery.

Three different tilting disc mechanical prostheses were developed in short succession by Lillehei and his team. The most successful was the Lillehei-Kaster valve which employed a single free floating pyrolytic carbon disc that opened to 80° within a ring of titanium. The valve, made available commercially in 1967, offered greatly improved central flow with relatively low profile rapid disc closure and for the first time a rotatable Teflon sewing cuff. This helped with optimum positioning so the moving discs would always be unimpaired with blood flow directed towards the coronary arteries. Lillehei boasted of lifetime durability and low risk of valve thrombosis, and a remarkable sixty-five thousand prostheses were implanted in patients between 1971 and 1990. In this enormous series there were just three reports of a worn disc escaping from the housing and fortunately two of the patients were rescued by urgent surgery.

The novel design concept for the Kalke-Lillehei bileaflet prosthesis originated from the one-way lock gates in the land irrigation system in India. Work began on the valve in 1965 and initial prototypes, though crude, provided the best hydrodynamic performance of any prosthetic valve. As the two discs opened within the titanium housing, they moved apart to create a quadrangular orifice with central lamina flow. This design would emerge as the forerunner to the enormously successful St Jude prosthesis.

Many other valve developments emerged by chance. Don Shiley the first Chief Engineer at Edwards Laboratories met Viking Bjork informally at the 1964 annual meeting of the American Association for Thoracic Surgery.

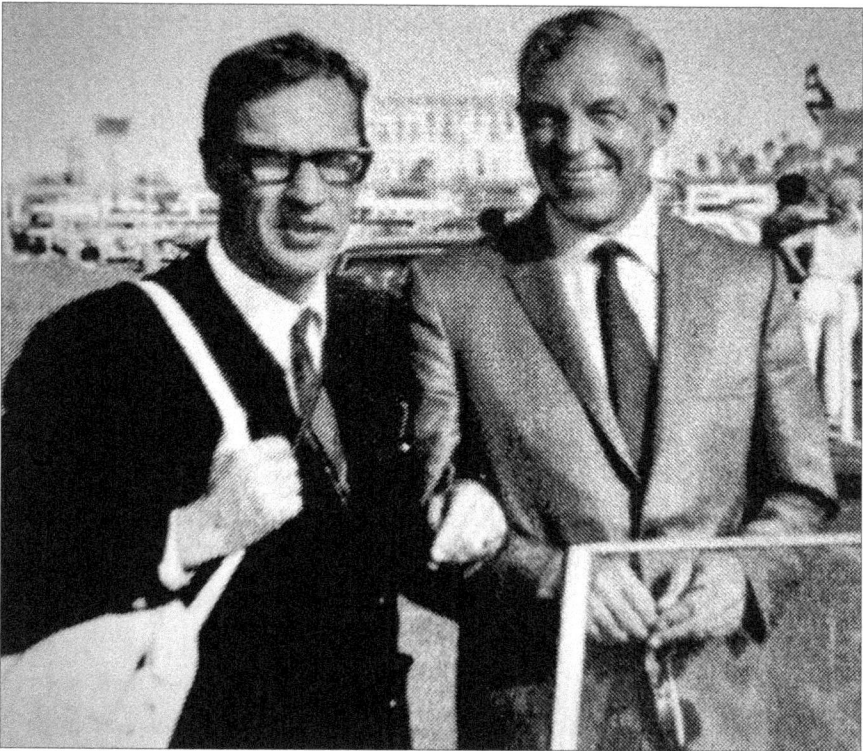

Fig 8.8 A. Bjork with Don Shiley.

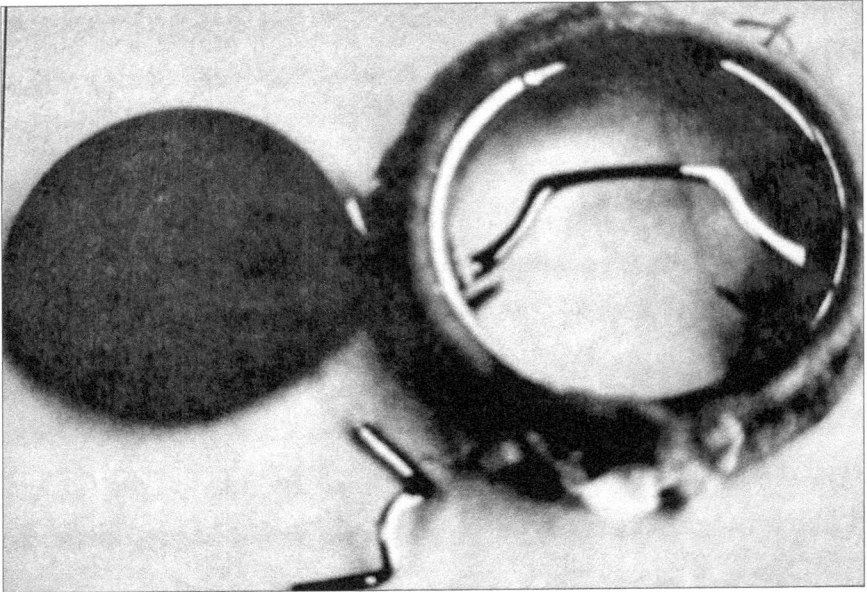

Fig 8.8 B. Fractured Bjork-Shiley Valve.

Shiley had recently left Edwards to establish his own company in the garage of his California home and was working on a mechanical mitral prosthesis with surgeons in Los Angeles. At the time the valves were crudely assembled with cloth sewing rings produced by his wife in the family bedroom. Bjork was persuaded to try out these prostheses at the Karolinska Institute in Stockholm but after a number had been used in both the mitral and aortic position it was clear that the pressure gradient across the valve orifice was unreasonably high. When Shiley travelled to Stockholm to review the findings Bjork shared with him the data on patients whose symptoms had been slow to resolve. Many had been subject to catheter investigation at rest and on exercise and it was clear that the design was unsatisfactory. Recognising an opportunity, Bjork persuaded the engineer to work with him on a new tilting disc valve, not dissimilar to a model designed by Juro Wada in Japan that was already being implanted by Cooley in Houston. Small world, cardiac surgery.

Shiley switched his attention to Bjork's vision of a slim single tilting disc held in place by two struts. The open valve had a major and minor orifice with flow resistance and pressure gradient being directly related to the shape of the disc itself. Shiley modified this into a convexo-concave shape made from Delrin that partially lifted out of the valve housing as the valve opened. This aspect was a critical detail that significantly increased the flow path through the valve orifice.

Within weeks Shiley had constructed the prosthesis in five sizes and dispatched two of each dimension to Stockholm. They were originally tested for aortic valve replacement then the same valve used upside down for the mitral position. Within a year Bjork was able to show impressive results for one hundred aortic and fifty mitral valve replacements. Nevertheless, tinkering with the design continued in an increasingly competitive market. When Delrin was found to retain water and swell, pyrolytic carbon was used to replace it for the disc. Then the conical disc was replaced by a more spherical shape with a radio opaque marker which could be non-invasively imaged within the chest to monitor valve function.

Cardiac surgical conferences were soon dominated by discussions on the merits of mechanical versus tissue valves. Fundamentally it was a balance between indefinite durability with the constant need for anticoagulation versus a valve that could be implanted and forgotten but would require re-replacement in ten years. The patients would be advised on the relative merits but given their own choice. At one meeting Denton Cooley recalled a discussion with the mother of a 12-year-old boy whose tissue valve had calcified and degenerated rapidly. He joked, 'About six months earlier this patient had had a porcine valve placed in the aortic annulus in a city in Louisiana. The poor bewildered mother knowing her son had received a pork graft, asked me what type of valve we would replace it with? I told her we would use a Bjork valve. She asked: 'What kind of animal is a Bjork?'

So much better were the flow characteristics of the tilting disc design over the ball valve that some surgeons, including Bjork, decided to risk withholding anticoagulation with warfarin. We tried that at the Brompton in 1974 but the outcome from valve thrombosis and stroke was catastrophic.

In March 1976 the entrepreneur Manuel Villafana, a former employee of the Medtronic company and developer of the lithium-powered pacemaker, was approached by the Minneapolis surgeon Demetre Nicoloff with a bileaflet heart valve design. Villafana saw merit in the approach and proposed that his company Cardiac Pacemakers Incorporated should refine and produce it. The board rejected the idea so their founder decided to go his own way with a separate company, St Jude Medical Incorporated. There was a story behind the name. St Jude is the Patron Saint of Lost Causes and Villifana had named his son Jude having survived serious medical problems in infancy.

A bileaflet design had already been pursued individually by Lillehei and Wada but before the introduction of pyrolytic carbon as a thrombo-resistant surface. Pyrolytic carbon is highly durable but expensive so Villifana chose to construct the two semi-circular leaflets with tungsten then coat them with the carbon which rendered them radio opaque. Within the valve housing the leaflets opened to 85° allowing near laminar blood passage. With its Dacron sewing ring this was an impressive design, thoroughly tested and first implanted clinically in 1977. Because of the excellent haemodynamics the patients were prescribed a lower than usual dose of warfarin with reduced bleeding risk, but no increase in thromboembolism.

Then amidst the thriving valve market came disaster. In March 1978 there was news of a Bjork Shiley valve strut fracture with escape of the disc and rapid demise of the patient from heart failure. In response the opening angle of the disc was promptly adjusted from 60° to 70° hoping to lessen the forces on the welded outlet strut. But then Bjork had two fatal fractures in his own patients. Realising the seriousness of the situation, he stopped using the valve until a modified strut variant was made available without the welded component. But now the unfortunate part of the story. Despite representation from Bjork himself and the Shiley engineers, the company kept the faulty valve on the European market until 1986. Of course other surgeons had lost patients but were not aware of the design issues at the time.

By June 1987 there had been 213 fatal outlet strut fractures reported from a total of 83,000 implanted valves. Others, particularly the elderly who died suddenly may not have had the true cause documented by post mortem examination. Whilst the proportion of valve failures was small, the model at risk was sold for a further four years after the early deaths. It was a commercial decision.

When the origin of the problem was scrutinised in detail, 76% of the strut fractures had occurred in the largest sizes of the mitral prostheses, manufactured between February 1981 and June 1982. Laboratory testing of this batch demonstrated excessive force on the outlet strut during closure of the valve, and for some reason the high-risk models had never been sold in the USA. Investigation by the Food and Drug Administration revealed many irregularities in the handling of the affair though Bjork himself was found blameless.

The worst and morally destitute aspect was that when the regulatory authorities banned sales in America, the Shiley Company continued to dispose of their stocks in other countries. This generated severe anxiety when the valve recipients and their families were made aware. I was faced with that problem myself in Oxford where Alf Gunning had implanted many of the valves at risk. Threatened with sudden death many patients requested re-operation to remove it simply for peace of mind. Eventually the monumental legal fees and compensation claims led to the disintegration of the company. The scandal was compounded by premature failure of the Ionescu-Shiley stent mounted pericardial valve resulting in thousands more re-operations within five years. The Texas Heart Institute alone implanted more than two thousand of these then faced the dreadful prospect of wholesale replacement. Much tighter medical industry regulation was introduced and the episode increased focus on valve repair techniques rather than routine replacement.

The Shiley affair was a tipping point in the evolution of cardiac surgery and for its supporting environment. Risk taking was justified in the pioneering days otherwise the specialty could never have progressed. But by the 1970s, it was no longer acceptable to promote medical equipment that might shorten lives. The brakes were on.

Lillehei was persuaded to leave Minneapolis and become Professor and Chairman of Surgery at the New York Hospital and Cornell Medical Centre. Yet the move failed to provide him with the opportunities he craved, and perhaps fuelled what had become a flamboyant, somewhat reckless personal life. He reflected on those heady days as we worked through the bottle of whisky at Culzean. As Medical Director of the St Jude valve company he had a penchant for Jaguar sports cars, gold jewellery and late nights in the jazz dives of Minneapolis. Nor was he inhibited when discussing the valve scandals and his fall from grace. 'Not all cardiac surgeons are saints,' he told me. 'Some of us are sinners.' I found him hugely charismatic and suspected that surviving cancer at a young age had spurred him on to live life on the edge. Despite being labelled the father of cardiac surgery and a distinguished Lasker Award winner, the tax man eventually caught up with him.

On February 16th 1973 Walt was convicted of five charges of income tax evasion by Judge Phillip Neville in St Paul Federal court after the Government produced more than 150 witnesses and 6000 exhibits. He had claimed deductions relating to four extramarital affairs including a $100 dollar cheque for 'typing' to a Las Vegas call girl who was summoned to give evidence in court. Many of those called as witnesses were patients of Lillehei or their relatives. Some refused to testify. 'I just couldn't do it', said one woman. 'If it wasn't for Dr Lillehei, my husband wouldn't be here today!' Lillehei's own attorney Jerome Simon acknowledged that he had made some incorrect deductions on his returns but insisted that this was nickel and dime stuff. The result of an overworked scientist trying to keep his own books.

Walt was sentenced to community service with a fine and chuckled cheekily when he told me that. What might have ruined anyone else simply caused envy and distain amongst some of his peers, and was soon forgotten. By the time of the court case his eyesight had deteriorated markedly so his surgical days were numbered. Intensive head and neck radiotherapy for his lymphosarcoma had caused cataracts so the great innovator could not see well enough to operate. That was the main reason he stopped in 1974 and took up the role in the valve industry.

When I staggered across the castle cobbles to the taxi at 1 a.m., I had a real sense of privilege having spent those hours with him. Manny Villifana who arranged the evening was still at the bar at Turnberry with surgeons attending the meeting. He asked me how it went. 'Very special' was all I had to say at that point. Villifana is a gentleman and a pioneer in his own right. He still had more in the tank, moving on to design another mechanical valve and funding the company ATS Medical, which stands for 'advancing the standard'.

Over the past forty years both tissue and mechanical valves have continued to improve whilst debate over their relative merits continues. Contemporary mechanical prostheses have an indefinite life span with little risk of structural failure. Nevertheless the need for anticoagulation persists, whilst biological tissue can be implanted and forgotten so to speak. That said, for the last few years of their lifespan, they have rigid, obstructive leaflets. Degeneration, with calcification, occurs particularly early in growing children and young adults. For the young with aortic valve disease, Ross's use of the patient's own pulmonary valve has provided persuasive long-term results with indefinite durability, central non obstructive flow, zero risk of thrombosis and no requirement for anticoagulation. But few surgeons are willing to perform the intimidating double valve procedure. By 1995 fewer than one hundred surgeons worldwide had attempted a Ross operation, and many that did have now retired.

Of those valves available to surgeons since the outset which has lasted the longest in a patient? The answer might surprise some in our profession, but I encountered that valve myself in Oxford. Here is a tongue in cheek passage from my paper, *The longest functioning heart valve prosthesis* published in the *Journal of Thoracic and Cardiovascular Surgery* in 2007.

'We present the case of a 32-year-old man who was referred to the Hammersmith Hospital in 1965 with a severely regurgitant bicuspid aortic valve and heart failure. Before his operation the heart-lung bypass pioneer Denis Melrose expressed concern that the Hammersmith machine had not previously supported such a large patient (98.5kg). During the operation the patient vividly recalls his surgeon, Professor Hugh Bentall saying "give it to him again", followed by three further shocks from the defibrillator! Eventually cardiopulmonary bypass and the valve prosthesis proved more successful than the anaesthetic and the patient survived.'

Consistent with the natural history of bicuspid aortic valves, the patient presented again in 2006 with central chest pain and an enormous ascending aortic aneurysm. Transoesophageal echocardiographic scanning showed a normally functioning ball valve prosthesis with a peak gradient of 24 mm Hg, and well-preserved left ventricular function. Both investigations indicated that the wall of the aneurysm was adherent to the posterior sternal table. At that point I would add that a huge thin-walled blow out of the aorta stuck to the back of the breast bone is a serious challenge. My objective was to replace the whole ascending aorta and the arch of the vessel that gives rise to the arteries to the head and arms. But the sternal saw was bound to burst the aneurysm on chest re-entry, resulting in immediate exsanguination with blood splattered on the ceiling and floor. Of course there was a way round that.

What I did was to place cannulas in the large artery and vein to the right leg, perfuse the patient on the bypass machine and cool the blood to 18°C. That allowed me to stop the circulation entirely whilst the saw opened the breast bone for the second time. As predicted the hugely dilated aorta was rent asunder but without any flow, no blood was lost and the brain was protected by cooling. I then proceeded to repair the aortic root around the old prosthesis and coronary arteries. The slightly discoloured silicone ball remained spherical and secure within the stainless-steel cage.

That much-maligned Starr Edwards ball valve had performed in an exemplary fashion for forty-two years, nor had the patient suffered a single valve-related complication. The case is remarkable because the patient sought help for heart failure in 1965 and having since followed him in the out-patients clinic, we knew him to be alive fifty years later with the same valve. Albert Starr was 80 years old when I performed that re-operation. We wrote to inform him, after which Edwards Laboratories confirmed it to be the longest functioning artificial valve.

Following a distinguished career at Karolinska Hospital from 1966 to 1983, Bjork left Sweden and emigrated to the USA. He became Director of Research at the Heart Institute of Desert Rancho Mirage, California until a second retirement, then died in February 1990 at the age of ninety. Walt Lillehei was still medical director at St Jude when he died of cancer aged eighty in 1999.

Having worked tirelessly on valve surgery in Paris Alain Carpentier shifted his attention to the development of a total artificial heart. Manufactured by the Carmat company this life-saving device has been implanted in patients since 2013. Moreover the Carpentier Edwards pig valve remains as the biological valve against which all others are measured.

Mending the Pipes

If I have seen further than others, it is by
standing upon the shoulders of giants.

—Isaac Newton

It was the weekend before Christmas in 1945, when Blalock's resident Denton Cooley was asked to review a post-operative patient on the Johns Hopkins thoracic surgery ward. The gentlemen had been operated on by the senior surgeon Grant Ward who had removed virtually the whole sternum for a malignant bone tumour. To stabilise the chest wall the sizeable defect had been filled with a stellite vitallium plate but now Cooley found the man in shock. When he informed Ward, as residents are meant to do, the surgeon came in and together they returned to the operating theatre to determine the cause.

With Cooley as first assistant, Ward dismantled the repair but on shifting the metal implant, they were confronted by brisk bleeding. In short the metal plate had eroded through the aortic wall but the resulting haemorrhage had been contained by the adherent tissues or inflammatory adhesions. They were now faced with a 'false aneurysm', a problem without an established solution in times preceding the heart-lung machine.

Ward initially stemmed the bleeding with a finger through the defect but was himself debilitated following surgery for a spinal cord tumour. Cooley was obliged to take over leaving Ward like 'the little Dutch boy with his finger in the dyke'. At first Cooley mobilised a pedicle of muscle from the chest wall and sewed it over the hole with some success. Nevertheless he was concerned that the patch would give way when normal blood pressure was restored by transfusion. Undoubtedly stressed by the experience the senior surgeon quizzed his resident on what might be done next? 'I believe I should put a clamp on the side of the aorta, then oversew it', said Cooley boldly. A fitting response from the junior whom Blalock had chosen to manage blood transfusion during the first shunt operation.

It was a pivotal moment because no one had operated on a leaking aneurysm in the chest before, not least a trainee. It was less than a year since the Swede, Clarence Crafoord, had managed to repair coarctation of the aorta in a 12-year-old schoolboy and of course the vessel was smaller. So the predicament facing Cooley at the dawn of his career was much more intimidating. Irrespective of that, the plan succeeded and the success received great acclaim at Hopkins where Ward sang his praises.

That wasn't the last of it. In the spring of 1949 when Cooley returned to Baltimore from war service, Blalock went on vacation and left his chief resident to preside over the Hopkins cardiac service. Soon afterwards one of Blalock's patients who had undergone coarctation repair was readmitted to the hospital with severe left-sided chest pain. The only investigation possible, a plain chest x-ray, showed what Cooley believed to be a massive false aneurysm at the site of the previous surgery. By that stage of his career, Cooley had performed a number of coarctation resections himself and believing the pain to portend imminent aneurysm rupture, he decided to operate. It was a good decision. The blood sac was paper thin but he managed to close the defect in the aorta successfully.

On Blalock's return the whole hospital was gossiping about the famous aneurysm case. This caused the Chief to remark: 'If you are confronted with a serious surgical problem that has no proven solution, take a trip to Hawaii and your resident will handle it for you.'

The normal aorta is an intimidating pulsating blood vessel about the same size and thickness as an old fashioned bicycle inner tube. Through it pass five litres of blood each minute, without which the organs of the body cannot survive. Given a minimum average internal pressure of 100 mm Hg, any damage to the wall is likely to cause rapid exsanguination. It is not surprising therefore, that the surgery of major blood vessels began hesitantly with life-threatening trauma and was restricted to that role until sufficient experience provided the confidence to tackle aortic aneurysms. Cooley's two cases were 'false aneurysms'.

A 'true' aneurysm occurs when the wall of an artery weakens causing it to balloon out. Then from the Laplace law of physics, as the diameter of the lumen increases so does the pressure on its wall. That is why aneurysm rupture occurs spontaneously whilst narrower segments remain intact. In truth, there had been one aneurysm operation the year before Cooley's, but because it happened in wartime it wasn't widely discussed.

Alton Ochsner was an eminent thoracic surgeon at Tulane University, New Orleans, who with his trainee Michael DeBakey, recognised the link between tobacco and lung cancer. In 1944 Oschsner explored the left chest of patient whom, on x-ray, he believed to have had a malignant tumour, but it was the wrong diagnosis. What he found at the back of the chest was an aneurysm of the descending aorta, probably caused by a tear sustained during a car accident. Again a 'false aneurysm', Ochsner simply placed a side clamp across the entrance to the blow out, stitched the aorta closed beneath the occluder, then excised the sac in an operation that Cooley would unknowingly replicate.

World War II generated a huge number of penetrating vascular injuries but despite having blood transfusion, antibiotics and more efficient ways to evacuate the wounded, the results were no more impressive than during World War I. In a monumental study, Michael DeBakey reviewed 2471 patients with penetrating wounds involving arteries of which only 81 were treated by suture repair. Following full ligation of the vessel to stem bleeding half of the limbs involved were amputated. After being Chief of the US General Surgery Service in Europe, DeBakey returned to Tulane University but was soon appointed Chairman of the Department of Surgery at Baylor Medical College in Houston. A very prestigious position.

Foreseeing widespread interest in the new specialty, cardiovascular surgery, DeBakey sought to recruit the charismatic young Denton Cooley on return from his adventures at the Brompton. Although the two had met fleetingly in war-torn Europe, their first professional encounter was during a ward round at Houston's Old Jefferson Davis County Hospital. The patient under consideration was Joe Mitchell, an emaciated 48-year-old with a large syphilitic, saccular, aortic arch aneurysm which DeBakey planned to wrap with cellophane. Wrapping was the only known treatment for aneurysms at the time with the intention of preventing further enlargement and rupture.

As DeBakey examined Mitchell he paused, somewhat provocatively, to quiz his new colleague on how he might approach the problem. Cooley's contrary response that he 'would excise the aneurysm' produced a stunned silence until DeBakey asked him to elaborate. Cooley explained that he would put a clamp across the neck of the aneurysm, cut it out, then over-sew the wall of the aorta, and undoubtedly that was the patient's best chance for survival. The bemused DeBakey naturally asked whether it had ever been done before and to everyone's amusement Cooley told the chief that he had done it twice.

Two days later Cooley operated on Mitchell, removing the aneurysm from the aortic arch and making him safe.

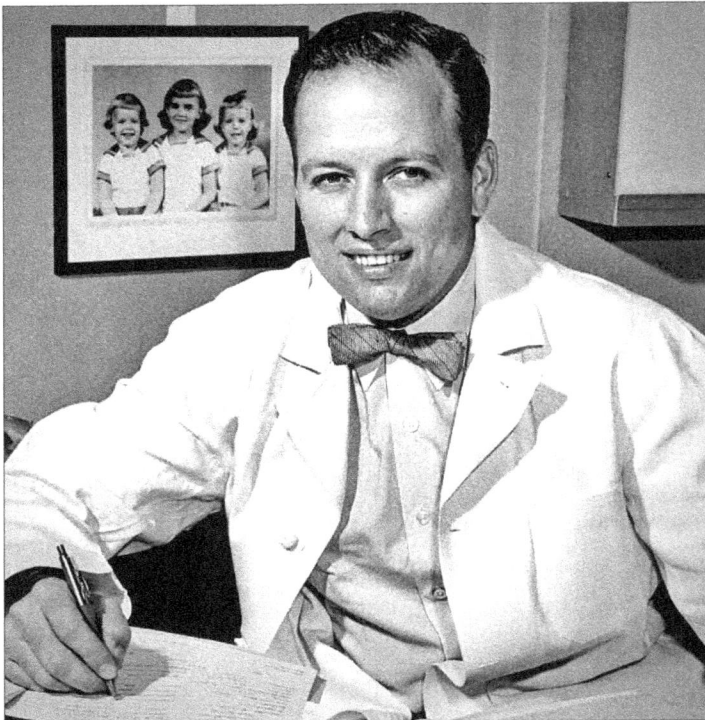

Fig 9.1 A. The young Denton Cooley.

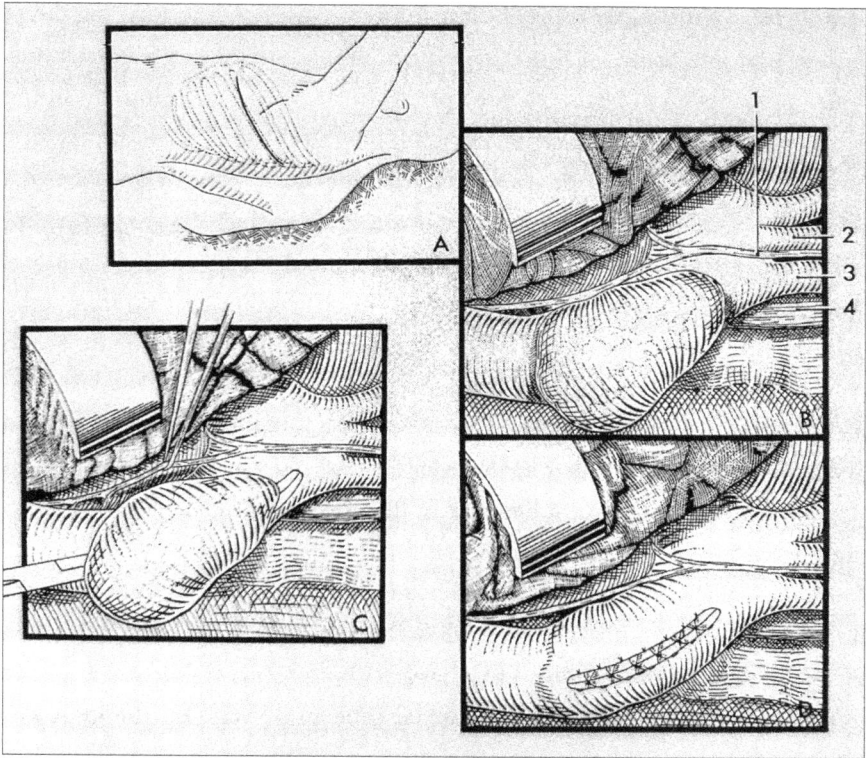

Fig 9.1 B. Diagram illustrating his first aneurysm resection.

It was claimed to be the first operation of its kind in the world, performed long before the heart-lung machine was introduced. Nevertheless it was DeBakey who personally presented the case at the Southern Surgical Society later that year. Cooley, a non-member, sat silently and resentfully in the audience. That's the way it is. The chairman of any surgical department had the option of stamping his name on whatever work emanated from the institution. DeBakey was immediately recognised as *the* aneurysm surgeon, and patients with aneurysms were referred from the whole of North America. Overnight Baylor emerged as the leading centre for vascular surgery.

This was an important beginning for surgery of the intimidating tube, but something was missing. Most aneurysms were not saccular. The vast majority of 'blow outs' affected a substantial length of the aorta which needed to be replaced. Short segments, as in coarctation, were dealt with simply by mobilising an adjacent portion of the wall and performing direct end-to-end anastomosis. But that proved impossible for larger aneurysms. Vain attempts were made to precipitate thrombotic occlusion by filling them with wire but interruption of blood flow to the lower half of the body usually spelled disability or disaster. Often but not always. In one case of a 19-year-old college student with a fusiform or rugby ball shaped aneurysm, distal to a coarctation, the surgeons simply ligated the aorta above and below the enlarged segment to prevent rupture and certain death. Despite the fact that this was high in the chest the lad recovered with adequate blood flow to the lower body through what we call collateral vessels that had developed during the life-long narrowing. Very high blood pressure associated with the coarctation helped in those circumstances.

Robert Gross in Boston began to collect segments of human aorta from trauma victims in the mortuary intending to use them to repair aneurysm patients. They were preserved in the fridge at 4°C in a mix of human serum and salt solution. Cell culture studies showed homograft cells to remain alive for more than a month after harvest though this was irrelevant. The grafts were simply intended as a vascular tube and bridge for the ingrowth of the patient's own cells. Moreover it soon became clear that 'dead' homografts were preferable because they didn't generate an immunological response within the recipient.

Gross began to employ these grafts to replace short segments of aorta in coarctation patients in 1948. That same year his associate Henry Swann used one to repair a traumatic aortic aneurysm in a 16-year-old boy and it was soon obvious that replacement tubes were simpler to use than mobilising and stretching the aorta for direct end-to-end joins. In turn other hospitals established homograft banks, sterilising and storing the tissue in formalin, alcohol, glycerine, ethylene oxide or beta propriolactone. Some irradiated the tissue or subjected the tubes to freeze drying in liquid nitrogen. They were then stored in plastic packets with dry ice.

A major landmark occurred on 5th January 1953, when DeBakey assisted by Cooley performed the first resection and homograft tube replacement of a long fusiform aortic aneurysm in the chest. DeBakey described the circumstances in a letter to his friend Viking Bjork: 'We were working on aneurysms of the abdominal aorta with homografts and there were several people, other surgeons, who had tried to resect an aneurysm of the descending thoracic aorta but all had failed. The only previous success was the one Dr Ochsner did, almost as an accident, in which he had a small sacciform aneurysm of the descending aorta, which he thought was a tumour, so he pinched it off at the neck, side clamped and removed it. So when I had this patient in 1953, I told him that nobody had done this successfully, but I thought that the principles were the same as they were in the abdominal aorta. We didn't know that at the time, that you ran the risk of spinal cord ischaemia you see. We found that out later. Fortunately he didn't get it, but before the surgery he had very, very severe pain. The aneurysm was eroding the spinal cord and vertebral bodies. He was from Arkansas, a very unusual character, an old sheriff. He died fifteen years later of carcinoma of the lung. He was a pioneer, he became a very successful case.'

As it happened that the eccentric sheriff returned to Houston's Methodist Hospital in August 1962 with lung cancer. On September 11th DeBakey operated to remove the left lung and found the homograft tube to be functioning well though solidly calcified. It was very reassuring follow-up.

As intimated in DeBakey's letter to Bjork, surgeons soon found that clamping the descending aorta in the chest for thirty minutes or more conveyed a serious risk of permanent paraplegia. This became the dreaded complication of aortic surgery. Goodbye aneurysm, but the patient could never stand or walk again. Once again, cardiovascular surgeons had to be expedite, confident and highly competent technicians. Unlike other specialties, slow and cautious didn't cut it. Nor did reticence or introspection.

Within two years of their first aneurysm resection Cooley and DeBakey between them had performed 245 similar cases, far more than any rival centre. In August 1955 they toured Europe together, lecturing, demonstrating their operations and popularising vascular surgery, just as Blalock and Taussig had done ten years before. The safety of aortic cross clamping for less than thirty minutes was accepted but by then they had introduced whole body cooling in a water bath as a spinal cord protective strategy for more complex aneurysms. They also developed a long temporary plastic shunt to divert blood flow from above the surgical site to below in order to maintain oxygenation of the abdominal organs. But whilst tubes of homograft aorta were satisfactory for a while, the complications of tissue degeneration, occlusion by thrombus and dilatation of the biological tube itself were eventually too frequent. Now the major challenge was to devise a more durable alternative with synthetic materials. But what properties would those materials need to have?

First and foremost, they had to prove biocompatible with a surface that would not provoke blood clotting. In turn they must be strong and durable in order to meet the life expectancy of the patient, yet easy to handle and pass stitches through. Not as straightforward as one might imagine.

Arthur Blakemore was a bold and accomplished vascular surgeon at Columbia Presbyterian Hospital in New York. With an interest in cirrhosis of the liver, he had already devised innovative methods to treat the bleeding varicose veins, known as oesophageal varices, in the gullet. Moreover he found abdominal aneurysms frustrating. The patients came to the hospital in pain, were treated with morphine, then the aorta would rupture and they exsanguinated. Blakemore tried coiling lengths of wire in the aneurysm hoping that the lumen would thrombose and occlude whilst collateral circulation developed. But it rarely did. Just to ligate the neck of the aneurysm as Astley Cooper had done at Guy's Hospital in 1817 starved the abdominal organs and legs of blood and usually proved fatal. And until Charles Dubost resected an aneurysmal abdominal aorta and used a homograft to restore continuity in 1951, no one even thought of intervening.

Blakemore was a phlegmatic heavily set Virginian who spoke with a drawl and moved slowly. He once commented wryly 'the only time I worry about bleeding is when I can hear it'. In contrast, Arthur Voorhees was a softly-spoken but determined young Quaker, who went to intern with Blakemore in 1946.

He was initially given a laboratory research project to develop an artificial mitral valve constructed from strips of vena cava from a dog. The fabricated structure was stapled into the mitral annulus and silk stitches used as substitutes for the chordae tendonae. Remarkably the skilled Voorhees was able to insert these Heath Robinson structures through a purse-string stitch in the left atrial appendage and whilst they never functioned well as valves they gave rise to an important discovery.

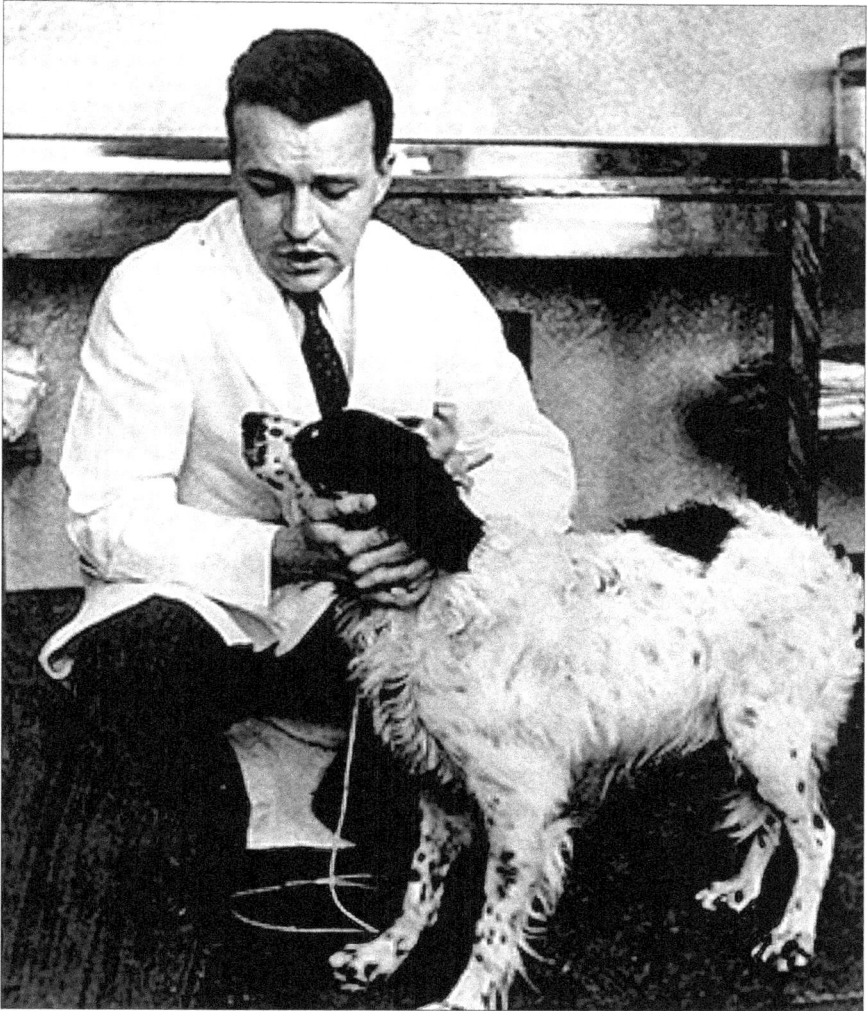

Fig 9.2 Arthur Voorhees with one of his dogs.

Voorhees elaborated on his finding as follows: 'During one of the early trials, I made an error in placing the ventricular suture, with the result that the stitch traversed the central part of the cavity. It would have been too difficult to correct, but I did make a note of my error so that several months later at autopsy I took pains to find the misplaced suture. To my surprise it was completely coated with what appeared to be endocardium (the natural cellular lining of the heart). It resembled a normal chorda except for the black core of the silk stitch. The appearance was sufficiently startling to make me wonder whether a piece of cloth might react in a similar way. From there I speculated that a cloth tube, acting as a latticework of threads, might indeed serve as an arterial prosthesis.'

Blakemore was impressed and curious about Vorrhees's vision of an artificial blood vessel. To test the hypothesis they fashioned a silk handkerchief into a tube and used it to replace the abdominal aorta of a dog. This functioned as a conduit for an hour before bleeding predictably terminated the experiment. And the animal. But soon afterwards, James Blunt an orthopaedic resident at Columbia, acquired a bolt of Vinyon-N cloth which for some unknown reason had been donated to the hospital by the Union Carbide Company. This faulty batch had failed to take up dye but consisted of the robust weave from which the army's parachutes were made. When Blunt tried to use the material as a tendon replacement it proved unsatisfactory, so he offered the cloth to Voorhees.

Using his wife's sewing machine Voorhees carefully constructed tubes of Vinyon though the tough material proved difficult to sew. Attaching it to arteries in a blood-secure fashion required painstaking dexterity but he succeeded in implanting tubes into the aorta of six dogs. Optimistically one survived for four weeks with a fully functioning graft.

Late one evening in February 1953, Voorhees as chief resident in the hospital, was paged to the Emergency Room to consult on a man in severe pain. The diagnosis was obvious. He had low blood pressure and a pulsating mass in the abdomen that heralded a ruptured aortic aneurysm. As it happened Dr Blakemore was the senior surgeon on call and within thirty minutes the patient was on the operating table. With the belly opened down the midline from sternum to pubis, the aorta was exposed and clamped above the leak. Whilst this immediately stopped the haemorrhage it soon became clear that the aneurysm extended down beyond the bifurcation of the aorta into the main arteries of both legs. It was then that the circulating nurse on the telephone to the homograft bank announced: 'I have bad news.

Apparently there isn't a single homograft available in New York City.' So the ruptured aneurysm was exposed with the bleeding controlled but there was nothing to replace it with.

There was a pause with silence in the room until Blakemore responded in his usual calm drawl, 'Well, we'll just have to make one of our own.' With that, Voorhees was dispatched to the laboratory in the medical school building tasked with producing a bifurcated graft, something he had not done before. Meanwhile the clock ticked on a clamped aorta with zero blood flow to the lower half of the body. One of Voorhees's colleagues, Sheldon Levin, the second assistant that night, described the scene. 'It was 02.00 hours, dark and eerie in the lab, and we couldn't find the light switch. The wind was shaking the windows and we could hear the indignant mice rattling the wheels in their cages. We turned on the lights, went to the corner where the sewing machine was located, and put down two sheets of Vinyon. We sketched an upside down Y and sewed three lines, one in the crotch, as the clock ticked on. Redundant Vinyon was cut away, and we raced back to the operating room. The graft was handed to the float nurse, who flashed (sterilised) it, and we scrubbed back in. Dr Blakemore was still working away to isolate the whole length of the huge aneurysm. Finally it was removed and the Y graft sewn into place.'

Blakemore removed the clamps from the leg arteries first to allow what little collateral circulation there was to retrogradely fill the tubes. Worryingly there was bleeding through the material of the graft itself causing the clamps to be replaced. After five more minutes they were reopened and the oozing had stopped. The natural blood clotting process had sealed the pores. With trepidation the upper clamp was removed slowly to restore brisk pulsatile flow downstream. The total aortic occlusion time had been three hours after which everything started to bleed – except the graft! With groin pulses palpable the abdomen was hurriedly closed leaving a drain in place.

That was the first occasion that a synthetic graft had replaced the human aorta but there was no happy ending. The man had coronary artery disease and suffered a myocardial infarction during the prolonged period of aortic cross clamping. He died from heart failure several hours later, but death wouldn't detract from the technical triumph. At the American

Surgical Society meeting in Ohio the following year Voorhees presented sixteen cases of abdominal aneurysm replacement with Vinyon-N cloth tubes but Union Carbide then terminated production of the material. Alternatives had to be found quickly.

The Glasgow surgeon, William Reid, had an interest in vascular surgery and had listened to Voorhees at the Cleveland meeting. Returning home through London he visited a smart tailor in the West End and bought two expensive shirts. These he presented to his operating theatre sister, Jane McKenzie, requesting that she take them home to her digs, cut off the tails and create two tube grafts using her landlady's sewing machine. The home-made artificial tube grafts were crudely sterilised overnight and the first implanted into a patient with an abdominal aortic aneurysm the following day. Jane's husband Bill Lang happened to be Reid's registrar on the surgical unit and dutifully used his own blood to seal the fabric. This was the first vascular graft to be used in Britain and the elderly recipient survived for several years.

Michael DeBakey by chance found a new material called Dacron in a Houston department store.

His mother, a seamstress had taught him to sew cloth so he was able to fashion his own tube grafts which were soon introduced to the operating theatre at Methodist Hospital. Serendipitously it was one of his aneurysm patients who transformed Dacron grafts into a commercial proposition. Following a bedside discussion regarding the potential to knit vascular tube grafts, the man suggested that DeBakey visit a sock factory in Reading, Pennsylvania of which he had part ownership. DeBakey found them eager to help but they did not have a suitable sewing machine.

Undeterred and energised by the potential of Dacron, he then travelled to the Philadelphia Textile Institute where the engineer Thomas Edman designed a purpose-built knitting machine for Dacron grafts at a cost of $25,000. This not inconsequential price was paid for by the grateful patient and provided a prototype for the modern commercial machines used to fabricate Dacron grafts today. DeBakey neglected to patent the invention, nor did the commercial producer, who subsequently took a full-time job working for the Baylor Vascular Service. Significant improvements were then made in house. The University's patent engineer, Oscar Creech, pointed out that crimped Dacron was easily tailored to avoid kinking and should provide a lattice for cell deposition and a biological lining. With that in mind he suggested soaking the semi-porous tube graft in the patient's own blood in order to prime the surface for cellular deposits. Coincidentally Creech was also a necktie factory owner which gave him insight into the problems.

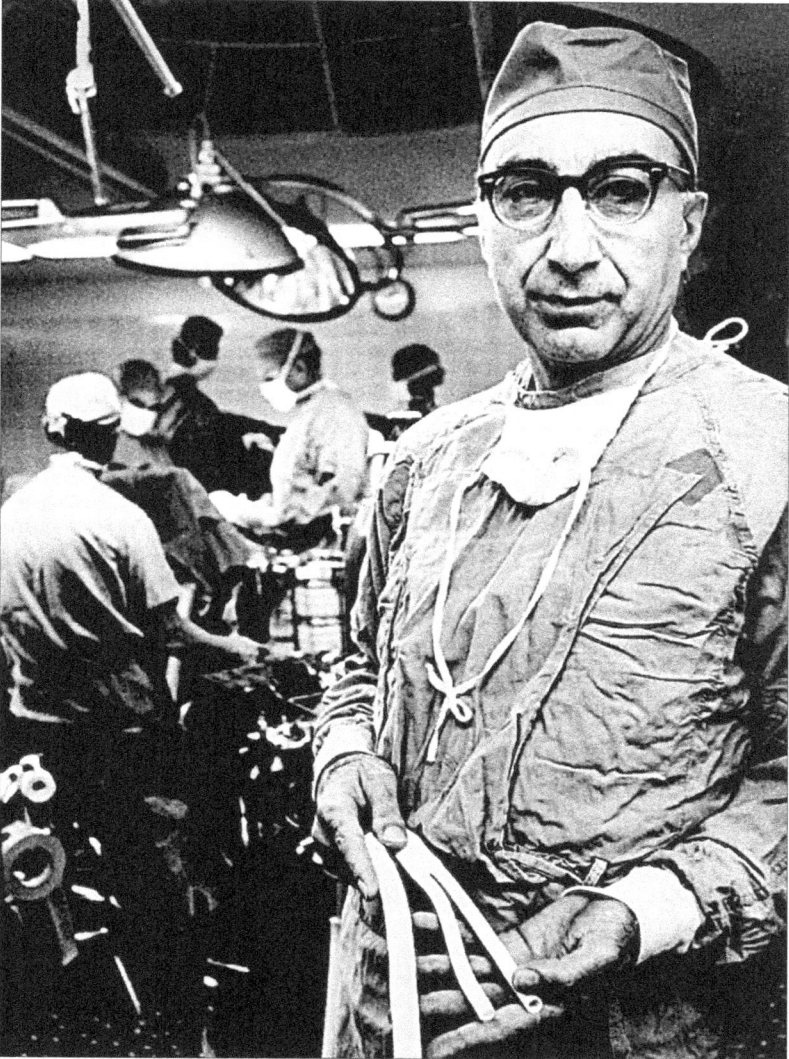

Fig 9.3 Michael DeBakey holding Dacron vascular grafts.

Given the technical advances, increasingly bold surgical techniques followed. The aorta in the abdomen has numerous important branches and with the advent of vascular grafts these could be mobilised from the aneurysm wall and reimplanted. The vessels to the kidney were first reimplanted in 1954 and in that same year a large aneurysm was resected from both the chest and abdomen in continuity. That time consuming operation at the Veterans Administration Hospital in Oakland California was performed with the use of an aortic bypass shunt to maintain blood flow to the tissues distal to the clamps.

DeBakey provided the first detailed description of the separate reimplantation of arteries to the kidneys, intestines and liver in 1958. Fifteen of the first twenty patients had syphilitic aneurysms, a common problem in soldiers after the war in Europe and the Far East. John Gibbon described this taxing procedure as 'one of the most brilliant technical achievements ever to be accomplished in the field of vascular surgery'.

Widespread adoption of the heart-lung machine combined with cooling then gave access to the ascending aorta above the heart, and to the curving aortic arch where it gives rise to the vessels of the arms and head. Syphilitic aneurysms were even more common in the proximal aorta as were the sequelae of the inherited Marfan's syndrome. As one might anticipate, Drs Cooley and DeBakey led the way by replacing the entire ascending aorta, amidst other world firsts in the late 1950s. Less than a decade later the Houston group reported on 138 patients operated upon for aortic arch aneurysms using a mix of temporary vascular shunts and cardiopulmonary bypass. Their mortality rate for these high risk cases was just 22%. Randell Griepp in New York described complete excision of the aortic arch with graft replacement and reimplantation of the head vessels for which he employed cooling to 18°C on the heart-lung machine then temporary arrest of the circulation for up to forty-five minutes. This reduced the brain's need for oxygen to the point where stopping blood flow for prolonged periods was tolerated.

Albert Starr became the first surgeon to replace the aortic valve and the ascending aorta at one sitting. Using his own ball valve he left the aortic sinuses immediately above the valve intact to spare the origins of the vital coronary arteries. However, the sinuses which accommodate the opening valve cusps can also dilate to aneurysmal proportions especially in Marfan's syndrome. That said, most surgeons regarded interference with the heart's own blood supply too great a risk. That is until an unanticipated but innovative procedure happened at the Hammersmith Hospital in 1968.

My old chief Professor Bentall took a young Marfan's syndrome patient to the operating theatre intending to replace the leaking aortic valve and then remove the aneurysmal dilatation from the ascending aorta as Cooley had done.

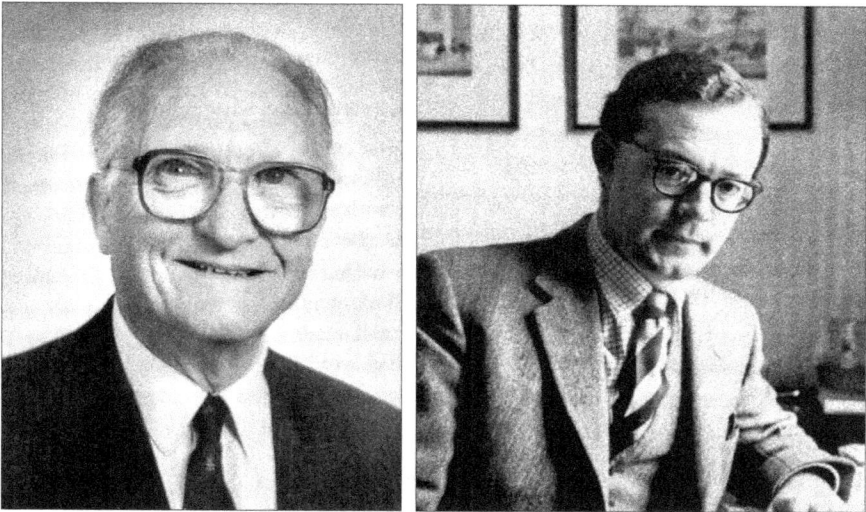

Fig 9.4 A. Hugh Bentall. B. Anthony DeBono.

Assisting him that day was Anthony De Bono, a bright Maltese trainee from a well-known academic family who would eventually return to Malta as Professor of Cardiac Surgery. What they discovered on opening the chest was a huge blow out of the very root of the aorta. The origins of the coronary arteries themselves were displaced well above the stretched valve annulus. As a result there was simply no proximal ring of aorta small enough to secure a vascular graft to. So the findings were concerning.

There was a 'what to do next' pause until De Bono made a brave suggestion as follows. 'Sew the Starr Edwards valve into one end of the Dacron tube.

Go onto the bypass machine, cool down and clamp the aorta as close to the head vessels as possible. Open the aneurysm widely, remove the leaking valve, and stitch the sewing ring of the Starr Edwards valve into the native aortic annulus. Then implant the origin of each of the two coronary arteries into holes cut into the sides of the graft.' Of course the final step was to join the distal end of the tube graft to the patient's transected aorta just below the clamp.

It was a brilliant concept but on the first occasion this was a technical nightmare for Bentall. At the end of the sewing when the cross clamp was removed and blood allowed back into the Dacron graft, the huge significance of the technique became clear. When the bleeding had stopped that is. The descriptive term for the operation is aortic root replacement though it is commonly referred to as the Bentall procedure. As Bentall's senior registrar in 1984 I wanted to report his long-term results for Marfan's patients but found fewer than fifteen cases in total. Like other trainees of the pioneers I went on to fly the flag for him performing more than three hundred Bentall operations in my own career, many on Marfan's syndrome patients. Anthony DeBono returned from Malta to the Oxfordshire countryside in his retirement. He lived close to me, and we remained friends. It should really have been called the Bentall-DeBono operation.

Cardiac surgery is in many respects analogous to the space programme. 'One small step for man, one huge step for mankind'. Marfan's syndrome is caused by a mutation in a gene called FBN1 which limits the ability to manufacture the proteins vital for the strength of the body's connective tissue. The patients are recognised through having a tall slender build with disproportionately long arms, legs and fingers. They often have a curved spine, high arched palate and crowded teeth, with extreme short sightedness. But the problem that limits life expectancy is the propensity for aortic root aneurysm formation and the predisposition of the lining of the aortic wall to split spontaneously. This allows blood under pressure to tear its way rapidly through the inherently weak middle layer, an agonisingly painful process called aortic dissection which usually proves fatal in a matter of hours. Lethal that is, unless the patient has access to a front-line cardiac surgical centre for urgent repair. And it's not just a problem for Marfan's patients. Those with persistently high blood pressure or other genetically based weaknesses of the aortic wall are also at risk. King George II is known to have died suddenly from aortic dissection at the age of seventy-six when his valet discerned a noise 'louder than the Royal wind'.

Yet again, the first successful repair of aortic dissection was performed at Baylor's Methodist Hospital, this time by Dr George Morris and the patient was a surgeon himself.

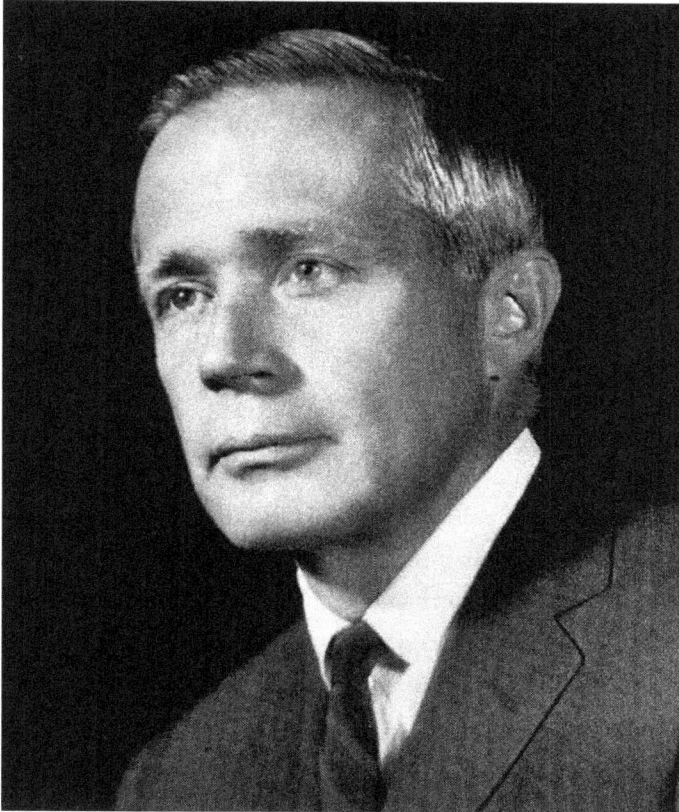

Fig 9.5 George Morris.

Some years afterwards Morris wrote this about the circumstances of the event. 'At the time of my operation, our group had abandoned the Creech re-entry procedure and were not attempting to treat this dreadful condition surgically. However, I had quietly planned a direct repair for several years if an appropriate patient and opportunity came my way. Interestingly the man was a senior fellow with Dr John Kirklin at the time of the catastrophic illness. He was on vacation in Louisiana when he collapsed in August 1962. Of further interest, Dr Kirklin, whom I consider the greatest gentleman in American surgery, was the speaker at the Houston Surgical Society just days after the operation and made rounds with me to visit his assistant.'

Morris replaced the leaking aortic valve with a prosthesis and repaired the torn dissected ascending aorta with a graft to exclude the initial tear. It was a great triumph. Twenty-nine years later the surgeon was referred back to Houston with a painful abdominal aortic aneurysm after which follow up studies also showed a huge ascending aortic aneurysm in the chest. On 3rd June 1991 the aortic root and the prosthetic valve were re-replaced first, then the following week the abdominal aneurysm was repaired too. A triumph for vascular surgery in that era, though aortic dissection remained a very high risk surgical challenge, and one that I took personal interest in.

One third of dissection patients die before reaching hospital either through free rupture of the aorta with cardiac tamponade or direct exsanguination into the left chest. Those who arrive alive are poleaxed by the sudden searing pain as the aortic wall rips longitudinally from valve to leg arteries shearing off vital branches on the way. Some present with stroke, others with abdominal pain through dead gut, or even a dead leg. Often they are short of breath when the aortic valve leaks suddenly, or suffer myocardial infarction through occlusion of the origin of a coronary artery. Can we save them from all that? Yes we can with an emergency operation to replace the part of the aorta containing the original tear as Morris had done.

For me the compelling nature of dissection surgery came from the fact that it brought together all the techniques and technology discussed so far. The patient is established on the heart-lung machine as a matter of urgency. Their whole body is cooled to 18°C after which the circulation is stopped altogether. Cardioplegic solution is given and the blood drained into the bypass machine. The dissected ascending aorta together with part, or the whole aortic arch, is cut away and replaced with a Dacron graft, whilst the leaking valve is either repaired or replaced with a prosthesis. Bleeding through needle holes in the fragile dissected aortic wall occurs as a matter of course but as Moshe Schein once said 'the best clotting factor is the surgeon!'

For decades the operative mortality rate for dissection surgery worldwide stood at a considerable 25%. So daunting a figure that cases in Britain are now directed to specific aortic surgery centres however long that takes. With expertise and experience that body count can be reduced. I published my own consecutive series of one hundred emergency operations in Oxford between 1988 and 2000 with just six deaths. Seven of those patients had Marfan's syndrome, and in total twenty-four had aortic arch replacement in addition to the standard repair. None succumbed to haemorrhage, though six required late re-operation for new aortic aneurysms or a leaking aortic valve. Fortunately each survived.

Cardiovascular surgery expanded rapidly in the 1960s alongside spectacular advances in blood vessel imaging using radio-opaque contrast medium. And there were important non-surgical advances. Thomas Fogarty, a surgical resident at the University of Cincinnati developed a catheter with an inflatable balloon to remove blood clots from the arterial system. Then the Oregon radiologist Charles Dotter found that forceful hydraulic balloon inflation was capable of dilating blood vessels narrowed by atherosclerosis. Up until this point radiologists and cardiologists made diagnoses and provided imaging for the surgeon to act upon. Fogarty and Dotter were about to change all that with interventions that had a huge impact on the whole medical profession.

Picture a modest setting at an obscure conference for radiologists in Czechoslovakia. Dotter had been invited to lecture on 'new developments in diagnostic blood vessel imaging', but he was about to reveal far greater ambitions. He harangued his audience with the claim that: 'The angiographic catheter can be more than a passive diagnostic tool. When used with imagination it can become an important surgical instrument.' This 'pen is mightier than the sword' moment was immediately greeted with rapturous applause. 'It was like a bomb had been dropped,' said one member of the audience. But just as Starr needed Edwards, Dotter needed Bill Cook, a small-time entrepreneur from Indiana destined to become one of America's wealthiest men.

The kindred spirits met at the annual meeting of the Radiological Society of North America in Chicago in 1963. Cook was busy making catheters on a table at his booth when he noticed a tall slim character watching intently. When the exhibition hall closed that evening Dotter approached Cook and asked to borrow a Bunsen burner and pieces of tubing he had seen the inventor working with. Cook acquiesced but insisted that the equipment be returned before the exhibition opened the next day. He was astonished when Dotter returned that morning with ten of the most perfectly formed angiographic catheters he had seen. Each was sold to a radiologist that day.

Dotter asked Cook to visit his home in Portland, an invitation refused by the salesman because he couldn't afford the travel. Undeterred Dotter bought him a plane ticket. Recounting the experience Cook recalled: 'We discussed guide wire and catheter manufacture and what he thought the future would be for angiography. Once started his mind went nonstop!' The two sat together in the kitchen, Cook taking the role of businessman and Dotter the scientist sprouting ideas at such a rapid pace that he broke half a dozen pencils scribbling notes and sketching possible ideas. There was no inhibitory regulatory environment in the 1960s so within a year they produced a functional commercial product. Dotter just needed an opportunity to use it.

Relatively speaking Fogarty's catheters to remove blood clots from the arterial system were still crude. He first constructed a long narrow hollow tube to which he attached a finger cut from a latex surgical glove to make the balloon. This was attached to a cylinder of compressed air which at the throw of a switch would inflate the balloon at the appropriate time. The clinical strategy was to make a small incision to expose the leg artery in the groin, insert the catheter beyond the obstructing blood clot, then inflate the balloon and withdraw it. This usually brought the clot slithering out and restored blood flow beyond. Sure enough the results were impressive with an immediate fall in the need for ischaemic leg amputations. Yet detractors were sceptical. When Fogarty tried to publish the results the first three peer review journals that the paper was submitted to declined to publish it. Why would they do that? The manuscript was reviewed by surgeons of course!

In 1962 Fogarty moved to the University of Oregon to complete his surgical training. There he met both Dotter and Albert Starr, but Dotter was in a different department so there was limited cross-fertilisation. Without doubt, Dotter was evangelical and a maverick. Starr said of him: 'I never saw him normal; he was always in a hypomanic state.' Irrespective of the controversy surrounding his pioneering endeavours Dotter, known as crazy Charlie, was made the youngest Professor of Radiology in the USA at the age of thirty-two. But sometimes unbridled enthusiasm pushed him to extremes.

As the German urologist Werner Forssmann had done decades before, Dotter catheterised his own heart using a mirror so he could watch the passage of the tube on the x-ray screen. He then engaged with students in the medical school, plugged the catheter into a monitor, and exposed his punctured arm, to illustrate that he was taking his own intracardiac pressure readings. Nonetheless, crazy Charlie was on the threshold of a massive advance in the treatment of vascular disease.

In January 1964 Laura Shaw an eighty-two-year old smoker with chronic bronchitis and severe peripheral vascular disease was admitted to the University Hospital. She had black gangrenous toes on the left foot whilst both legs were pale and cold. An angiogram in Dotter's department showed widespread atherosclerosis of the aorta and virtually complete obstruction of blood flow to the left leg. The pessimistic vascular surgeons asked to review the images felt that the compromised lower limb should be amputated. This did not sit well with the woman who despite being in pain, refused to consider the proposal. It was the perfect scenario for Dotter to test his new technique. After all, there was nothing to lose. One of his much vaunted aphorisms was: 'If a plumber can do it for pipes, we can do it for blood vessels.' And he did.

The practicalities of that first case were very much the same as they are now. After his assistant Melvin Judkins had cleaned the woman's skin with iodine, Dotter probed the groin until his hollow needle punctured the main femoral artery. Through this he passed a guidewire towards the aorta in the belly, then withdrew the needle over it. Under x-ray control he then negotiated a path through the craggy critical obstruction caused by the atheromatous plaques. Once satisfied it was time to railroad the balloon catheter over the guidewire to position the dilating section in the narrowest part of the lumen. This took just a few minutes after which he forcibly inflated the balloon and kept it inflated hard for a whole minute.

Dotter was nervous as he evacuated the compressed air then quickly withdrew the whole thing. Almost instantaneously anxiety was followed by elation as blood spurted out of the arterial puncture site. Then the foot changed colour to purple and the leg itself became pink. After a few minutes of finger pressure by Judkins over the small entry wound the arterial bleeding stopped and the procedure was finished. The outcome was nothing short of miraculous for its time. Pulses could be felt in the groin again and her pain disappeared. Within days the infected ulcer above the ankle had healed. Then three weeks after the intervention a follow-up angiogram showed the severe narrowing to have gone. Laura Shaw came into the hospital in a wheelchair but she walked out triumphantly with two legs instead of one. This single intervention triggered a complete revolution in the treatment of vascular disease.

Poor Fogarty could only watch enviously from the Department of Surgery where his colleagues remained hostile to the competition. But he did manage to collaborate with Dotter on one project in 1965, when the radiologist tried out his latex balloon. The conclusion? It was great for extracting blood clots, but much too flimsy to crush atheroma. That said I saved many ischaemic legs with a Fogarty catheter as a surgical trainee in Cambridge. As Dotter implied, it was great for removing clots, and that saved legs too.

Surprisingly for years to come the majority of radiologists in North America, ignored the therapeutic opportunities that catheters presented. It was different in Europe. Switzerland, Germany and the Netherlands, adopted transluminal angioplasty with enthusiasm. Even so, no one could foresee that prosthetic heart valves and even vascular grafts for aneurysms would eventually be deployed using catheter techniques. It was difficult to conceive that coronary artery disease could be conquered by an angioplasty catheter much to the disgust of my surgical colleagues. The radiological 'crazy man' started all that, and it was very much in the patients' interests.

Preserving the Pump

If I can stop one heart from breaking
I shall not live in vain.
—Emily Dickinson

Throughout the ages, coronary arteriosclerosis, the progressive narrowing of the heart's own blood vessels, accompanied by chest pain, has been the dreaded forerunner of either sudden death or inevitable heart failure. Epidemic in modern times, even Egyptian mummies were found to have coronary artery disease, though it took centuries to relate those obstructive plaques in tiny arteries to the symptoms that they caused.

How does coronary artery disease come about? Pathologists researching the problem noted that as soon as cholesterol and fat begin to accumulate in the lining of the vessel, smooth muscle cells that normally provide strength to the constantly moving arterial wall start to grow, multiply and obstruct the narrow lumen. Factors known to promote coronary artery disease include raised blood cholesterol levels, high blood pressure, smoking, diabetes and obesity.

When the great essayist and poet Samuel Johnson was asked whom his doctor was during his ultimately fatal illness, he replied, 'Dr Heberden ultimus Roman orium', the last of our learned physicians. As well as an astute doctor in London, William Heberden was an outstanding Latin and Hebrew scholar, much respected by his contemporaries. In 1768 he delivered a keynote lecture to the College of Physicians in London titled *Some account of a disorder of the breast.* During the talk he discussed what we now refer to as acute coronary syndrome for the first time.

'But there is a disorder of the breast marked by strong and peculiar symptoms, considerable for the kind of danger belonging to it, and not extremely rare. The sense of strangling and anxiety with which it is attended, make it not improperly called angina pectoris. They who are afflicted with it are stricken when they are walking, more especially if it be uphill, or soon after eating, with a painful and most disagreeable sensation in the breast, which seems as if it would extinguish life, but the moment they stand still all this weariness vanishes.'

There could barely be a more insightful description of anginal pain today, but Heberden became even more specific. 'The pain is sometimes situated in the upper part, sometimes in the middle and sometimes at the bottom of the os sterni, but more inclined to the left than the right side. It likewise very frequently extends from the breast to the middle of the left arm, but the pulse is not disturbed by the pain.' At least the pulse was not disturbed unless the patient drops dead, one might add, but at this point he was vividly describing exertional angina, not a heart attack. When asked whom angina was most likely to afflict he said, 'I have seen barely a hundred people with this disorder, of which there have been three women, and one boy of 12 years old. All the rest were men past their 50th year of age.'

In 1772 Heberden published his description of 'anger in the chest', or angina pectoris in the literary magazine *Critical Review.* Soon afterwards he was approached by a concerned reader who recognised the symptoms and wrote: 'I have never troubled myself much about the cause of it but attributed it to an obstruction of the circulation or a species of rheumatism.' Given that the pathological process underlying the symptoms had not yet been identified the man gave him permission to dissect his corpse after death. Heberden did not have to wait long. Only three weeks in fact. On hearing of the death he immediately arranged to collect the body and engaged the most experienced anatomist of the times to examine it for him.

Such a legend was the Scotsman John Hunter that his majestic statue still presides over the entrance of the Royal College of Surgeons of England where his collection of dissected zoological specimens and human body parts is named the Hunterian Museum.

With the imperative to keep his anatomy school supplied with cadavers he invested enormous sums in the sinister world of body snatching. He even managed to exhume and steal the corpse of the eight foot Irish giant Charles Byrne, much against the poor man's wishes. Irreverently, his skeleton remains on display in the college.

Disappointingly Hunter's autopsy inexplicably overlooked the pathological basis for angina in Heberden's case. His esteemed student, Edward Jenner, who went on to develop the smallpox vaccine, was troubled by that missed opportunity. Years later Jenner admitted that 'almost certainly the coronary arteries were not examined'. A pity because the pathology might have given Hunter some insight into his own problems.

Hunter's angina began in 1773 with low central chest pain behind the sternum. Jenner was with him on the first occasion and described him as so pale he had 'the appearance of a dead man'. But in forty-five minutes the pain had abated. Perhaps that experience focused his interest in a possible link with the heart and coronary arteries. Soon afterwards he performed an autopsy on a 54-year-old man who died 'in a sudden and violent transport of anger'. This time Hunter wrote 'from their origin to many ramifications upon the heart the vessels were becoming one piece of bone'. This was diffuse calcified coronary atheroma, yet he still seemed to miss the point, stating that although the man 'felt frequent pain in the arms, there was nothing very remarkable in this case worth taking notice of'. The link between blocked coronary arteries and dropping down dead seems to have eluded him.

Hunter's biographers identified him as a man of science with an obsessive tendency towards hard work driven perhaps through sibling rivalry with his surgeon brother William Hunter. He would 'commence his labours in the dissecting room generally before six in the morning and stay there until nine when he breakfasted. He then saw patients before returning to the autopsy rom and working on the cadavers well into the early hours. Others found him difficult however. A personal friend, Lord Holland considered him 'dogmatic and angry when crossed'. A man whose judgement was clouded by an irascible and tenacious temper. The physician Thomas

Pettigrew actually wrote of Hunter in the *Lancet*, 'he had no command over his temper', and that 'his speech was rude and he habituated himself to the disgusting practice of swearing'. His surgical rival Jesse Foot of St George's Hospital accused him of 'being embroiled in a continual war, exciting jealousies and quarrels amongst his colleagues'. Thus the psychological origin of Hunter's deteriorating health was readily apparent to those around him.

By 1785 Hunter was so disabled by recurrent angina that he left London for a period of rest and recuperation at Bath Spa. At that point his physician John Coakley Lettsom wrote: 'He can scarcely go upstairs, so much is he affected with shortness of breath on the least motion.' And by this time his close friend Jenner had recognised that the symptoms were those of progressive heart failure. Writing to William Heberden, Jenner confessed that he was 'fearful if Mr H should admit this, that it may deprive him of the hopes of a recovery'.

This was the first documentation of the natural history of coronary artery disease and unfortunately for the irascible Hunter, there would be no recovery. On more than one occasion he made the statement 'my life is in the hands of any rascal who chooses to annoy or tease me'. And indeed it was. On 16th October 1793 a full twenty years after the first onset of symptoms, Hunter was due to attend a board meeting at St George's. He had gone to the dissecting room in his basement before dawn and worked on the corpse until breakfast at nine. At noon he left the house in Leicester Square in a carriage bound for Hyde Park Corner. The discussions turned out to be frustrating and confrontational when the administrators refused to accept two young students from his homeland, Scotland. In the midst of a vitriolic verbal attack by a surgical colleague Hunter experienced 'a fit of anger', ceased speaking and abruptly left the room, allegedly struggling to suppress 'the tumult of his passion'. He had barely entered the adjoining room when 'with a deep groan he fell lifeless into the arms of a colleague'.

Hunter's own brother-in-law, Sir Everard Home, performed the autopsy, identifying the cause of death as angina pectoris, the coronary arteries being 'thickened and ossified', and the muscle 'unable to carry out its functions'. Yet whilst Hunter was shown to have severe coronary disease there was a separate problem in his ascending aorta which coincidentally narrowed their origin. Difficult to believe, but as part of his studies on venereal disease Hunter had inoculated his private parts with the syphilis organism obtained from a patient. Having developed full-blown syphilis himself he suffered neurological complications and developed an ascending aortic aneurysm with coronary ostial stenoses. As a result he suffered compromised blood flow to the heart muscle for very many years.

The first physician to attribute heart attack to sudden coronary thrombosis was Adam Hamer of St Louis in 1876. He correctly reasoned that the rapid onset of severe and persistent pain was caused by complete interruption of coronary flow in one of the major branches. Inevitably this deprived a substantial territory of muscle of its vital blood supply. In Hammer's own words: 'I mentioned my convictions to my colleague at the bedside. He, however had a nonplussed expression and burst out, "I have never heard of such a diagnosis in my life", and I answered, "Nor I also".' But the patient died and a carefully conducted post mortem examination proved him to be correct. Ruptured atheromatous plaque, blood clot in the occluded vessel, and dead muscle in the territory supplied. Conclusive.

Why was it so difficult to shake down the relationship between prolonged chest pain and coronary thrombosis with myocardial infarction? Perhaps because the findings after death don't always reveal the cause, at least in those days. Normal coronary arteries are small vessels of around three to four millimetres in diameter at their origin from the sinuses of the aorta above the valve. There is a left main coronary artery which within an inch or so, bifurcates into two major branches. The left anterior descending branch courses down the front of the heart between left and right ventricles, then the circumflex coronary courses around the groove between left atrium and ventricle, and turns down between the ventricles on the diaphragmatic aspect of the heart. The distal branches are little more than two millimetres in diameter and give origin to even smaller branches that disappear into the muscle. Separately the right coronary exists from the front of the aorta and descends to the diaphragmatic surface of the heart between the right atrium and ventricle.

Heart muscle is highly metabolically active given its astonishing workload. Under resting conditions it receives five per cent of the total blood flow amounting to around 250 millilitres per minute. Inevitably this increases substantially both on exercise and when the heart responds to emotional, hormonal or neurological stimuli. Hence Hunter's angina when stressed.

In the presence of atheromatous plaques, in other words fixed narrowings of the vessel, the increased flow needed in response to a stimulus cannot happen. The upturn in muscle metabolism is not accompanied by adequate blood flow so lactic acid accumulates in what we call ischaemic muscle and causes angina. With rest or calm the limited flow becomes sufficient again so the pain abates. This cycle is termed stable angina, but when the obstruction worsens, any emotional response or increased heart rate, even without physical activity, can precipitate ischaemia. Then it becomes unstable angina with pain at rest.

What happens in a full-blown heart attack? Typically myocardial infarction occurs when an important coronary artery suddenly occludes through rupture of an atheromatous plaque. Cessation of blood flow leads to clotting in the vessel, hence the term coronary thrombosis. Muscle that is persistently deprived of blood flow will die and the ischaemic pain persists. Dying muscle also precipitates electrical instability that may result in ventricular fibrillation and sudden death. In time the dead muscle turns to scar and as we have said fibrotic scar tissue stretches to cause heart failure. Before the introduction of the electrocardiogram it was extremely difficult to correlate the nature of chest pain with temporary ischaemia or irreversible infarction. Not that it mattered since nothing could be done about it at that stage. Chest pain held dreaded connotations.

In 1889 Augustus Waller, an innovative general medical practitioner in London, attempted to measure the electrical impulses created by the heart but his equipment was not sufficiently sensitive. Willem Einthoven in Leiden, improved upon this by adapting a string galvanometer and connecting electrodes to the chest wall. The apparatus was cumbersome with the patient sitting with their feet in a tub of salt solution, yet in 1903 he succeeded in recording an electrical trace and named the characteristic features the P, Q, R and S waves. He received the Nobel Prize for the work in 1924, after which electrocardiography became an invaluable cardiological investigation tool both in the clinic and the laboratory.

Thomas Lewis, an acquaintance of both Waller and Einthoven, succeeded in combining the ink writing polygraph with the electrocardiogram in his studies of cardiac pathology and heart rhythm disorders. Attracting many visiting physicians from both Europe and the USA Lewis's work did much to establish cardiology as a specialty in itself. Bousfield first recorded the ECG during an episode of angina in 1918 after which James Herrick characterised myocardial infarction by comparing the clinical symptoms with electrical changes and then autopsy. Survival or death were unpredictable during heart attack even in those days, but Herrick's patient was particularly obliging. Harold Pardee reported survival after myocardial infarction even when the ECG traces showed deep Q waves and raised ST segments. These became the standard electrocardiographic findings that we rely on today.

Diagnosis was the first step, treatment another matter altogether. And as the public became aware of the significance of angina the more anxious they became. In 1867 the pharmacologist Lauder Brunton wrote in the *Lancet*: 'Few things are more distressing to a physician than to stand beside the bedside of a suffering patient who is anxiously looking to him for relief of pain which he feels utterly unable to afford. Perhaps there is no other class of case as in some kinds of cardiac disease in which angina pectoris forms at once the most painful and distressing symptom.'

Brunton introduced the inhalation of a volatile chemical agent, amyl nitrate, to dilate the coronary arteries. This proved very effective in the early stages in most cases, but it didn't change the outlook. That needed a substantial boost in myocardial blood flow, but how? Elliot Cutler argued that it would be simpler to reduce the heart muscle's oxygen requirement by reducing cell metabolism. Logically he felt that could be achieved by lowering the level of thyroxine the thyroid hormone, in the blood. Not a bad suggestion for a surgeon.

In 1927 Cutler was referred a 61-year-old woman with severe heart failure at the Massachusetts General Hospital. She was thought to be suffering from hyperthyroidism and he was asked by her physician to perform thyroidectomy. Certainly the gland appeared to be normal both during the operation and under the microscope afterwards, but her symptoms of breathlessness and fatigue 'were surprisingly improved'. So Cutler next carried out a partial thyroidectomy with the specific remit to treat angina. This patient also claimed symptomatic relief, and a series of other angina patients followed. Unfortunately many were reduced to a vegetative existence through the opposite of an overactive thyroid that we call myxoedema. Some suffered accidental damage to the nerves supplying the voice box and others lost their parathyroid glands so within a decade the strategy was abandoned. Indeed, physicians such as Sir James McKenzie reasonably argued that angina should be allowed to persist untreated to prevent over exertion and ventricular fibrillation.

By now it was clear that angina was caused by restriction in coronary blood flow so surgeons schemed how they might improve it. And it was a curious case that led to the first attempts. Claude Beck, a Professor of Neurosurgery at Western Reserve School of Medicine in Cleveland, Ohio was asked to attend an autopsy on a patient found to have longstanding complete obstruction of the two main coronary arteries. Whilst that should have caused death months before, the pericardium around his heart was inflamed and densely adherent. Moreover the fibrous adhesions contained blood vessels that connected with the muscle itself. Beck therefore wondered whether the deliberate creation of adhesions between the pericardium and cell layer on the surface of the heart might form the basis for treatment in ischaemic heart disease patients. So he tried it out in the lab.

Encouraged by dog experiments the adhesions principle was first tried on a 48-year-old angina patient on 13th February 1935. Operating through an incision between the fifth and sixth ribs of the left chest, Beck roughened the internal surface of the pericardium with a burr then denuded the external membrane, or epicardium of the left ventricular muscle. But key to the intervention was the grafting of a well vascularised strip of chest wall muscle between the two. Gradually the patient's angina receded and after a year he had no symptoms. Spurred on by this, the brain surgeon who had now become a leading heart surgeon, began to use fatty omentum from around the guts instead of strips of muscle. This technique originated through the awareness that the English surgeon Laurence O'Shaughnessy had wrapped the gullet with omentum to improve blood supply after removing the stomach. And sure enough O'Shaughnessy went on to use Beck's approach for the heart. Through journal articles medical advances were at last beginning to be adopted on an international level.

A simpler method to create vascular adhesions in the pericardium was to promote chemically-induced inflammation using talc. Other irritants tested were carborundum sand, powdered beef bone, asbestos, iron filings, iodine and even human skin. Dwight Harken used carbolic acid to destroy cells on the surface of the heart as well as talc within the pericardial space. Some patients claimed immediate improvement but this was much too soon to be the result of new blood vessel formation. This was the good old placebo effect, though carbolic may have destroyed all the nerve endings too. That said, denervating the heart was a suggestion explored by Charles Mayo, one of two brothers who established the Mayo Clinic. Others tried it, including Sampson Handley at the Middlesex Hospital in London. Some patients claimed to experience symptomatic relief but their coronary occlusion progressed inexorably.

Running down within the chest wall on either side of the breast bone is a two millimetre diameter blood vessel called the internal mammary artery. From the name, as you might imagine, these give origin to branches called the intercostal arteries that course along the underside of the ribs and supply the breasts. In 1946 the surgeon Arthur Vineberg of McGill University in Montreal, argued that the internal mammary vessels could be mobilised from the chest wall and relocated to bring blood to the heart muscle. Would the breasts drop off? No one knew yet.

What Vineberg did initially in dogs was to dissect the left internal mammary artery from the chest wall, ligate it close to the diaphragm, then implant the bleeding end into a tunnel of ventricular muscle close to the left anterior descending coronary artery.

His co-workers reasonably expected the method to cause a bruise within the muscle, after which the artery itself would clot off. But remarkably no haematoma formed. And after sacrificing more than two hundred animals, it was possible to demonstrate by injecting dye, that connections had formed to blood vessels within the heart muscle in the majority of experiments.

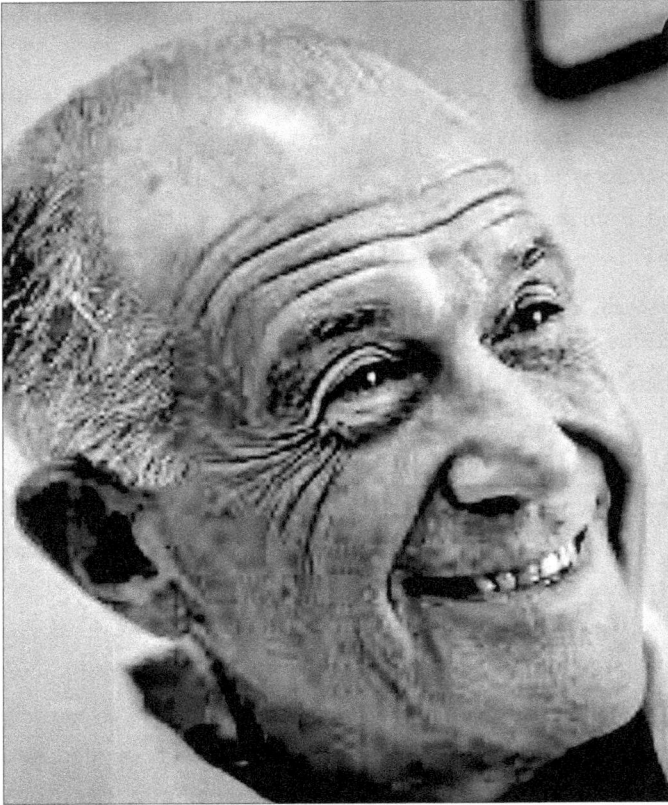

Fig 10.1 Arthur Vineberg.

Why should this work? If a bleeding artery were to be implanted into any other muscle it would simply cause a large clot, but heart muscle has a sponge like quality. In early embryonic life the sponge is soft and loose, extracting its oxygen from blood squeezed in and out of it. This is the mechanism by which the hearts of many lower vertebrate animals such as fish obtain their nutrition. During development of the human embryo, the sponge tightens and the coronary blood vessels and capillaries condense out of the spongy network. However, when collateral connections open up under the stress of heart muscle ischaemia there is the tendency to revert towards the sponge state. This was the complex theoretical basis that Vineberg presented to justify his operation on patients in 1950. Butchers were evolving into surgical scientists. At least some were.

The McGill group were cautious to select their first candidates very carefully. As Vineberg stated in his paper the following year: 'We have to date only operated upon patients who are unable to carry on because of the severity of their anginal pain. Patients with an enlarged left ventricle and myocardial decompensation are considered poor risks for surgery and have not been accepted.' There was no direct coronary artery imaging at that stage but electrocardiograms were performed at rest and after exercise to confirm coronary obstruction. Then exercise tests were performed by climbing the stairs to precipitate angina. Not satisfied with that, radiological investigations were undertaken to rule out pain mimicking angina from the gullet, peptic ulcers or gall stones.

Vineberg's first patient on April 28th was a 53-year-old tailor who had been crippled with angina and virtually unable to walk for three years before admission to the Royal Victoria Hospital. The poor man even suffered a severe anginal attack through anxiety in the anaesthetic room. The surgeons opened the left chest between the 4th and 5th ribs and mobilised the internal mammary artery from the chest wall for about twenty centimetres, ligating the branches with catgut. Manipulating the position of the left ventricle with a stitch through the apex, a short tunnel was made within the muscle itself with the scalpel and the artery introduced with a traction stitch. The heart was disturbed for no more than three minutes, following which blood pressure returned to normal and the chest was closed. Blood loss was minimal.

Post-operatively the patient's condition was described as excellent so he was removed from the oxygen tent in twenty-four hours. Unfortunately two days later, in the late afternoon, he attempted to use the bed pan. This precipitated an abrupt fall in blood pressure with elevation of his pulse rate to 160 beats per minute. Later that same evening he developed severe central chest pain, a precipitous fall in blood pressure and died. Autopsy showed that his main coronary arteries were calcified with multiple areas of critical narrowing. The right coronary was occluded long term whilst the left had recently blocked with thrombus. The left ventricular muscle showed acute myocardial infarction. Perhaps the only good news was that the internal mammary artery was patent throughout with no haematoma at the site of the implant. It was that frequent cardiac surgery thing - 'Great operation but the patient died!'

Things could only get better, and they did. The next two patients, men aged 54 and 49 respectively survived and were discharged home after prolonged periods in hospital. Their symptoms gradually improved and Vineberg hypothesised that, like the dogs, they had developed collateral blood flow to the coronary arteries. In 1954 he reported 140 heart operations for angina with an overall death rate of one in three. Subsequently between 1954 and 1963 only two per cent of the patients died and the vast majority reported some relief of their chest pain. Was the operation used in Britain? Rarely.

At the Cleveland Clinic, Mason Sones who had already performed the first ever cardiac catheterisation of a newborn infant, was asked to investigate one of Vineberg's patients. On 12th January 1962 under radiological guidance, the brilliant Sones succeeded in manipulating a catheter into the mouth of the left internal mammary artery and injected dye. This showed conclusively that the relocated vessel had established a connection with the blocked left anterior descending coronary and had relieved the patient's ischaemia. When the finding was shown at the clinic's thoracic surgical meeting, the surgeons discussed more direct alternatives but without direct visualisation of the sites of blockage, and the concept of meaningful coronary revascularisation remained only a remote possibility. Sones, a chain smoker, was tantalised by the transient glimpse of the coronary arteries he often saw when contrast medium was injected into the ascending aorta. But even when the dye was released directly into the aortic sinuses above the valve, the coronary images were not conspicuously better.

On October 30th 1958, Sones was investigating a young man with congenital heart disease when after reaching the ascending aorta with his catheter, he decided to take a break for a quick cigarette before injecting the dye.

In the meantime the tip of the catheter unknowingly flipped into the orifice of the right coronary artery which went unnoticed. Catastrophically the full volume of contrast material meant to visualise the whole aorta was shot unintentionally into the small vessel. Disaster. Sure enough the heart stopped beating immediately and Sones thought he had killed the man.

He recounted: 'I was sure he was going to die and when I looked over at the oscilloscope the ECG was flat. The guy's heart just wasn't beating at all. Well, I knew there was plenty of blood in the aorta so I yelled 'cough' figuring that would push in some blood and force out the dye. The guy coughed three or four times and thankfully his heart resumed beating. There were no defibrillators then.'

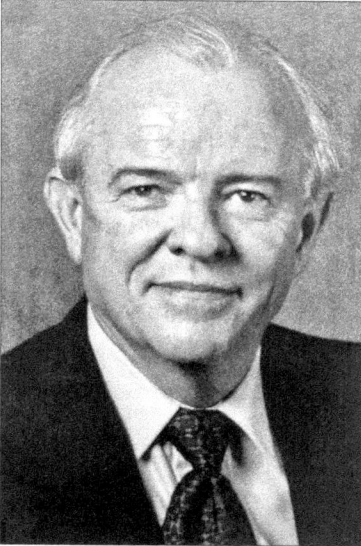

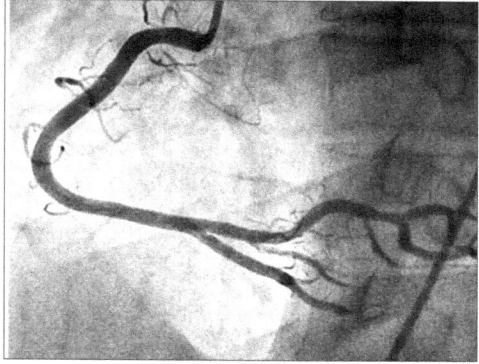

Fig 10.2A (left) Mason Sones.

Fig 10.2B (above) Angiogram of the healthy right coronary artery.

When the images were reviewed there was perfect visualisation of the right coronary artery in question. This was the breakthrough needed to initiate meaningful coronary artery surgery, albeit with much smaller doses of contrast medium. For Sones and his cardiology colleagues this was a revelation and thankfully the pioneering patient suffered no adverse effects.

Sones soon designed a catheter and fluoroscopic screen specifically for coronary angiography but did not rush to publish the advance in the scientific literature. He first aimed to collect one thousand coronary angiograms to correlate the radiological findings with the patients' symptoms and was obsessional about dictating the catheterisation reports and filing them in the patients' notes. Often he would still be in his smoke-filled office at two or three in the morning scrutinising the images and contemplating surgical referrals. As his eminent colleague Floyd Loop declared: 'Collectively, all of the cardiological advances this century pale in comparison with this priceless achievement.' One of the biggest killers on the medical curriculum could now be conquered.

During the early 1960s direct coronary angiography was undertaken on angina patients at the clinic and if a major branch was occluded, a left internal mammary artery was implanted into the muscle of that territory. In time when the right coronary was diseased, the right internal mammary was used instead. More often than not the vessels were implanted through a midline sternal incision, yet the results were difficult to assess. No breasts fell off, but a leading article in the *British Medical Journal* in 1967 stated that: 'The operation has yet been shown to increase the patient's life expectancy.' And indeed the natural history of coronary artery disease seemed to vary greatly. One patient without previous angina would suffer an acute myocardial infarction and die instantly. Another might complain of stable angina for many years, then suffer an acute myocardial infarction but still be alive and active twenty years later.

Given Sones's reliable visualisation of the pattern of coronary disease a direct surgical approach to improve flow in the vessels followed rapidly. On the whole critical narrowings occurred within the first few centimetres of the artery so why not simply open it and core out the disease? That is precisely what the intrepid Charles Bailey did in Philadelphia for the first time on 29th October 1956 but without imaging. It was guesswork stimulated by autopsy studies. The procedure termed coronary endarterectomy was undertaken by incising the artery beyond the suspected blockage then passing a curette retrogradely to scrape out the obstruction. Not performed without difficulty on the beating heart before the advent of cardiopulmonary bypass. When this first patient recovered somewhat surprisingly Bailey tried again several times giving heparin to prevent thrombosis. When he obtained a Gibbon machine in the late 1950s he switched to opening the aorta and coring out the atheroma through the coronary ostium. Somewhat unpredictable and high risk but Bailey was used to disappointment.

As is often the case, the first direct anastomosis of the internal mammary artery to a coronary artery was not a planned procedure. William Longmire was now Professor and Chairman of the Department of Surgery in Los

Angeles having been Chief Resident with Blalock the year before Cooley. Vivien Thomas wrote of him: 'Dr Longmire was one of the very best to go through the surgical residency programme at Johns Hopkins during the Blalock era. He had superb natural technical skill, his hands moving deftly, smoothly and swiftly so he usually completed the procedure (the shunt) in less time than was required by the professor.' And it certainly needed to be a great surgeon to achieve what Longmire did on that occasion in 1958.

From Bailey's early efforts it was apparent that when an endarterectomy crossed the mouth of a large branch, the sheared-off atheroma rapidly retracted from the main channel, occluding the branch by clot. Longmire was in the midst of that problem with a struggling heart when he decided to introduce a new source of blood supply altogether. He wrote: 'Repeatedly we would do the coronary thromboendarterectomy procedure and the vessel disintegrated. In desperation we were forced to anastomose the left internal mammary artery directly to the distal end of the right coronary artery and later decided it was a good operation.'

What must be acknowledged is the degree of difficulty that these pioneers faced. The blood vessels were tiny, diseased and fragile. The heart was in constant movement so the surgeon had to perform with extreme accuracy on a moving target. Worse still the needles were too large and the stitch material too crude for microvascular surgery. Even the surgical instruments were cumbersome. So these were courageous men. The only woman in the game was Nina Braunwald.

Similar desperate circumstances led to the first coronary bypass operation using the saphenous vein harvested from a patient's leg. Michael DeBakey's colleague, Edward Garrett, was having difficulty in separating a patient from the bypass machine and suspected it was due to obstructed coronary arteries. In desperation a segment of leg vein was used as a bypass graft directly from the aorta to the left anterior descending coronary artery. This turned the case around, yet unfortunately and unusually for surgeons, the outcome was only reported ten years later in 1974.

It was the unusual friendship between Mason Sones and a talented young surgeon from Argentina that launched coronary bypass as a routine procedure. When Rene Favoloro arrived in Cleveland in 1962 at the age of thirty-nine, he could barely speak English.

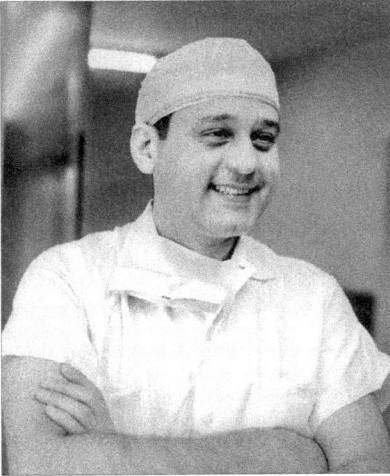

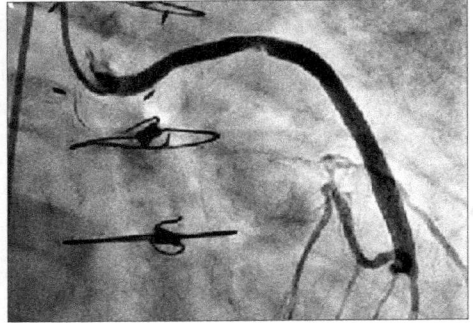

Fig 10.3A Rene Favaloro.

Fig 10.3B Angiogram showing saphenous vein bypass supplying an occluded left coronary artery.

Nor was he licensed to work as a surgeon in the USA, but recognising his technical expertise, Donald Effler, the Chief of Thoracic Surgery, was prepared to help with that. Until that point the clinic's whole thoracic department consisted of Effler with one partner, Harry Groves, and two residents. Initially Favaloro was only acceptable at the clinic as an unpaid observer in a team that mostly performed lung and oesophageal surgery.

Just prior to Favaloro's arrival Effler, encouraged by Sones, had employed a patch graft of pericardium to enlarge the lumen of a left main coronary artery as it emerged from the aorta. This they considered safer than Bailey's endarterectomy approach and proved moderately successful in a small number of cases. Of necessity, the department's heart-lung machine was used for the purpose and on arrival Favaloro inherited the responsibility for cleaning and reassembling the equipment to gain experience. And from the beginning he spent hours in the catheter laboratory with Sones, fascinated by the images of hearts and coronary arteries. It became clear to him that patients fell into two groups. Some have diffuse disease that involves most branches, but the majority have localised obstruction in the proximal part of a vessel with good distal run off. Surely this category of patient would benefit from a bypass of that narrowing.

Favaloro had vascular surgery experience with vein bypass grafts for obstructed leg arteries which caused him to wonder whether the saphenous vein might be similarly used for the coronary arteries. Logically the pressure and flow should prove adequate if the origin of the bypass grafts was placed on the ascending aorta. Moreover Effler's patch grafts were not working out that well. So it was time to try something different.

In 1964 Favaloro passed the Educational Council Foreign Medical Graduate Examination and given his advanced surgical skills he could now be made Chief Resident in the Thoracic Surgery Department. Once the midline sternal incision, or median sternotomy, became the preferred access for most heart operations Favaloro considered performing Vineberg's operation using both internal mammary arteries. Sones cautioned him not to. Reviewing the chest wall vascular anatomy he felt that the sternum deprived of its blood supply could be at serious risk from necrosis. So Favaloro had to be patient until he was taken on as a full staff member. He then performed 38 bilateral implants without a death or life-threatening complication. The sternum healed fine as it happened.

In May 1967 Favaloro was referred a 51-year-old woman who had suffered from angina for three years. Sones images showed the left coronary to be free from critical narrowing but the large right coronary artery was completely occluded in its proximal third. Sones regarded this as the perfect opportunity to attempt a vein bypass since graft failure was unlikely to result in fatality. So on 7th May Favaloro took the woman to theatre, resected the occluded portion of the artery and interposed a segment of saphenous vein from the thigh to restore continuity. Clearly the simpler concept of joining the proximal end of the vein to the ascending aorta, and the other end to the side of the coronary artery hadn't yet occurred to him. Nevertheless re-catheterisation ten days after the operation showed a perfectly functioning repair and her angina was gone. When followed up ten years later the findings were the same.

The next ploy was a bypass graft from the ascending aorta to the distal end of the resected coronary segment using end to end anastomosis. This was performed in a further fifteen patients before finally settling on the simpler end-to-side join to the coronary artery beyond the blockage, the splendidly enduring coronary bypass technique used today. It is the world's commonest heart operation by far, performed hundreds of times each year in every adult cardiac unit. Why? Because it works. Delicate new instruments, fine suture materials and tiny needles were designed to facilitate the techniques. Then Melrose made his monumental contribution by stopping the heart from moving. Suddenly microsurgery for diseased arteries on the surface of the heart became a practical proposition for surgeons less skilled that Favaloro.

Now there was a real buzz around the Cleveland Clinic. Coronary artery disease was common. Many thousands of patients converged on the hospital for Sones to investigate, then Favaloro to cure them. The first vein bypass grafts to the left coronary artery followed in spring 1968. The inaugural case had tight obstruction of the left main coronary so a single bypass graft was placed on the dominant left anterior descending branch. That filled the whole left coronary territory as demonstrated graphically by Sones a couple of weeks later. By the end of the year 170 similar operations had been performed and, following on, areas of aneurysmal scar tissue were excised from the left ventricle in patients who were developing heart failure. Left ventricular aneurysmectomy was the technical name for that.

Sones would state modestly that twentieth century cardiology could be separated into the pre-Favaloro and post-Favaloro eras, yet scepticism prevailed in the surgical community. Many simply didn't believe that a mortality rate less than five per cent could be achieved with any type of heart operation. But the key in coronary bypass surgery was that the instantaneous boost in myocardial blood flow rapidly improved ventricular contraction. Because the heart muscle contracted better after the procedure than before, the patients didn't die. This was a revelation helped by improvements in cardiopulmonary bypass and cardioplegia.

Soon afterwards, new developments in microvascular stitching techniques allowed George Green in New York to join the left internal mammary artery directly to the left anterior descending coronary artery. One two millimetre vessel to another two millimetre vessel. Green had spent many hours in the New York City morgue examining the hearts of patients after fatal infarction. He needed to convince himself that the distal segments of diseased coronary arteries were sufficiently free from atheroma to allow the exacting anastomosis. They were indeed, and David Tice, the Director of Surgery at the New York Veterans Administration Hospital encouraged Green to proceed. This was an important step because the internal mammary artery in continuity with its origin from the chest wall would eventually be shown to have better long-term patency than saphenous vein grafts. As a result patient survival was demonstrably improved.

The next challenge for Favaloro was to attempt bypass surgery in those in the midst of a heart attack, aiming to preserve the threatened muscle and prevent heart failure. Again serendipity played its part. It happened that a booked patient awaiting admission in the Bolton Square Hotel across the street suffered sudden severe chest pain causing the hotel desk to call the surgeon's secretary. Favaloro went directly to Sones's office to review the angiogram performed earlier that week. It showed a severe narrowing of the left anterior descending coronary with normal left ventricular function. But it wasn't normal now. The critically ischaemic territory no longer contracted and the lungs were filling with fluid. Favaloro rushed to the hotel and found the man 'in pain, sweating, short of breath and very pale'. The electrocardiogram confirmed extensive anterolateral myocardial infarction, and again Favaloro consulted Sones in what would evolve into the multidisciplinary team meeting. A collective view to formulate the best medical decisions. Predictably Sones said 'go ahead and operate', which triggered the inaugural emergency bypass operation for acute myocardial infarction.

It was a brave decision to tackle a lethal problem. That said the technical aspects were no different from elective surgery and the man recovered. So did the dying muscle. His left ventricular function was preserved and the long standing anginal symptoms gone. Within a year Favaloro and Sones had treated thirty similar cases and published their results in the *American Journal of Cardiology*. They showed that if coronary bypass can be performed within six hours of the onset of symptoms virtually all the muscle can be saved.

In 1970 Favaloro and Arthur Vineberg were both invited to speak at the 6th World Congress of Cardiology meeting at the Royal Festival Hall in London. The presentation took place in a hall that was packed to over-flowing and to an audience who listened in disbelief. After the discussions Donald Ross persuaded Favaloro to visit and demonstrate his new opera-tion at the National Heart Hospital. This first coronary bypass operation in Britain was proceeding calmly with Ross assisting, until Favaloro opened the right coronary artery and inserted his first stitch. At that point the somewhat inattentive scrub nurse accidentally avulsed the vein and ripped the stitch through the wall of the diseased vessel. At least she didn't drop it on the floor. Favaloro later reflected warmly on the events: 'Most of the outstanding cardiovascular surgeons from Europe watched the operation from behind us, some almost on top of our shoulders. We participated in informal discussions between operations, most of them held in the pub op-posite the hospital, where we exchanged knowledge and friendship.' I spent many happy hours in that pub too.

Soon after the European trip a delegation of cardiologists from Argentina appealed to Favaloro's patriotism and put pressure on him to return home. Reluctantly he capitulated when they insisted that his homeland needed him more than the Cleveland Clinic did. This was an emotional time as he subsequently described. 'In 1970 I decided to return to my home country. It was a difficult decision. I gave serious thought to the request and finally considered that my work and duties were needed in Latin America. One day in October, late in the afternoon, I wrote my letter of resignation to Effler. I closed the envelope with tears in my eyes and left it on his desk. I wrote: As you know there is no real cardiac surgery in Buenos Aires. Destiny has put on my shoulders one more difficult task. I am going to dedicate the last one third of my life to building them a new centre. At this particular time the circumstances suggest that I am the only one with the possibility of doing it.'

Favaloro relinquished great personal wealth in making that decision. Every operation he performed in Cleveland made him at least $10,000. Sones was distraught, thought him crazy, and refused to accept the de-cision. So difficult a time was it that Favaloro felt it necessary to accept an invitation to lecture in Boston, take his wife with him and then leave for Argentina without returning to Cleveland. Only his secretary Candice knew about the impending departure and Sones was inconsolable.

Favaloro was very successful in Argentina, at least initially. He returned to Cleveland a number of times and on one occasion took Sones on holiday to France and Italy. Recalling the occasion Favaloro wrote: 'I think Mason was in direct communication with life for the first time. It was the end of summer. He was amazed by the wheat prairies, the corn fields, the vineyards and the fruit trees. This giant of modern cardiology was bathed in sun instead of by the lamps of the cardiac laboratory where he spent all his life.'

That was a realistic assessment. Sones spent his days in a dark room lit by the glow of the projector, clad in T-shirt and old trousers and constantly puffing on a cigarette. He dictated his findings there, often interrupted by eager visitors including the author who were enthralled by his descriptions of sick coronary arteries. At night he was known to sleep on the catheterisation table. When Favaloro learned that his old friend was dying from lung cancer, he immediately flew to Cleveland to be with him. Ultimately Favaloro's own life was destined to end miserably amidst the financial woes of Argentina in the 1990s. His clinic and Favaloro Foundation came to owe huge debts and on 29th July 2000, when deeply depressed, he took his own life at the age of 77.

Under Donald Effler's guidance, Favaloro had established the Thoracic Surgery Department of the Cleveland Clinic as the world's leading centre for myocardial revascularisation. When Effler retired Floyd Loop became Chief of Cardiac Surgery and, with his associates Delos Cosgrove and Bruce Lytle, the Clinic continued to push the boundaries. As effective as it was in relieving symptoms, coronary bypass surgery was subject to numerous clinical trials where patients were recruited to compare surgery versus continued medical treatment. This was justified because the introduction of Beta blockers and calcium channel blockers for angina and heart failure improved outcomes in tandem with the surgical advances. And whilst bypass grafts relieved angina in most cases there was no proof initially that the patients lived longer. After all, coronary bypass amounted to a huge operation on both the chest and leg. Frequently saphenous vein harvest was needed from both thigh and lower leg, amounting to a thirty-inch incision, before satisfactory segments were obtained.

The first comprehensive study report was published by the Veteran's Administration Hospital's Cooperative in the USA. This enrolled 686 volunteers who were randomly assigned to either medical or surgical treatment. When the patients were stratified according to the number of grafted vessels their mortality was an impressive zero for a single bypass graft, six percent for two vessels, and seven per cent for three. Follow-up catheter imaging of the grafts showed 69% to be patent at a year, meaning that virtually one third had rapidly thrombosed. Interestingly the only group to demonstrate survival advantage were those with a severe narrowing of the left main coronary artery. However, looking at those who had suffered previous heart attacks with a scarred left ventricle, 76% were alive at seven years following surgery versus just 52% who remained on medical therapy.

In Europe a multicentre randomised study included 768 men under the age of 65. They were selected for mild to moderate angina, with greater than 50% narrowing of two major coronary arteries and normal left ventricular function. Operative mortality was 3.6% but bypass grafting modestly improved survival overall. For patients with narrowing of all three major vessels the five-year surgical survival was 94% versus 90% on medication. Later, single-centre studies of higher risk patients demonstrated clear superiority of surgery over medical treatment. For those with three vessel disease and a previously damaged ventricle, the difference in survival came close to 90% versus 50% in favour of surgery. Consequently coronary bypass grafting emerged as the most frequently performed of any surgical procedure in the USA and heralded widespread expansion in cardiac centres to cope with the influx of hopeful candidates. And eventually we went back to doing it without the heart-lung machine. I called that 'scratching around on the surface', not open heart surgery, but it worked.

But back to Dotter. Recall that in 1964 Charles Dotter with Melvin Judkins had employed a guide wire and catheter technique to dilate arteries in the leg. Unfortunately 'Dottering' was never widely applied because the production of balloon catheters stalled through lack of appropriate materials. Within ten years however, catheter technology had improved and so had the ideas for its deployment. Andreas Gruntzig, a German-born cardiologist at the University of Heidelberg devised his own inflatable balloon catheter which he could miniaturise to pass within the coronary arteries. The work was instigated by a patient who asked him: 'Is it possible, instead of using drugs or a complex bypass operation, to just "clean" my obstructed arteries like a plumber uses a wire brush?' Gruntzig was taken by the idea. As reported in his unfinished biography, this was the moment when he began to contemplate coronary interventional techniques.

As Gruntzig recalled he received little encouragement locally. 'It was at this time my chief invited me to attend an afternoon meeting in Frankfurt. For the first time I listened to Dr Zeitler speak about peripheral recanalization of arteries using Dotter's method. I recall he was very upset that someone would try to interfere with diseased arteries by forcing catheters into areas of narrowing. He made it clear that he never wanted such a treatment to take place in his own hospital.' Disappointing. Gruntzig regarded this as an overly conservative lack of vision, so in 1971 following a fellowship at St Thomas' Hospital in London, Gruntzig moved to the Department of Radiology at the University of Zurich. There, whilst performing angioplasty of the leg vessels using Dotter catheters, he worked on producing a dilating catheter with a 4 millimetre balloon suitable for the coronary arteries.

He wisely chose to test his device on a 67-year-old man, Fritz Ott, with pre-gangrenous leg ischaemia and continuous pain in the calf. Within hours the man was able to walk comfortably again. Despite this encouraging start, Gruntzig was unsure that the balloon was sufficiently robust. As he explained: 'I spent the next two years contacting manufacturing plants in an attempt to solve the problem. Especially fruitful was the cooperation of a factory which produced shoelaces and provided me with silk meshes which I planned to wrap around the balloon to limit its outer diameter. I then needed a very thin balloon to insert within the mesh. It was at that time I met a retired chemist Dr Hopff, a professor emeritus of chemistry at the Federal Institute of Technology. He introduced me to polyvinyl chloride compounds. After hundreds of experiments mostly in my own kitchen, I was able to form a sausage-shaped distensible segment. When I mounted this on normal catheter tubing and applied pressure to distend the balloon, I realised that the strength of this material was so great that the silk mesh was unnecessary. This was a great breakthrough that enabled me to reduce the size of the catheter.'

Again he tested the product on leg arteries with each catheter custom-made for the individual on the Gruntzig kitchen table. He would obtain the patient's angiogram, take it home, measure the length and width of the narrowed segment and construct the balloon accordingly with his wife Maria. This was personalised medicine in the early 1970s and continued until the Schneider Company was founded and built the balloon catheters for him.

By 1975 Gruntzig felt ready to tackle the coronary circulation. It was a big step, but when he approached Zurich's Chief of Cardiac Surgery, Ake Senning for support, he was pleasantly surprised. Senning responded: 'Mr Gruntzig, you will be taking away my patients but get started right away.' With Senning's blessing and the help of the Croatian surgeon Marco Turina, Gruntzig began testing smaller balloon catheters for coronary arteries in dogs and human cadavers.

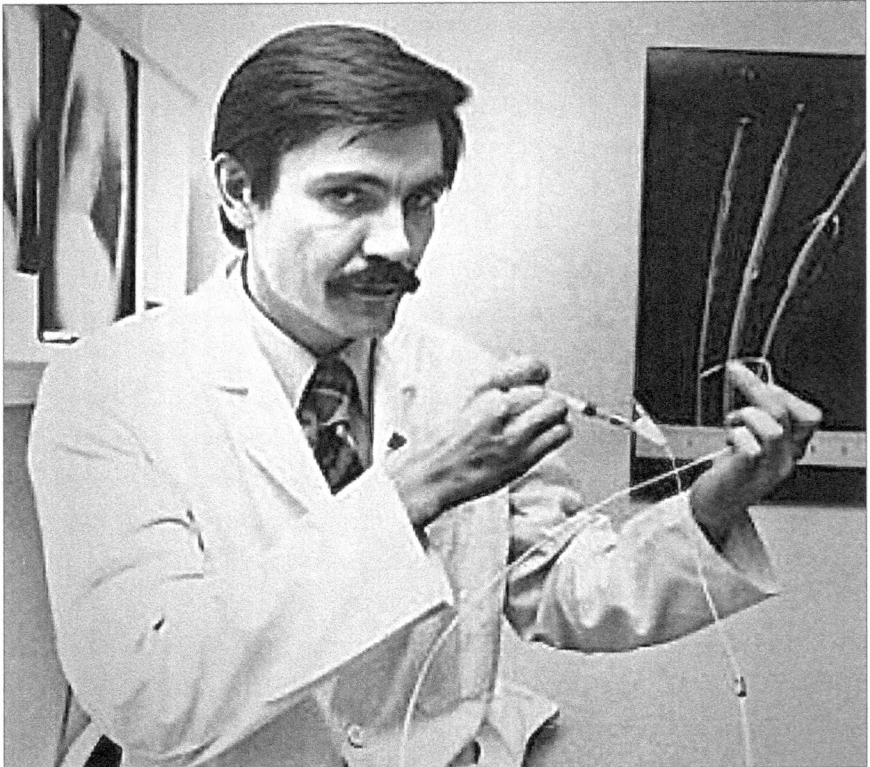

Fig 10.4 Andreas Gruntzig.

Turina recalled: 'He had the sacred fire, as the French call it. It was what he thought about constantly. I have never seen somebody so focused on a single idea as Andreas was. Everyone was telling him his idea wouldn't work and that he was going to fail, that there were pitfalls at every turn. But the concept was consuming him all the time.'

In truth, Gruntzig couldn't have had better surgical colleagues. By 1975 Turina was creating artificial coronary stenoses to practise on in the laboratory. Gruntzig's new catheter succeeded and the work was presented to great acclaim at the American Heart Association meeting in Miami the following year. It was the right time to move on to patients. On March 22nd 1977 Gruntzig was shown a difficult case with unstable angina. The angiogram showed severe disease in all three major coronary branches but a particularly tight narrowing of the left main coronary artery. The man was in heart failure and deemed inoperable by the surgeons.

This is how Gruntzig described the stressful events that day. 'I agreed to try, eager to enter the area of competition with the surgeons. Unfortunately the patient was so diseased that every attempt to puncture the groin arteries failed because of occluded femoral arteries. Only the left brachial artery had discernible flow to allow passage of the catheter into the aorta. From this route the catheters were unable to guide the coronary dilatation balloon into the orifice of the left main so we had to abandon the procedure. The patient died several days later from a final myocardial infarction. The case taught me that when you start a technique, you should start with an ideal case and not with end stage disease.'

Whilst that last statement made sense the whole episode typifies the beginning of high-risk cardiac interventions. The pioneers always had to take the worst possible cases, and in the light of this first failure Gruntzig adopted a completely different strategy. He decided to take his catheter into the operating theatre and try it under direct vision in patients undergoing coronary bypass operations. Unfortunately yet understandably, the plan was opposed in Zurich. The surgeons feared that retrograde dilatation of an atheromatous narrowing would create competitive blood flow for the vein bypass graft and early thrombosis. In other words it was an experiment regarded as having the potential to cause harm, so Gruntzig looked elsewhere.

Elsewhere happened to be far away in California. Dr Elias Hanna, a cardiac surgeon at St Mary's Hospital in San Francisco was willing to help. As Gruntzig put it: 'Dr Hanna did not have the same fear. He indicated that his bypass grafts would always be better than what was accomplished with a catheter.' So on May 9th 1977, Gruntzig assisted by the local cardiologist Richard Myler, performed the first of a number of balloon angioplasties undertaken during coronary bypass operations. Hanna opened the diseased vessel beyond the obstructive lesion, then Gruntzig inserted his catheter retrogradely through the vessel to dilate the narrowing. Hanna then sewed on his vein graft and the results were studied by angiography days afterwards. The angioplasties proved safe and successful and the bypass grafts functioned appropriately. Everyone was happy including the patients.

Four months after the San Francisco cases Senning in Zurich encouraged Gruntzig to perform his first direct angioplasty on a conscious patient. Thirty-eight-year old Adolf Bachmann had originally been scheduled for surgery but with an isolated narrowing of the left anterior descending artery. And sure enough the balloon angioplasty cured the problem. Soon afterwards a report in the *Lancet* established the catheter intervention as an alternative to surgery. And inevitably the technique was not restricted to coronary disease. Balloon catheters were designed to dilate coarctation of the aorta, then obstructions in the bronchial tree, the bile ducts and the gut. Open vascular surgery was decimated by catheter techniques much to the comfort of the patients and the beneficial effects on hospital costs.

By April 1979 Gruntzig had treated sixty patients in the catheter laboratory, six of whom had to be rescued by urgent coronary bypass for inadvertent coronary occlusion. As such, an operating theatre always had to be held open in case of adverse events and one in ten patients needed it in the early years. Scepticism persisted amongst cardiologists in Switzerland, so many of the patients were actually referred from abroad. Meanwhile several institutions in the USA offered Gruntzig a position including Harvard and the Cleveland Clinic. He eventually accepted an offer from Emory University in Atlanta, Georgia who had received $105 million from the Coca-Cola Foundation to fund a new interventional cardiology programme. Gruntzig was appointed Professor and Director. Dotter wrote congratulating him:

'You proved to be one of the most skilled catheterisers I have seen; not only that but a superb teacher and doctor who never forgot his patient. We will be happy to have you in this country.'

In less than five years at Emory, Gruntzig had treated more than three thousand coronary disease patients without a death. Then tragedy. He was killed together with his second wife, Margaret-Ann, when his own plane crashed in Georgia on the night of October 27th 1985. Crash investigators were unsure why.

Following Dotter's original concept, Gruntzig's pioneering use of balloon catheters and coronary stents to maintain vessel patency, produced one of the most successful medical interventions of all time. The arguments as to which patients derived superior survival benefit from coronary bypass versus transluminal angioplasty raged on for years. Surgeons fought back with 'off pump' revascularisation without the heart lung machine or fewer grafts through smaller incisions. In March 1996 we held the first international meeting on 'Less invasive coronary surgery' in Oxford with huge attendance. So we followed with 'Cost Containment in Cardiac Surgery' conferences in Washington DC and San Francisco, in a concerted attempt to stay in the game. Yet what would any rational patient prefer? A saw up the sternum and a leg filleted for vein harvest, or catheterisation under local anaesthetic, with a couple of stents, then safely home that same evening? Both have been shown to preserve the pump. So you decide. And long may it last.

New Hearts for Old

Nothing helps a broken heart like having
someone wonderful give you theirs.
—Rita Stradling

There is a line from the Old Testament (Ezekiel, Chapter 36,verse 26): Thus sayeth the Lord God, 'A new heart also will I give you and a new spirit will I put within you; and I will take away the stony heart, and I will give you a heart of flesh.'

Undoubtedly, Ezekiel was speaking metaphorically, but perhaps he had insight into the stony nature of valve and coronary artery calcification which causes some of the conditions for which transplantation is the only treatment. Aristotle considered the heart to be the seat of the soul, all emotions and intellect. Despite some counterarguments Aristotle's views prevailed and made it difficult to debate the fanciful idea of heart transplantation dispassionately.

Legend has it that in the 3rd century BC, Pien Ch'iao, a Chinese physician, slipped a hypnotic potion into the drinks of two soldiers. Whilst they slept, he removed and swapped a number of internal organs, including their hearts. The soldiers awoke three days later, none the worse for their experience. Further fictitious transplants were attributed to the twin brothers Cosmos and Damian, who after their martyrdom in the 3rd century AD, became the patron saints of surgery. They are said to have removed the cancerous leg of a European and replaced it with the leg of a recently deceased

Moor dug up in the local cemetery. The following morning the patient had trouble convincing friends about the transplant despite the darker colour of the leg. But taken to the Moor's grave they found the patient's cancerous limb to be buried there.

Heart failure is a desperately miserable condition. One in five people will develop symptoms during their lifetime and all age groups may be affected. This amounts to twenty-six million people worldwide of whom half will die within five years of diagnosis. To begin with, as the left ventricle fails, comes shortness of breath. This progresses to breathlessness at rest and being unable to lie flat. Then the feet, ankles and lower legs swell, followed by abdominal distension as right ventricular function deteriorates. A distended liver is painful, and a belly full of fluid weighs them down. Most patients eventually become housebound and unable to fit into their shoes. As breathlessness worsens they sit propped up by pillows on the bed or must sleep in a chair. Eventually fluid, pulmonary oedema, fills their lungs. Blood-stained froth pours from their mouth and nostrils during which they turn blue and cold and die. No one knows that better than I do.

Organ transplantation had been contemplated in principle since the turn of the 19th century, but to join together small blood vessels required tiny needles and fine stitches. Catgut really didn't fit the bill and threaded needles used for stitching guts left holes in the vessel wall that bled. A poor anastomosis spelled thrombosis, vessel occlusion and inevitable organ death.

By 1905, Alexis Carrell at the University of Chicago began to use tapered needles of polished steel together with fine silk thread or human hair to join small blood vessels. Working alongside Charles Guthrie, Professor of Physiology and Pharmacology at the University of Pittsburgh, the pair transplanted kidneys, endocrine glands, ovaries, loops of intestine, then whole legs, arms, heads and even the lower half of a body in the laboratory. Their aim was to study transplant physiology in the recipient animal and attempt to define the mechanism of organ rejection.

Remarkably, fowl and guinea pigs gave birth after receiving new ovaries, whilst cats and dogs survived for several weeks after kidney transplants. What's more they transplanted hearts into the necks of recipient animals by joining the donor aorta to a head artery and the stump of the donor superior vena cava to the central end of the recipient's jugular vein. Usually circulation could be re-established in the donor heart around seventy minutes after removal and an hour later the ventricles would be beating vigorously though at a much slower rate than the recipient's heart. The experiments were usually terminated a couple of hours later when blood clotted in the donor heart's chambers. The pair even managed a heart and lung transplant from a week-old kitten to an adult cat.

Carrell considered rejection of the transplant tissues to be due to 'biotoxins', and wondered whether preliminary immunization of the recipient with donor blood might overcome the problem. Guthrie went on to transplant the head of a dog to the neck of another. Remarkably this disgusting experiment worked in some respects. The grafted head responded for a short time to light and sound with an element of consciousness. Others were destined to take the same route.

It was 1943 when the Oxford zoologist Peter Medawar showed that rejection of skin grafts was due to an immunological response, after which the same mechanism was found in transplanted organs. Medawar conducted extensive studies of skin grafts in rabbits characterising the timing, microscopic features and immunological changes during rejection but he still failed to identify the antibodies responsible.

The stimulus for human kidney transplants began with the remarkable achievements of Wilhelm Kolff who developed renal dialysis during the Nazi occupation of Holland in 1944. Kolff assembled an artificial kidney and saved many lives using a crude dialysing membrane of sausage skins. Once the technical imperfections of his early machine were overcome he used it to improve the condition of end-stage kidney failure patients to render them fit enough for a transplant operation.

On December 23rd 1954 Joseph Murray at Brigham Hospital in Boston bypassed the barrier of aggressive organ rejection by using a kidney patient's identical twin as a donor. With a well-functioning organ without rejection the impact of this first human transplant was enormous, and others were keen to follow. But how to avoid the rejection response in non-identical recipients? Two scientists, Joan Main and Richmond Prehn suggested a radical approach after weakening the immune system of mice with intense radiation, then priming them with bone marrow from the donor. A single dog transplant to test that process appeared to work so in 1958 Murray adopted the Main-Prehn strategy for human transplants. Twelve kidney failure patients were conditioned with lethal total body irradiation and given injected bone marrow from the donor. Eleven died within a month. The good news was that the single survivor who did not receive bone marrow maintained excellent function in his twin brother's kidney for twenty years.

In the 1950s cancer specialists began work with drugs such as nitrogen mustard and 6-mercaptopurine (6-MP) to treat malignancies and documented a degree of immunosuppression in their patients. When shown to extend the lifespan of skin grafts, Roy Calne a surgical trainee in London, tested the effect of 6-MP on kidney transplants in dogs and found it to significantly improve survival.

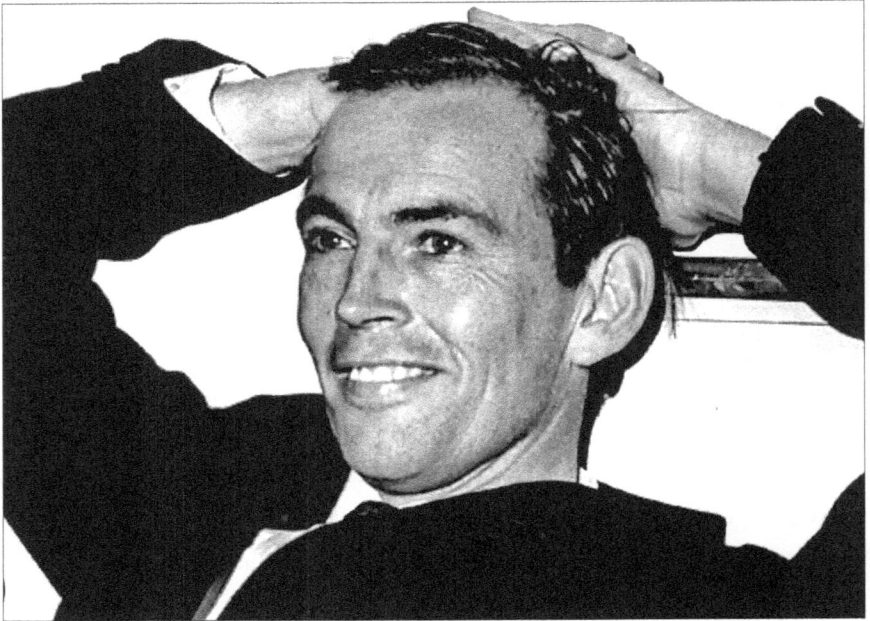

Fig 11.1 A. Christiaan Barnard in relaxed mode.

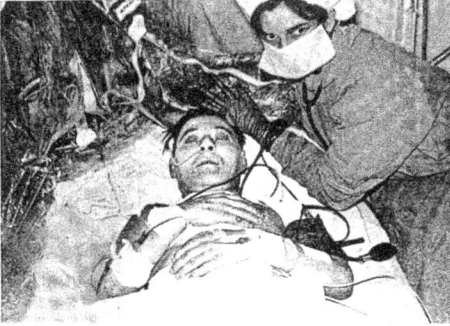

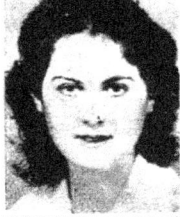

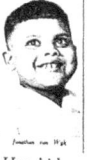

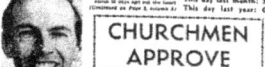

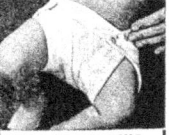

Fig 11.1 B. Front page of the Cape Town Argos
the day after the first heart transplant.

In 1960 Calne published his findings in the *Lancet* thereby launching the science of immunosuppression in the transplant world. Unfortunately when he treated three human kidney recipients in the same way their organs failed rapidly and they all died.

Undeterred, Calne obtained a research fellowship with Joseph Murray in Boston who encouraged him to continue the work with radiation. But he didn't, instead opting to experiment with a derivative of 6-MP, azathioprine, in dogs. The finding that kidney transplant rejection could be delayed substantially with azathioprine prompted Murray and the Brigham Hospital transplant team to begin using 6-MP and azathioprine for human kidney recipients. When Murray reported on his first ten patients at a transplant conference in Washington in 1963 one had survived for a year, though at the time of the conference the kidney was already failing. All of the others had died within six months so the results were barely better than with whole body irradiation. In fact the mood at the meeting was so gloomy that many questioned whether continued attempts at human transplantation could be justified.

Fortunately it took just one presentation to let the genie out of the bottle. Tom Starzl from Denver described a new immunosuppressive regime combining the steroid prednisone alongside azathioprine which provided consistent success in reversing kidney transplant rejection. Reporting seventy percent one-year survival the less well-known researcher had more success than all the leading surgeons combined. The audience was sceptical but he had brought with him the charts detailing the day-to-day progress of each patient. These included the laboratory tests, urine production by the transplanted kidney and drug doses. And although rejection episodes occurred with azathioprine alone these were usually reversed by introducing a dose of prednisone. Of course there were detractors and the formal conference report seemed to obfuscate the importance of Starzl's findings. But almost half a century later some of the patients were still alive and off immunosuppression altogether with the same functioning organ.

Before this conference there had been only three kidney transplant centres in North America. Within a year fifty new programs began in the USA alone. All of them adopted the Starzl cocktail for immunosuppression, which remained the standard for almost two decades. Then it would be Roy Calne who changed it, when they both pioneered liver transplants. Calne became Professor of Surgery at the University of Cambridge where I had the privilege to train with him in general and transplant surgery. The technicalities of implanting a kidney were relatively easy – but what about hearts?

Concealed from the West, a considerable amount of cardiac transplant research was happening at Moscow State University. The prolific Vladimir Demikhov began his experiments in the 1940s but was inevitably interrupted by war service. His original concept was to use the donor organ as an auxiliary pump within the chest, rather than remove the patient's sick heart and to that end he carried out more than 250 laboratory transplants using many different methods. The longest survivor was a dog called Borzoi who received a second heart on 4th October 1956. The hound resumed as active a life as possible within the laboratory environment until termination at thirty-two days when the donor heart fibrillated.

Demikhov did not have a heart-lung machine and was perturbed by the time taken by multiple vascular anastomoses that often resulted in brain injury. He therefore changed tack and with remarkable ingenuity began to transplant the heart and both lungs as a unit. With two dogs side by side on a table he used rubber tubing and temporary joins to achieve his goal without completely interrupting the circulation to either animal or the donor organs. In 1951 after sixty-seven attempts he achieved post-operative survival for six days in a bitch called Damka.

Impressive though that was at the time, other aspects of his experiments were a little off piste and pissed off many who learned of them. He performed a series of operations transplanting puppies' heads onto the necks of adult dogs. Within minutes the transplanted heads reacted to their surroundings and would lap up water when thirsty. He also managed to transplant heads in continuity with the spine so that all four legs made running movements. The longest survivor of this bizarre undertaking was twenty-nine days, but he went on to transplant the whole of the gastrointestinal tract including pancreas and liver, and then the whole of the lower half of the body. Whilst a surgical *tour de force*, these procedures made little scientific contribution because he had no method with which to immunosuppress the recipient animals. It was a 'Why? Because it was there endeavour.'

Demikhov wrote a book, published in Russian in 1960, which made the work accessible to researchers and indeed the public in the West. David Wheatley, a medical student in Cape Town at the time, recalls being in the surgeons' changing room at Groote Schuur hospital when Demikhov's head transplants featured in the *Cape Argos* newspaper. Someone commented on the article to Christiaan Barnard who was clearly put out. He stormed out of the room with the retort 'anything those Russians can do we can do too!' The same afternoon Barnard transplanted the head of a dog in his own laboratory and it survived seemingly with consciousness for several days. News travelled fast and the animal rights lobby was justifiably incensed. The medical students built a papier mâché two-headed dog for their rag parade and in the eyes of the University Barnard had already walked the tightrope between genius and vulgarity.

In the late 1950s Webb and Howard applied the Melrose cardioplegia solution to excised canine hearts which were stored at 4°C for several hours and then transplanted. They anticipated long distance donor heart procurement, should human transplants ever be undertaken, and correctly presumed that it would take long periods to access the heart, prepare the recipient and perform the operation.

In 1959 Donald Ross and Sir Russell Brock at Guy's Hospital described six different methods to remove the heart and transplant it into a recipient. This work was particularly significant because it introduced the principle by which the heart was separated from both the venae cava and pulmonary veins by simply cutting through the walls of the left and right atrium. This formed wide cuffs of both right and left atrium and was the first method to reduce the need for time-consuming multiple individual joins of donor and recipient veins. Two large cuffs instead of six smaller anastomoses.

The following year Richard Lower and Norman Shumway in Stanford, California published their seminal paper pulling together the optimal transplant technique and most favourable donor organ preservation methods integrated into a single definitive approach. All eight consecutive dogs treated with their regime survived the operation using cardiopulmonary bypass. Five lived between six and twenty-one days and were rehabilitated to eat and exercise normally. Yet no immunosuppression was given, so each soon died from organ rejection. Examination of the transplanted hearts under the microscope showed massive cellular infiltration with the white blood cells (lymphocytes) on which acute rejection is based. Lower and Shumway predicted that if the immunological system of the heart-failure recipient could be stopped from destroying the donor organ, in all likelihood it would continue to function for a lifetime. Optimistic, but optimism was certainly needed in the hostile sceptical environment.

Lower moved to become Professor of Cardiac Surgery at the University of Virginia in Richmond where he began to use a different immunosuppressive drug, methotrexate, with encouraging results. Many of the dogs exceeded one-year survival without rejection, an extraordinary achievement at the time. One transplanted bitch gave birth to a litter of puppies, the father of which had also had a heart transplant. In tandem, Adrian Kantrowitz at Maimonides Hospital in Brooklyn performed transplants in 3-month-old puppies using whole body cooling. One of these survived for 213 days without immunosuppression, a somewhat unexpected outcome attributed to the immunological incompetence of very young animals. Kantrowitz showed that the transplanted hearts steadily grew with time keeping pace with normal animals. Moreover the autopsy specimens showed none of the lymphocyte infiltration found in adults. But when he tried to repeat the experience using the heart-lung machine, all the animals died. Those damaging effects of blood-foreign surface interaction were largely responsible, but Kantrowitz's overall experience gave him optimism towards heart transplants for babies with congenital heart disease.

As the science moved forward in the 1960s cardiopulmonary bypass was well established, protection of ischaemic heart muscle with cardioplegia was improving, and intensive care units were becoming skilled in cardiac post-operative care. Many thousands of dogs had been sacrificed to the cause but when would someone take the gigantic leap and transplant the heart in a human? It happened that one substantial and rather obvious barrier remained. Someone had to die first and donate their precious heart, the logistics of which were undoubtedly controversial. An understatement. The honoured definition of death was when the heart eventually stopped. Utilisation of kidneys was already compromised by the prolonged lack of blood flow and oxygen deprivation in the process. The concept of brain stem death to suit transplant surgeons still remained in the ether.

In one notorious case in Newcastle a young man suffered serious head injuries from an assailant. Placed on a ventilator his condition was deemed irretrievable and his wife wanted to donate her husband's kidneys for transplantation. Doctors discontinued life support in accordance with her wishes but charges brought against the assailant were subsequently dismissed. The court ruled that the victim had died at the hands of the doctors who turned off the ventilator. The murderer could only be convicted of common assault and it was against the background of these dubious conditions that the first human cardiac transplant had to take place.

At the University of Mississippi Medical Centre, James Hardy and his team had performed mock transplants on human cadavers so that the group were well prepared. He had already performed the first human lung transplant in 1963 and as a result had experience with both immunosuppressive drugs and cobalt radiotherapy. In January 1964 Hardy was made aware of a potential recipient. The 36-year-old man was admitted to the Medical Centre in severe heart failure one year after being operated on for a cardiac knife wound that severed his left anterior descending coronary artery. In addition he had suffered multiple blood clots to the brain with permanent right-sided paralysis, severe mental impairment and both urinary and faecal incontinence. Amputation of the left leg for embolic gangrene had been followed weeks later by removal of the right leg, and he had recently needed urgent gut resection for ischemia. Otherwise he was fine.

Hardy was hoping to find a young donor with brain injury as there were an abundance of gunshot wounds in Jackson. The issue was how soon after cardiac arrest in the victim could the heart be removed? If it could not be done promptly, ischemic damage might ruin this landmark event. In an attempt to stage-manage the situation the team planned to insert catheters into the potential donor's leg arteries before death and use the by-pass machine to maintain blood flow to his heart muscle afterwards. Hardy presumed that if the relatives were willing to donate the organ for transplantation they would not object to their loved one being resurrected by a machine then terminated by the heart's removal. However, since he and his colleagues were too worried to turn off the donor's ventilator in case of prosecution for murder, they formulated a contingency plan. They had already purchased two large chimpanzees.

How did the size of the chimpanzees compare with the legless recipient? The larger of the two monkeys weighed 44 kilograms and had a measured cardiac output of 4.25 litres per minute whereas the man weighted just 33 kilograms. Perfect except it was an entirely different species! Ultimately it was decided that the brain-injured potential recipient was not in a fit state to provide written consent. Nor were the monkeys for that matter.

Not to be deprived of the chance of being the first, Hardy soon found another candidate. This was a 68-year-old man with high blood pressure and lower leg gangrene who had been admitted pulseless and comatose, but was resuscitated. He went on to have a tracheostomy and below knee amputation. Why Hardy had this penchant for amputees is difficult to explain but simultaneously in the hospital was a young man dying from severe brain injury. Unfortunately not quickly enough. The transplant team was therefore faced with the same legal and logistical problem as before. The chances that the donor would enter terminal decline before it was too late for the recipient were considered slim.

The 68-year-old soon lapsed into cardiogenic shock and it was clear that if a transplant was going to happen it had to be now. But the donor wasn't playing ball. So Hardy took the dying man to theatre and placed him on cardiopulmonary bypass to sustain life. The larger chimpanzee was brought to the adjacent operating theatre and anaesthetised. Shumway's transplant guidelines were followed and the relatively small monkey heart used to replace the patient's hugely dilated and terminally failing organ. The operation was described as technically satisfactory but the patient died from acute rejection one hour after weaning or rather creeping, from the heart-lung machine. Surprise, surprise and for obvious reasons, the morally destitute operation was not openly discussed at the time.

In 1966 Lower performed mirror-image experiments of Hardy's transplant, whereby human hearts were resuscitated from dead kidney donors and implanted into baboons. Clever stuff though the baboons weren't very pleased about it. One heart sustained the circulation of the animal for several hours until acute rejection. Again this work was not reported in the medical literature but Shumway was aware of it and at least it confirmed that the heart could be stopped, excised, resuscitated and successfully transplanted. What's more Christiaan Barnard was visiting Lower in Richmond at the time.

By the summer of 1967 Shumway considered that the three most crucial problems associated with heart transplantation had been addressed and solved. These were the evolution of a workable surgical procedure, then reliable cardiopulmonary bypass to maintain the recipient's circulation and lastly an effective drug regime to modulate the body's immunological response. In an interview for the *Journal of the American Medical Association* he stated that the time was right for human heart transplantation should a potential recipient and organ compatible donor be found simultaneously. This remained the major stumbling block without a legal policy on brain death. Indeed there was a 35-year-old man in the hospital at Stanford awaiting transplantation at the time. This patient had undergone extensive chest radiotherapy for Hodgkin's disease and Shumway knew him to have a depressed immune system, so that was a good starting point.

The interview was published in November and shortly afterwards Adrian Kantrowitz in New York sent out five hundred telegrams to other hospitals searching for a heart donor. Who would be first past the post given the secrecy behind Hardy's bizarre case? Nobody could have predicted it.

I was a second-year medical student when the news emerged. The explosive impact was of no less magnitude than the landmark moon landing or the Kennedy shooting in Dallas. The world's first heart transplant had been done in Cape Town. Christiaan Barnard's handsome profile graced front pages from Scunthorpe to Stanford, much to the disgust of those who had published numerous scientific articles on the subject beforehand. Yet as Barnard repeatedly pointed out, published work is for others to learn from, and in his case, act upon. Not only that, after spending three months with Lower in Richmond, he had gone back to Cape Town and performed forty-nine dog heart transplants himself. Controversially and generating much local criticism, he had also transplanted a kidney from a coloured donor to a white Afrikaans, Edith Black, who survived for thirteen years. So it was difficult to describe him as opportunistic.

Life and death were indeed simpler in South Africa. The law allowed organ harvest if the donor was declared dead by two doctors, one of which had to be qualified for more than five years. Neither should be members of the transplant team. Death itself was not defined in detail and it was possible to use the concept of irreversible brain injury. In that respect the legal issues surrounding organ removal were much more liberal in South Africa than in the USA. Permission to harvest the organs was needed from either the donor's relatives or the coroner.

At this point I should state that my deep insight into the circumstances of the transplant came from Chris Barnard himself, whom I knew well, and from members of his team who were present that night in the operating theatre. On the fiftieth anniversary of the event, long after the surgeon's death, I was asked by the BBC to make a program about the circumstances and succeeded in contacting all those present who were still alive. So my account comes from within the establishment not from what was written about it.

The recipient, Louis Waskansky was a 54-year-old diabetic who had suffered three previous myocardial infarctions, and had an irreparably damaged left ventricle with intractable severe heart failure. All conventional treatment options had been exhausted and his cardiologist Professor Schrire had some weeks before being asked by Barnard to look out for potential transplant candidates. Washkansky's angiograms had even been sent to the Cleveland clinic for consideration of coronary bypass surgery but rejected, Schrire decided to offer him to Barnard on one condition. He insisted that the donor must be white. This emanated from the negative press coverage about Cape coloured's organs being used to save the privileged white community following the kidney transplant on Mrs Black.

In many respects Waskansky was a poor candidate. His diabetes was difficult to control with insulin, he smoked heavily and his abdomen was grossly distended with fluid. Besides that he had spreading infection in both legs where metal tubes had been inserted to drain oedema fluid. Very dangerous for someone whose immune system was about to come under attack.

On the 22nd November, Waskansky's wife Ann was summoned urgently to the hospital because he was being prepared for surgery. A coloured boy had fallen from a lorry and sustained severe head injuries but the intensive care unit staff were nervous about switching off the ventilator to benefit a white patient. Mindful of Schire's feelings on the matter, Barnard called the Afrikaans Attorney General of the Cape who was ambivalent. He simply reiterated that the decision as to when someone was dead enough to become a donor was best left to doctors and side stepped the race card. However, he did confirm that he would not prosecute Barnard whatever the eventual decision. Although the boy's organs were wasted, this opened the door to a safer decision-making process for the surgeons on the next occasion. But it almost cost Washkansky his life. Politics, racial discord and medicine make poor bedfellows.

On the sunny summer afternoon of 2nd December 1967, disconsolate Ann and her sister left Louis in the hospital and set off to drive home. Within five minutes they drove past two badly injured women lying in the road. At 3.40 p.m. Denise Darville and her mother had been hit at high speed by an inebriated police reservist who missed the red light at a crossing. Mrs Darville suffered severe chest injuries and was killed instantly. Denise was hurled through the air and her head smashed against the wheel of a parked car. The base of her skull shattered and blood poured from her ears, nose and mouth. It was group O rhesus negative blood whilst Washkansky was O rhesus positive. They were compatible so Barnard had his donor. Ann drove by shocked but oblivious to the unfolding disaster. For some reason the significance of the tragedy was lost on her.

Edward Darville collapsed in despair outside the emergency room when told that his wife was dead. He was stretchered into the hospital and looked around for his daughter Denise. When he found her she was still moaning and he hoped she might be saved. What he didn't notice was the pulped brain oozing from her right ear. The brain surgeons examining her were pessimistic, so Darville in his distressed state was asked to donate her organs. Denise was a Christian who liked to help others. Under duress therefore, he felt that it was his duty to give permission so that part of his precious daughter would live on.

Schrire had to investigate the heart first. It looked fine on the chest x-ray and the ECG was normal apart from some early changes associated with brain death. With the stethoscope there were no audible murmurs so there was no reason not to take it. At 11 p.m. they alerted Barnard and the rest of the team who were scattered all over the city. They came from fancy-dress parties and romantic dinners for two, whilst others were already in bed. The chief heart-lung technician was rushing in when his car broke down. He ran the remaining kilometre to the hospital.

Chris confessed to being very anxious at that point. Many things were going through his mind. What if the organs are not compatible, or that the family refuse permission to use the heart? What if the heart has been damaged during the accident? Even more concerning – what if she fails to die as the brain surgeons promised? Then when he saw Denise on the hospital trolley he felt a surge of pity. As well as the open skull fracture, she had a fractured pelvis with internal bleeding and a horribly distorted right leg with all its bones shattered. He explained in vivid terms, the disbelief that no one had bothered to straighten the limb or put it in a splint. Everything seemed to be focused on organ donation, nothing on the poor broken victim. Others present that night recall him walking in and out of both donor and recipient operating theatres asking, 'Are you ready yet? Are you ready yet?' He was facing the most critical hours of his career and the sheer magnitude of the challenge did not escape him.

When Peggy Jordaan, the senior theatre sister, walked in on Barnard in the surgeons' changing room, he was on his knees praying audibly. 'God, don't let me make any mistakes. Make me do the best I can. Let me be your favourite son just for a little while. Give me a hand tonight.'

Rodney Hewitson, a first class technical surgeon, was scrubbing up in theatre A, ready to open Washkansky's chest. He had absolutely no experience of the laboratory work and in that sense was totally unprepared. Later he admitted: 'Chris gave the wrong impression that the whole team had been through it together and knew exactly what had to be done.' The petrified Washkansky was still sitting bolt upright on the operating table of theatre A grasping for breath. Joe Ozinsky, the principal anaesthetist had to coax him to lie down so that he could dispatch him into oblivion. Once done, an aura of calm descended over the room. Hewitson said 'you could cut the air with a knife', as he began to open the chest. All that could be heard was the hiss of the ventilator, the sizzle of the electrocautery and the buzz of the saw.

In theatre B the surgeon designated to harvest the heart was Terry O'Donovan, assisted by Barnard's brother, Marius. Poignantly someone had left a bunch of violets in a drinking glass beside Denise's bed. Her dark hair was spread on a clean pillow even though most of her head was heavily bandaged. She looked so young and innocent, the sight upset many of the team who were unaccustomed to the gruesome reality of organ donation. Some asked whether she was really dead. Was it reasonable to remove her heart when it was beating away so strongly? Absolutely not they were told. It would have to stop first.

The accepted definition of death in South Africa was when the heart stopped beating. Consequently O'Donovan refused to lift the scalpel until Denise's ECG flat lined. Marius and Ozinsky both wanted to stop the heart with cold cardioplegia, to preserve the muscle. Barnard concurred with this but O'Donovan with his strong religious beliefs made them hold back. This was a dilemma which should have been sorted out beforehand and was ultimately damaging. For a heart to stop naturally it has to be metabolically damaged and die. Yet no one felt confident enough to mess with the legal system.

The artificial ventilation was switched off by Barnard himself at 02.20 a.m. Then they waited. Ten minutes later the heart still had a regular ECG. At twenty minutes it finally fibrillated and stopped beating. Marius said 'what a shame, we are killing this heart'. And he was right. Yet only then did O'Donovan open the sternum. Clearly a damaged donor heart was a problem for the transplant recipient whereas waiting to flat line had no impact whatever on Denise's future. She was dead anyway.

Newsweek wrote of the moment of death: 'They (the surgeons) will not say whether they took Miss Darville off the respirator before the heart stopped. That's considered to be an impertinent question! They claimed to have taken full resuscitative measures until the time of death.' Of course they did but did anyone believe it?

Marius spoke out honestly afterwards: 'My feelings before the operation were that we should remove this heart in the best condition possible. Our responsibility was to the patient not this girl whose heart was beating but whose brain was dead. The problem on the night was confusion. It hadn't been thought through and ultimately it risked Washkansky's survival.'

Chris described to me the way he felt when removing that small sports car of a donor heart followed by Washkansky's clapped-out wreck of a rubbish truck. He was really concerned that they had waited too long and that Denise's heart would never start again. If so the political fallout would be dire. As he walked through the scrub room which connected the two theatres, Sister Jordaan followed, thinking to herself: 'Whatever you do, don't drop it.' (Later Marius did drop a donor heart on the floor). In order to minimise the time without blood flow the heart was quickly connected to a side line from the heart-lung machine and perfused with Washkansky's blood. At first purple and cold in the kidney dish, it finally began to beat. Feebly at first but stronger with time.

The practice of sewing together similar-sized dog hearts in the laboratory was hardly preparation for the extreme donor-recipient size mismatch. A tennis ball replacing a rugby ball with a garden hose connected to drain pipes. Tense surgeons, taxing operation, and total silence in the room. Apart that is from the quiet hum of swivelling blood pumps and the surgeons' heavy breathing. The huffing and puffing ventilator was switched off during cardiopulmonary bypass. Every so often the anaesthetists would quietly pass on blood results to the perfusionists. Curious night staff alerted on the grapevine stared down through the condensation of the glass-domed viewing gallery, scarcely believing what they were witnessing.

Chris had described the events of that night on innumerable occasions, but one thing he rarely mentioned was the perfusion accident. Geraldine 'Dene' Friedmann, a young trainee perfusionist and personal friend of Barnard's daughter Deirdre, told me the story years later. In those days it was customary to pump blood to the body from the heart-lung machine through a plastic tube inserted into the main leg artery in the groin. It happened that Washkansky was a severe arteriopath and his femoral arteries were occluded by fatty atheromatous plaques. Hewitson hadn't been warned of this when he originally inserted the cannula and Chris hadn't checked the lines himself because he was removing the donor heart in theatre B.

As they prepared to remove Washkansky's quivering heart Chris instructed the chief perfusionist Johan van Heerden to 'Go on, bypass'. Blood drained from the venae cavae into the circuit and was in turn pushed on by a roller pump towards the diseased femoral artery. But this was virtually blocked. Young Dene was calling out the pressure in the arterial line to van Heerden. Up and up it went to alarmingly high levels until Ozinsky screamed at Barnard to stop the pump. Realising that he would have to switch the cannula from the diseased femoral artery to aorta above the heart, the surgeon instructed Sister Jordaan to clamp the arterial line, which she did. But in the panic of the situation, no one said 'pump off' to the perfusionist. With the flow still at 4.5 litres per minute, the occluded line pressure rose precipitously, and the circuit burst open at the connector. Suddenly bright red blood sprayed around the operating theatre like a fire hose prompting the circulating nurses to rush for mops and buckets. Alarming to say the least at that stage of the adventure.

According to Dene: 'Barnard stood resolute, cold as steel and completely in command of the situation.' He shouted 'pump off' and quickly clamped the venous drainage pipe to avoid more blood loss. But now there was an air lock in the circuit which could cause a massive stroke if the pump was turned on again. Washkansky had no circulation at this point but Chris calmly joined the disconnected arterial and venous pipes together so the circuit could be refilled with donor blood and de-aired until safe. The system was restored and bypass established again within the critical four minutes of brain vulnerability. Otherwise Washkansky would have suffered significant neurological injury. New heart, buggered brain, piss poor publicity. This operation could never had been kept secret.

It was an episode that Barnard would repeatedly blank out when explaining to everyone how well prepared the team were and how the whole procedure went like clockwork. Others were less sanguine. As Dene put it: 'Johan and I found the experience terrifying. We had shaking knees until everything was under control again. When Chris quietly asked Peggy Jordaan why she had done such a stupid thing, she replied, 'But you told me to, Sir!'

The sight of an empty pericardium without a heart was strange indeed. Like a car without an engine under the bonnet. At the time Hitchcock was more impressed by the rapid pulsations in Barnard's neck. He had a heart rate twice normal through the sheer stress of it all. He was pouring adrenaline, the same hormone that Denise Darville's heart would need to propel Washkansky from the bypass machine.

By 05.43 a.m. the final stitch lines were complete but the neat little donor heart looked lost in Washkansky's capacious pericardium. The cross clamp on the aorta was released to allow warm blood back into the flaccid organ which soon started to squirm in ventricular fibrillation. At 05.52 a.m. the defibrillating paddles were gently squeezed onto it. The first 20 Joule shock caused electrical standstill. Yet the power was sufficient to stiffen Washkansky's spinal muscles and jolt his body from the table. More to the point, Denise's heart soon began to flap about like a goldish in a bowl. Barnard gave the order to 'leave some blood in' her circulation and partially clamped the venous pipe. As the pulsating organ visibly expanded, Ozinsky noted flickering on the arterial pressure trace. The new left ventricle, just one fifth the size of the old one, began to eject blood against the flow of the heart-lung machine. An encouraging sign.

The first attempt to wean from the bypass machine failed. Washkansky's blood pressure drifted down as Denise's little heart distended like a balloon. Anxiety rippled around the room and rained down from the viewing gallery. Was this the price for waiting too long for the heart to stop? Perhaps. But given ten more minutes of supportive perfusion the heart looked better, so an impatient and tiring Barnard tried to come off again. It was still too soon and failed once more. Someone suggested that the struggling piece of meat may have suffered blunt injury in the accident? Having relaxed once the heart was sewn in, the operating theatre became extraordinarily tense again.

Ozinsky gave a shot of calcium, then a potassium infusion, and finally turned up the stimulant drug isoprenaline. At 06.13 a.m. they attempted to discontinue cardiopulmonary bypass for the third time. No one dared speak but this time the left and right ventricles continued to pump. Not exactly powerful but good enough. The blood pressure held at a miserable 70 mm Hg for a few minutes then started to improve spontaneously. Ozinsky and Barnard stared hopefully at the screen. As the African dawn broke over Table Mountain the fog began to clear in theatre A. Four short words from Barnard shattered the bleak silence, 'Jesus, dit gaan werk!' The translation from Afrikaans is obvious. A wave of relief swept through the theatre and viewing room. This was history in the making.

As one of the nurses hugged Barnard his face lit up with sheer exhilaration. He had been desperate to be first and had done it. An onlooker in the gallery later confessed: 'The atmosphere was fantastic. I felt slightly hysterical and hardly dared breathe. The tension was terrific.'

But this wasn't the end, it was only the beginning as Washkansky's white blood cells met the foreign proteins in Darville's heart. The macrophages and lymphocytes took note of the intruder and told the bone marrow to get moving. Irrespective of the optimistic cross match, this heart was like a rat in a hornets nest. The hornets would immediately try to get rid of it.

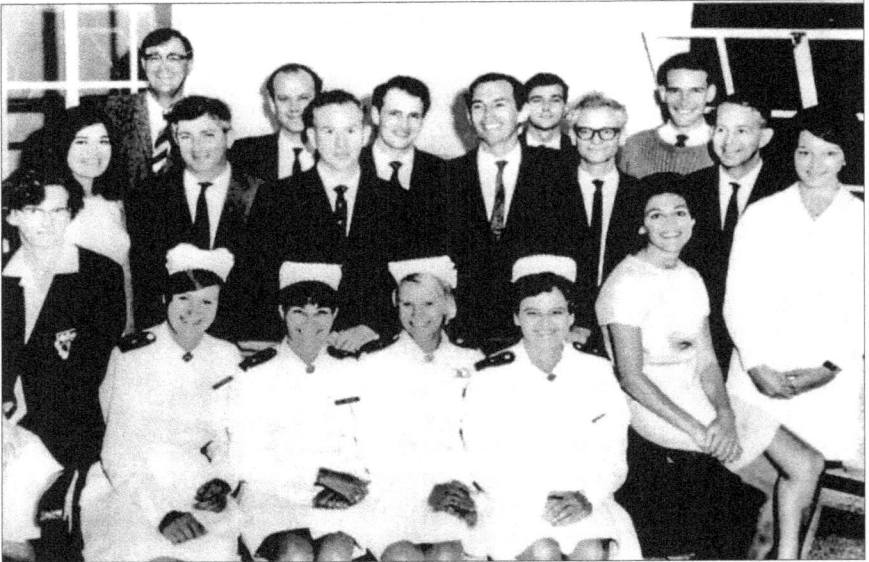

Fig 11.2 A. Barnard and his team on the steps of Groote Schuur Hospital.

Barnard left Hewitson and Hitchcock to close the chest and went for a cigarette. Brother Marius joined him in the surgeons' room and recorded his pulse rate at 140 beats per minute. Two calls were made. The first woke the hospital's medical superintendent with the short sentence: 'Sir, we have just transplanted a heart and the patient is well.' Next was a call to Lapa Munoik of the Executive Council for Health for the Cape, as a result of which the Prime Minister, John Vorster knew about the transplant within the hour. After that Chris talked with his wife Louwtje who had little insight that this spelt the end for her marriage. Within hours the world's press descended upon Cape Town. Their first question – did the donor heart come from a black or white person?

The post-operative care was meticulous. After the perfusion incident it was a relief to see Washkansky open his eyes again. Immunosuppression was started on the day of surgery with steroids and azathioprine. Cobalt irradiation was applied to the heart on the fifth, seventh and ninth post-operative days. He was kept in isolation within the operating theatre for the first days to minimise the infection risk.

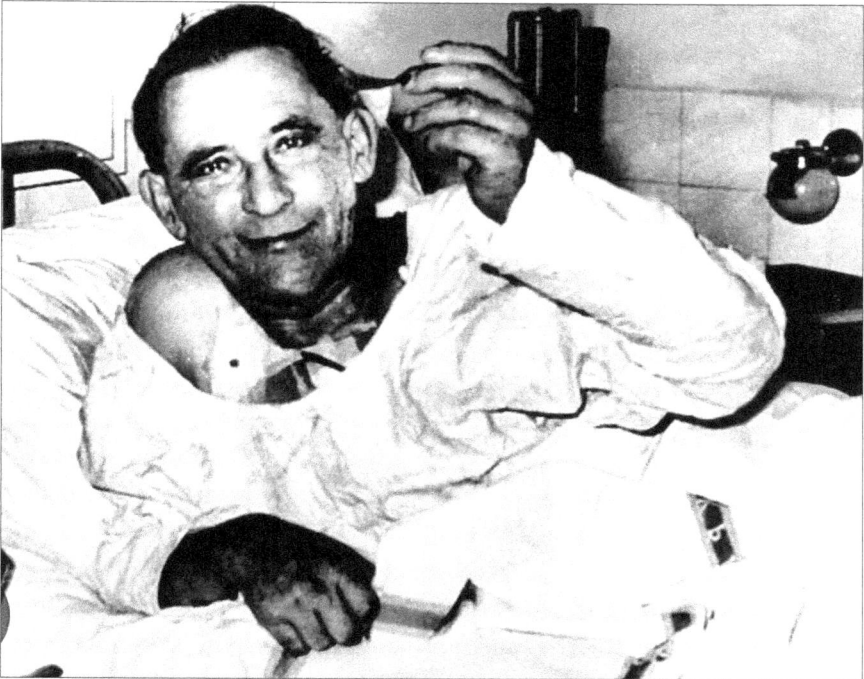

Fig 11.2 B. Louis Washkansky recovering whilst nursed in the operating theatre.

For those charged with looking after Washkansky this was a voyage of exploration. 'Worrying' might be a better word. The first anxiety was an abnormal and rapid heart rhythm which they treated with digoxin. But life was different for Louis too. He told Ann: 'When I woke up I could breathe again. I was not gasping for air. I could breathe because my heart was fixed up.' In fact Louis' heart was already pickled in a jar of formalin. It was Denise's youthful organ that made him feel good. Their two hearts now sit side by side on display in the museum at Groote Schuur Hospital.

By suppressing the immune system to avoid rejection the risk of infection is inevitably increased. Those visiting or attending him had to wear protective clothing and bacteriological samples were taken from all over his body on a daily basis. The initial effects of the transplant were remarkable. His kidneys passed gallons of fluid and the grossly oedematous legs and liver shrank down. The diabetes was easier to control and he could breathe without panting.

Then on the third post-operative day swabs from his mouth and nostrils grew a particularly dangerous organism called Klebsiella. Twenty-four hours later he was mildly febrile with a raised white blood cell count of 28,000, more than four times normal. To add to the difficulties, there was an obvious drop in the voltage of the electrocardiogram from 15 to 9 millivolts. Barnard was aware of a report by Shumway which correlated rapid heart rate and decreased ECG voltage with organ rejection in dogs. Because there were no overt signs of infection, such as a swinging fever, an inflamed surgical wound or chest x-ray signs of pneumonia, the team decided to increase the immunosuppression. The raised steroid dosage immediately made Louis feel much better, but it worsened his diabetes, a secondary risk factor for infection. Then sure enough the ECG voltage improved again, so it looked as if the problem was rejection. It was expected

The following week was filled with optimism and excitement, for both Barnard and the Washkansky family. Perhaps injudiciously the strict quarantine was relaxed. International journalists flew in and television crews besieged the hospital. On the twelfth post-operative day he was visited by a South African government official and interviewed by Stern, CBS and BBC television. The BBC reporter was crass beyond belief. His two questions were 'what is it like to be famous', and 'how does it feel to have a female heart?' Frankly, Louis wasn't well enough to answer.

During that night he complained of griping abdominal pain. Besides that he was sleep-deprived and worn out by the constant questioning. The team had concerns about pancreatitis or a duodenal ulcer because of the high doses of steroids, then the following morning the chest x-ray showed a shadow on the left lung. He felt generally unwell and spiked another temperature.

On Saturday 16th December, the thirteenth post-operative day, Washkansky's pulse and blood pressure remained stable but his temperature soared to 103.5°F and his breathing was laboured. He developed pain in the left chest and the x-ray now showed what appeared to be pneumonia in both lungs. This time, culture of the sputum grew the bacterium pneumococcus. The physicians suggested that the lung shadowing could be from blood clots breaking off from his leg veins – pulmonary emboli. So to cover both bases the daily ward round decided to prescribe the anticoagulant heparin together with high doses of penicillin to which the pneumococcus was sensitive. By now Washkansky felt terrible so for the first time the cameras were kept away.

Monday 18th December, now the fifteenth post-operative day, and penicillin hasn't helped. The white blood cell count and temperature remain elevated. Louis won't talk or eat and is now incontinent. The same caring nurses remain with him constantly, whether on duty or not, because they know that he is sinking fast. Barnard is concerned that the chest x-ray shows transplant lung not infection. In desperation he orders more aggressive anti-rejection therapy whilst appreciating that this will further reduce any chance Louis has to combat infection.

I asked Chris why he didn't take the bull by the horns and biopsy the lungs. If it was infection they would have found the bacteria. If it was rejection they would have identified those characteristic lymphocytes that attack the tissues. Easy for me to suggest this thirty years later when transplantation was routine. His answer was that they were overtaken by septic shock before registering the fact that Washkansky was dying. On the following morning his blood pressure fell precipitously, and the white blood cell count plummeted from 22,200 to 6,000. Both his feet and hands were cold and mottled. This was total body failure now. In the end Denise Darville's heart was the best thing about him. It kept pumping on whilst the rest of his body disintegrated.

Blood donors were brought in to provide fresh white blood cells but it was all too late. Soon the chest x-ray showed widespread consolidation in both lungs. A complete white out. There was nothing left to breathe with and he was put back on a ventilator.

Barnard assembled an experienced team of cardiologists, bacteriologist, haematologists, immunologists and radiologists in a desperate last ditch attempt to turn the ship around. They went round in circles. It could be infection or it might be an immunological complication. The haematologists favoured infection. Under the microscope they saw toxic changes in the white blood cells but where were the bacteria in the sputum? With the severity of the chest x-ray changes the bronchial secretions should be teeming with organisms. The consensus was that it must be transplant lung, something rare that none of them had seen before. So they prescribed even more hefty doses of immunosuppressive drugs.

On Wednesday twentieth December the hospital Christmas parties were in full swing, but not for the cardiac team. Chris received a call from bacteriology. 'Professor, I think you'd better come over right away. We have just grown Klebsiella and pseudomonas from yesterday's sputum samples. We are certain that he has pneumonia.' It happened that Klebsiella had been detected in his nose and mouth several days before. There it did no harm, but in immunosuppressed lungs it was devastating. Both bacteria were sensitive to a specific cocktail of antibiotics but not to the penicillin prescribed.

A desperate rearguard action followed. High doses of targeted antibiotics, an increase in ventilation pressure, then high doses of isoprenaline to support the circulation. Still the oxygen levels in his blood continued to fall. Both lungs were teeming with an infection that he had no white blood cells left to flight. Denise's heart kept supplying the blood but there was little oxygen to carry. In a last-ditch effort they considered putting him on the heart-lung machine but Schrire and Ozinsky knew that to be fruitless. During a 03.00 a.m. phone call Schrire who had referred Louis in the first place, made his feelings clear.' Listen Chris, Washkansky is clinically lost. Everybody knows it except you.'

Thursday 21st December at 05.00 a.m. Septic shock completely wiped out Washkansky's blood pressure. His blood is black through lack of oxygen yet the donor heart is as slow to die as it was in Denise. Finally it went into fibrillation and intensive care sister Papendieck started to cry. Most of the dedicated nursing team were weeping, not because they had lost the world's first heart transplant but because they cared about Louis, the way it should be. Then a whole nation's pride turned to despair.

There had to be an autopsy, after which Barnard addressed the world's media. It was a simple statement. 'Louis Washkansky, the first man to live with a transplanted human heart, died this morning at Groote Schuur hospital in Cape Town. He lived eighteen days with the heart of a 25-year-old girl.' By now everyone knew that he had been lost through a diagnostic error and too many anti-rejection drugs.

The autopsy revealed that lungs, chronically damaged by smoking, now oozed with blue green pus. The little heart lay blue and dead floating on old blood in the capacious pericardial sac. Remarkably there was no sign whatever of organ rejection. No myocardial swelling or lymphocyte cell infiltration. They were confronted with the fact that with the correct diagnosis the death was entirely preventable. Too many interviews at the expense of clinical focus? It was a learning experience at best, yet devastation would rapidly revert to determination. It's what cardiac surgeons do. Bury the dead and move on.

Three days after the Cape Town operation Adrian Kantrowitz took the tiny heart of a severely brain-deformed infant and implanted it into a 2-day-old baby doomed by a hypoplastic left heart. The child died on the operating table but the floodgates were now open. Barnard's next candidate, Phillip Blaiberg was already in the hospital.

Even before Washkansky's death an international panel of prominent cardiac surgeons assembled in the Plaza Hotel in New York to discuss the ethical implications of the Cape Town experience. Charles Bailey who had dabbled in transplantation himself, declared the operation to be ten years premature. Jacob Zimmerman a colleague of Bailey's at St Barnabas Hospital agreed, adding: 'It is medically and morally wrong for doctors to stand by a dying patient's bedside hoping he will get it over with quickly so we can grab his organs.' In contrast, Donald Ross, a former classmate of Barnard in South Africa, together with Ake Senning from Sweden, both said they would perform transplants and were optimistic that 'heart banks' would be established where a supply of on-demand organs could be stored.

In Houston Michael DeBakey set up a committee to deliberate whether Baylor should begin transplanting whilst Cooley immediately set out to find donors.

Virtually as soon as Washkansky had died the television company CBS brought Chris and Louwtjie to New York City for their *Face the Nation* show.

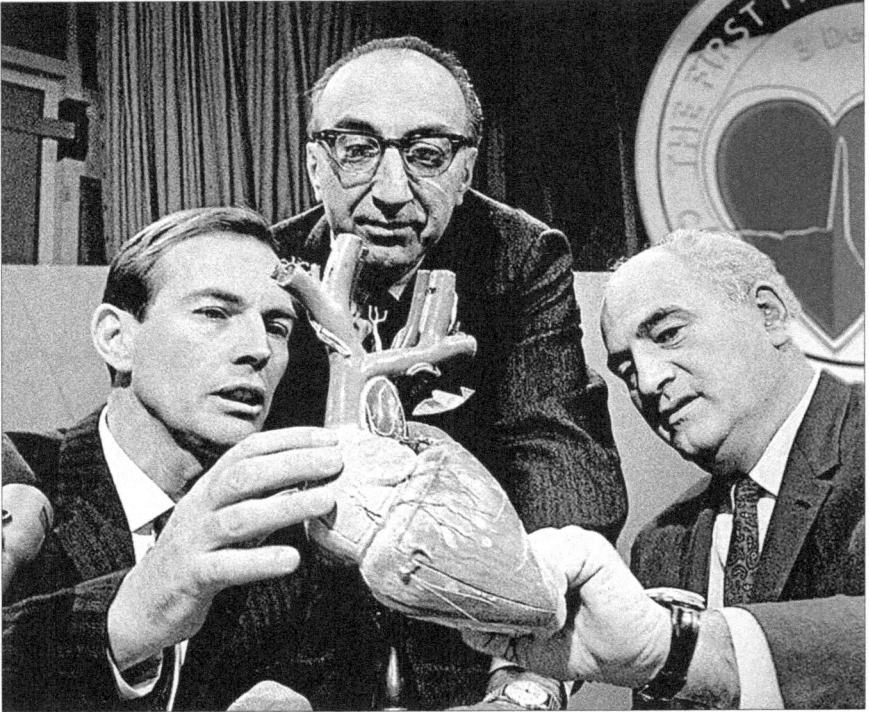

Fig 11.3 Barnard with DeBakey and Kantrowitz in New York.

There he succeeded in dismissing accusations of stealing Shumway's ideas and unexpectedly received praise from both Cooley and DeBakey for making the political breakthrough. Shumway eventually commented begrudgingly on the brain death issue stating that: 'It was a monumental advance, more societal than medical because it applied to all organ transplants.' Sour grapes dismissed, CBS took the pair on to Texas to meet President Lyndon B. Johnson at his ranch.

Immediately on return to Cape Town, Barnard carried out his second and more successful transplant on the local dentist Philip Blaiberg, using the heart of a black man. It seemed that fame had instantly overcome the controversial race issues, though the operation on 2nd January was no less dramatic or controversial than Washkansky's. Clive Haupt was a 24-year-old factory worker who had suffered a massive cerebral haemorrhage whilst sunbathing on a Cape Town beach. When his condition was declared hopeless he was transferred from Victoria Hospital to Groote Schuur pending the transplant.

This time the American television network NBC had signed a $50,000 deal with the Blaibergs for exclusive rights to film the surgery, but Barnard was struggling with a flare-up of his arthritis. As he threw the final stitch to secure the new heart the hospital suffered a catastrophic power cut shutting off the operating lights, the heart-lung machine and the movie cameras. The pumps had to be hand-cranked to keep Blaiberg alive until the auxiliary generator kicked in. Nevertheless the operation transformed Blaiberg from a breathless 'cardiac cripple' to an independent man, able to drive a car and swim in the sea. He spent 73 days in the hospital but then survived for eighteen months before chronic organ rejection caught up with him.

This second landmark operation gave the world's press the ammunition they had waited for. In London, the Daily Mail announced that what remained of the black donor's body would be buried in the non-white section of a segregated cemetery. But if it was of any consolation to the young man's widow his heart would rest in a white man's grave. That would be the nearest Clive would ever become to being a first class citizen in South Africa. I read that in 1968 and thought what a load of rubbish. And they were wrong. The heart was pickled in a jar of formalin for the Groote Schuur museum – just like Washkansky's two hearts. You can still visit them. What's more, when Barnard compassionately attended the donor's funeral he was mobbed by thousands of blacks who tried to touch, kiss or talk with him. Adoration was what he received not hostility.

On January 6th 1968, just four days after the Blaiberg operation, Norman Shumway transplanted the heart of 43-year-old Virginia May White into a 54-year-old steelworker, Mike Casparak.

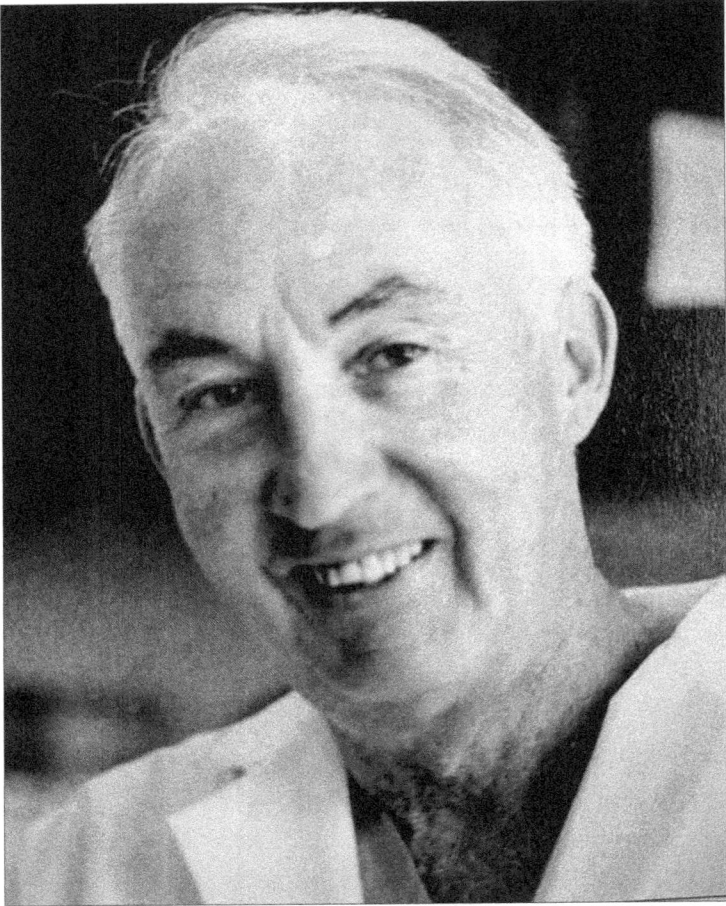

Fig 11.4 Norman Shumway.

Mrs White had collapsed with a cerebral haemorrhage during celebrations for her 22nd wedding anniversary whilst Casparak was dying from viral myocarditis. Misfortune dogged the operation from the start. First the heart sizes were a serious mismatch causing technical difficulties. Then the recipient suffered post-operative bleeding requiring further surgery. As a result his kidneys and liver failed and he suffered a large gastrointestinal bleed. A staggering total of 288 pints of transfused blood were used, then he required kidney dialysis. On the eighth post-operative day he underwent removal of an inflamed gall bladder under local anaesthetic but lapsed into liver failure with coma and died on 21st January. The hospital bill of $28,845 caused a barrage of criticism from many who felt the money could have been better spent. This was an unfortunate start for the surgeon who had done more than anyone in background research.

Within three weeks of the second transplant and with Blaiberg still in hospital, Chris was on tour again. This time he was travelling through Europe, accompanied by Louwtjie. That didn't stop him being photographed in a compromising position with Sophia Loren in Italy and having a passionate fling with Gina Lollobrigida who rapidly succumbed to his magnetic charms. I first saw him when he presented in London. On his first public appearance he and Louwtjie posed for photographs in Trafalgar Square when a pigeon landed on his head and did what pigeons tend to do. The pictures adorned the front pages the following day. Typically the BBC arranged a programme entitled *Barnard faces his critics*, the automatic inference being that the transplant was a trigger for abuse not praise. And this was clearly the message from the hostile surgical fraternity in Britain. Leading doctors wrote open letters to the *New Scientist* and *British Medical Journal* accusing him of ignoring the risk of organ rejection and shamelessly seeking publicity. In *The Times* the cartoonist Gerald Scarfe depicted Barnard as a sharp-beaked African vulture ripping the heart from the chest of a living patient.

Yet some surgeons took a more positive view. Russell Brock praised Barnard's courage for bringing heart transplantation into the clinical arena. So did my old mentor Roy Calne who was destined to make the next big step in anti-rejection therapy. But the curtain fell on the criticism with an act of pure theatre. Donald Longmore, a surgical associate of Donald Ross at the National Heart Hospital, pushed in a wheelchair-bound heart failure patient, Bill Bradley, causing the raucous audience to fall silent. Panting for breath and with visibly swollen legs and abdomen the man gasped that he would accept a transplant without question should a donor become available. That was the key phrase unfortunately.

As a humble medical student at the Charing Cross Hospital on Strand, I tentatively raised my hand from the back of the room, and when invited to speak made this provocative comment. 'I wish all this had happened sooner for the sake of my own family. But how can a treatment that needs someone else to die first ever become mainstream?' Perhaps the audacity to make that statement in austere company later led to both Calne and Ross eventually taking me on as a trainee.

The floodgates were now open. Kantrowitz had already attempted another paediatric transplant in New York. The operation took longer than the patient survived and he gave up. Sen in Bombay had a go and lost the patient on the operating table. Then Cabrol at the Hôpital de la Pitié in Paris transplanted a truck driver who died without gaining consciousness. Bizarrely, Ross conceived a different approach which could only end in disaster. He planned to save the patient using a pig's heart implanted alongside the patient's own failing organ. A booster pump so to speak, but the plan backfired when the feisty beast bolted and ran through the streets of central London in the early hours of the morning. Longmore chased the porcine athlete in hot pursuit but a senior nurse was awakened in her hospital accommodation by the high-pitched squeals. Having complained bitterly of the outrage to the hospital management she found a plate of pork chops on her doorstep the following morning. And of course the operation when it did happen was a farce. The patient died within an hour of separating from the heart-lung machine and the experience was not repeated in London. That is not to say that others wouldn't pursue pig hearts.

On 3rd May 1968, Ross at the National Heart Hospital and Cooley at St Luke's in Houston, performed their first human heart transplants on the same day, both surrounded by intense media coverage. It was easy for journalists to question the surgeons' motives. As one newspaper put it: 'They seemed to be working in competition with each other using a high-risk expensive procedure for the gratification of their own egos.' In his forthright and honest manner, Cooley revealed his own thoughts on the matter. 'My first concern was saving the lives of sick people, but it would be untrue to say that I was not eager to take part in this, the most exciting development in cardiac surgery. The delay of my entry into heart transplantation is easily explained. We couldn't find any donors, and we suspected that they were being purposefully denied us.' That said, the Texas Heart Institute would soon overtake the experience of all other centres combined.

Forty-seven-year old Everett Thomas had been bedridden for five months with rheumatic valve disease before Cooley met him. He also had blindness and paralysis following blood clots to the brain. The only conventional surgical option was a high-risk triple valve replacement which Cooley scheduled for 3rd May. But on 1st May a fifteen-year-old girl, Katherine Martin, was offered as a transplant donor after a self-inflicted gunshot wound to the brain. Coincidentally, Cooley had operated on her to repair a coarctation of the aorta six years before and she still had a thickened powerful left ventricle in response to that condition. Whilst explaining the substantial risks of the conventional operation to the Thomas family, Cooley proposed a heart transplant as backup in the event that he could not be weaned from the bypass machine.

On the day of the surgery, Thomas and the potential donor were brought to adjacent operating theatres and from then onwards the outcome was somewhat predictable. Cooley's colleague Grady Hallman removed the donor heart without cooling or myocardial protection. It just kept on beating as it was implanted into Thomas, taking little more than half an hour. And it functioned well despite the size discrepancy with the recipient's huge heart.

Ross's case was not as straightforward. Nor was it the poor man that Longmore had wheeled into Barnard's lecture. He was already dead. Frederick West had chronic severe heart failure at the age of forty-five and was desperate for a new life. The previous day in South London a 26-year-old building worker, Patrick Ryan, sustained a severe head injury when a concrete slab fell on his head. He was taken to King's College Hospital for urgent brain surgery but the damage was deemed irrecoverable.

During the afternoon of the 3rd May Ross had the ventilated patient transferred across the Thames to the National Heart Hospital, but he suffered a cardiac arrest *en route* and needed external cardiac massage. A good bashing was the last thing the donor heart needed; yet West initially recovered after the transplant. One person who played a vital role in that was the recently appointed anaesthetist Alan Gilston. Such was his dedication that he spent the whole night of the operation sleeping alongside West who was kept in the operating theatre.

The day after the transplant, photographs of Ross and the surgical team posing proudly on the front steps of the hospital, graced all the front pages.

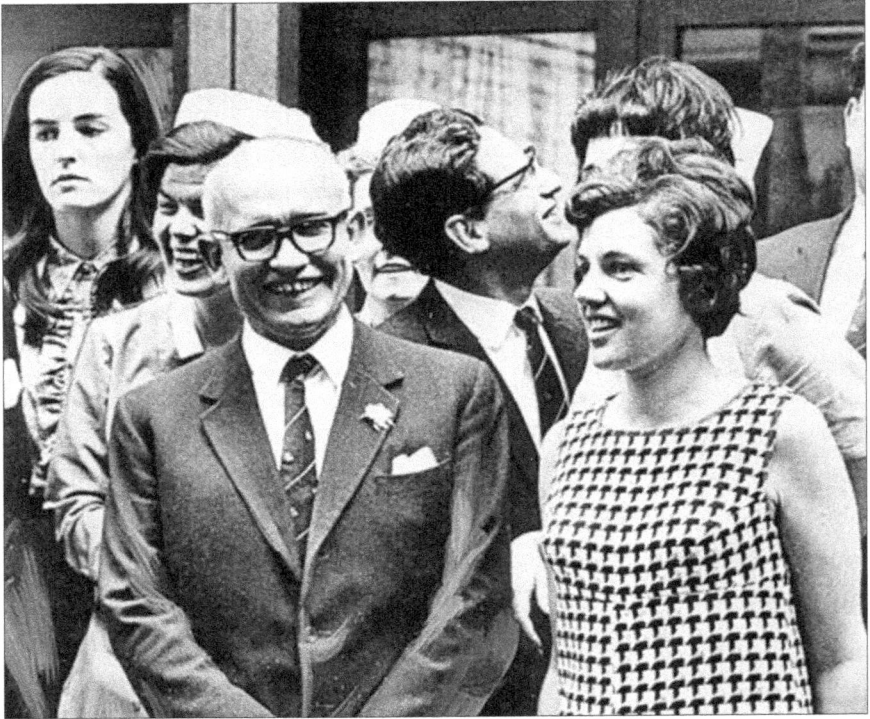

Fig 11.5 A. Ross with Jane Sommerville and his team
outside The National Heart Hospital.

Yet the responses were not always congratulatory. *The Times* article headlined 'British Heart Transplant May Be Too Early'. And true to form, West died from blood clots to the lungs forty-five days later.

The *Guardian* newspaper quoted consultant cardiologist Dr Donald Scott who used the words 'almost amounting to cannibalism' to describe the heart procurement process. Others were outrageous enough to suggest Ryan with his battered brain had been abandoned against his interest in order to take the heart. The malign inquest was heard in front of a jury and once again, it was Longmore who provided the impact. Threatened with the verdict 'unlawful killing' Longmore theatrically produced Ryan's smashed skull from a briefcase insisting that the original accident had pulped his brain and killed him. Shock, horror! Returning a verdict of accidental death the coroner accepted the transferring doctors' account of cardiac arrest and therefore death in the back of the ambulance.

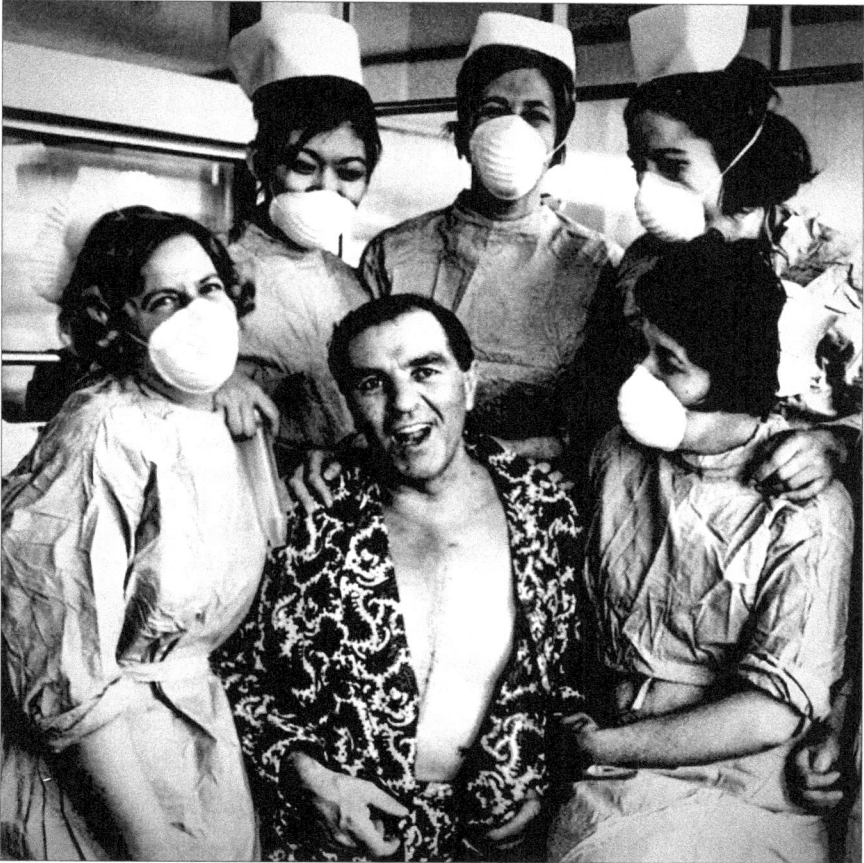

Fig 11.5 B. Fred West with his nurses.

After the Thomas case, Cooley performed two more transplants in Houston during the next forty-eight hours hours. The second donor was the 15-year-old son of a personal friend of Cooley's and the recipient a Houston hospital administrator. The next was a homicide victim whose heart was used irrespective of the fact that the County Medical Examiner expressly refused permission. Cooley simply claimed the victim met the legal criteria for death and proceeded. Whilst both recipients died within the week, Thomas eventually recovered to be discharged from hospital in good condition. He was one of the few successful transplants of the first tranche. And one thing was clear, the laws governing organ donation had to be sorted out.

On 5th August 1968, delegates attending the World Medical Assembly produced an influential document called *The Declaration of Sydney*. Fundamentally this recognised the concept of brain death, acknowledging that all other organs could continue to function as long as the heart kept beating. On the very same day Harvard University published a persuasive report requesting that a new definition of death relating to the central nervous system should be enshrined in law. In other words, dead brain, dead patient, organ donation allowed. Harvard stated that brain death could be confirmed if the patient was unresponsive, with fixed dilated pupils and absent reflexes. Under those circumstances, and only under those circumstances, could supportive treatment with the ventilator be withdrawn.

In the meantime the hotels in Houston filled with patients pleading for transplants whilst donor hearts remained scarce. On one occasion a sheep's heart was implanted into a dying 58-year-old man and rejected so rapidly that there was no time to resort to the pig heart held in reserve. On 17th August Cooley took the heart of an 8-year-old boy with severe head injuries and transplanted it into a 5-year-old girl with congenital heart disease. Besides Kantrowitz's abortive efforts, this was the first paediatric heart transplant though miserably she died in less than a week. Not to be outdone, at the Methodist Hospital, down the street, Michael DeBakey's colleague Ted Dietrich orchestrated a transplant fest from a single teenage suicide victim. On 31st August, the heart, a single lung and both kidneys were harvested from the victim and given to four separate recipients. All survived. The newspaper headlines read 'DeBakey team of sixty performs multiple transplant'.

So dismal were the results in general, however, that enthusiasm for heart transplantation waned rapidly. Sure it was technically possible but for most candidates it was actually shortening life. In December 1970 the American Heart Association reported that of 166 recorded operations in the previous two years, only 23 patients were still alive. The cover of *Life Magazine* in

September 1971 ran the story line: 'The tragic record of Heart Transplants: A new report on an era of medical failure'. The author had shadowed patients in Houston reporting that besides prohibitive early death rates, survivors suffered dreadfully from the side effects of immunosuppression. And they did, but the hopes of thousands of heart failure patients had been raised then dashed. In Britain Sir George Godber, England's Chief Medical Officer, insisted upon a moratorium on all heart transplants.

In the USA there was general agreement that further attempts should be restricted to established renal transplant centres with a research infrastructure. Such departments could ensure state of the art tissue typing and immunosuppressive therapy and cope with the two prominent causes of death, infection and rejection. These criteria favoured Shumway's unit at Stanford, Lower in Richmond, Virginia, and both the Baylor and Texas Heart Institute teams, though the latter never did transplant kidneys.

Barnard, needless to say, continued relentlessly in Cape Town achieving some of the best long-term results. In 1974 he began a programme using the donor heart as an accessory to the patient's failing organ, on the basis that two hearts were better than one. And interestingly, provided with support the patient's own heart function often improved. Over the next six years he performed thirty such implants without a death, achieving 60% one-year survival. These encouraging results were partly because rejection of the auxiliary donor heart didn't immediately kill the patient.

Early recognition of rejection was the key to a boost in immunosuppression but whilst it relied upon white blood cell counts, ECG changes and overall heart function, the diagnosis was often in doubt. That all changed in 1972, when a young surgeon, Philip Caves from Glasgow, took a fellowship with Shumway and devised a catheter-based device to biopsy the transplanted heart directly. This was introduced through the jugular vein in the neck and into the right ventricle to take a small bite of muscle. Examined under the microscope in the pathology laboratory these biopsies would immediately warn of rejection and have remained the standard means to monitor immunosuppressive therapy.

Caves returned to Glasgow as Professor of Cardiac Surgery but unfortunately had a family history of high cholesterol and premature coronary artery disease. In his mid-thirties he suffered a fatal heart attack whilst playing squash, tragically terminating what should have been a brilliant career.

The next advance came from a fungus found in soil, in a remarkable discovery that echoed the chance finding of penicillin. First isolated by the Microbiology department of Sandoz Laboratories, the substance cyclosporin A, was shown to directly inhibit the key blood cells responsible for the rejection process. Roy Calne and co-workers at Addenbrooke's Hospital, Cambridge then confirmed the ability of cyclosporin A to prevent the rejection of transplanted hearts in pigs and showed it to be sufficiently non-toxic to justify human trials. I was his registrar in 1978 when he first prescribed it in kidney transplant recipients and it certainly damped down the rejection process. Moreover it selectively spared other key parts of the immune system leaving it sufficiently competent to fight infection.

Within ten years, experienced centres that carried out more than fifty heart transplants each year, and used the powerful combination of cyclosporin A, azathioprine and steroid immunosuppression, were able to report a five-year survival rate of 80%. A massive turnaround. Progress sufficient to rekindle the miracle that was cardiac transplantation, but not always by the conventional route.

Baboons were plentiful in South Africa. Barnard saw a use for them and had a few on standby. In October 1977 the opportunity arose when a young woman couldn't be weaned from the bypass machine after a valve operation. Under the circumstances there was nothing to lose by trying the primate heart as an assist device, implanted with the same operative technique as the heterotopic heart transplants he had employed since 1974. Barnard argued that it might buy time until a human donor was found and, despite furious opposition from his brother Marius, went ahead with the attempt. The woman died when both hearts gave up a few hours later. He tried again a few weeks later, this time opting for a chimpanzee heart but the patient died after four days. Even so, others remained tempted to use animal organs given the paucity of human donors.

At Loma Linda in California Leonard Bailey had a laboratory research programme looking into the exchange of organs between different species or xenotransplantation. By now Ross, Cooley and Barnard had all tried it with dismal results but Bailey succeeded in keeping a goat alive with a sheep's heart for five months. He believed that the substantial improvements in immunosuppression justified further attempts but that the best chance of success would be in infancy before the mature immune system had a chance to develop.

In 1984 a paediatric cardiologist colleague of Bailey's presented the case of Stephanie Fae Beauclair born days previously with a hypoplastic left heart and whose main pumping chamber was virtually absent. The prognosis for the child was dismal since conventional corrective surgery was rarely successful in those days.

Bailey met with the parents for a frank discussion on the issues.

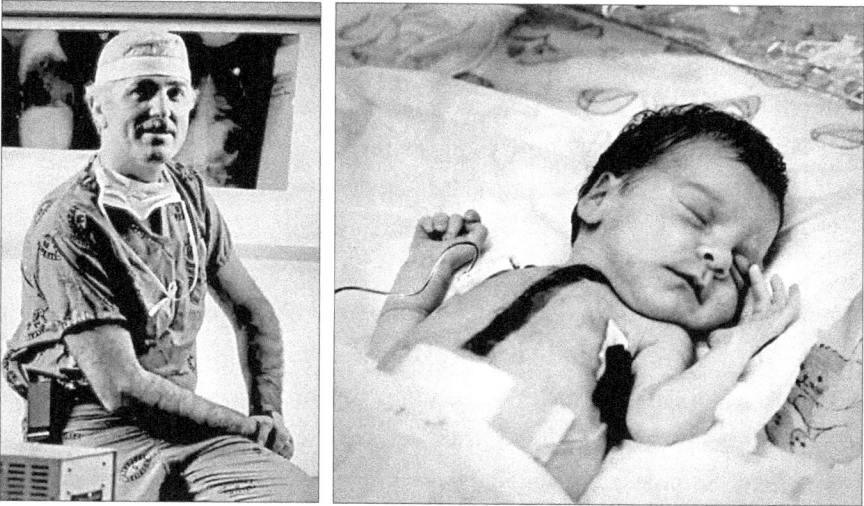

Fig 11.6 A. Leonard Bailey. B. Baby Fae.

The limited prospects with conventional surgery were reiterated and the possibility of a xenotransplant being their best hope explained in some detail. Did the parents understand the implications of the approach? We don't know but they willingly consented to the procedure. Anyone would have done the same for their child, and allegedly serum from the baboon had triggered less adverse reaction in the baby than samples from the parents.

Switching the hearts of new-born babies is always technically challenging but is the least of the problems faced in transplantation. Baby Fae received a tiny baboon heart, survived the operation and for the next week there was intense media coverage. At the end of that time her mother was able to hold and feed her and an element of optimism pervaded the medical centre. Early rejection was predicted and every effort made to combat the process. But in the end nature triumphed over hope and the inflamed lymphocyte infiltrated muscle gave up at three weeks. Every single xeno-transplant had been a disaster. Every new wave of optimism dashed, and so it would go on. It is the same forty years later.

Then came shock and anger when Bailey was confronted as to whether he had sought a human donor. He hadn't. He defended himself by stating that the new-born's immune system, was expected to tolerate an animal organ and claimed there was little sign of rejection at autopsy. Then someone pointed out that a potential human donor had indeed been available on the day. And Eric Rose at Columbia Presbyterian Hospital in New York had succeeded with a paediatric transplant just days before. So the animal rights folk had a field day. They picketed Bailey's hospital with placards stating 'Ghoulish tinkering is not science'.

Meanwhile Stanford remained resolute in its conventional efforts. With the use of cyclosporin, cardiac transplants were firmly established so attention turned to using both heart and lungs together. Many conditions such as cystic fibrosis and congenital heart disease affect both organs and whilst the surgery sounds daunting it is no more taxing than isolated cardiac transplantation. Shumway's associate, Bruce Reitz had achieved long-term survivors with monkeys in the laboratory, some treated with cyclosporin living for five years. Additionally, it was reasonably believed that rejection episodes would affect both organs together so that endomyocardial biopsy would be sufficient to monitor the heart-lung bloc as a whole. That actually proved to be wrong. Clinical experience would show lung rejection to occur without the heart being affected. Curious.

In advance of Stanford's first human operation there had been three other abortive attempts. Denton Cooley had transplanted a two-month-old child with complex cardiac deformities and raised pressure in the lungs in

1968. The infant died soon after surgery. The following year Walt Lillehei in New York transplanted the heart and lungs of a 50-year-old woman into a 43-year-old male with end stage respiratory problems. That patient was taken off the respirator easily the following day and could soon walk around the hospital corridors. Great, but sadly he died a week later from pneumonia. Christiaan Barnard was the last to try, but not until the same year as Shumway's group. That said, he probably did it knowing that Stanford were about to do so. And some useful information was gained from the experience because the patient lived for twenty-three days.

What surgeons were mainly concerned about was disconnecting the heart and both lungs from their nerve supply. Nerves did not reconnect between transplanted organs and their recipients, so it was impossible to predict the outcome of denervation until it was done. Barnard's case also died from pneumonia and vigorous coughing to clear secretions broke down the join between the donor and recipient's windpipe. It eventually appeared that concerns about nervous control were unfounded, something that Reitz must have been aware of by the time of his operation. Cardiac surgery was a small world. Transplantation even smaller.

In March 1981 the superlative Stanford team made their move after four years of experimentation for which Reitz had done most of the surgery. A forthright academic Mary Gohlke had contacted the hospital having read about the research work. She described the course of events in her autobiography, *I'll Take Tomorrow*, beginning with her question to Bruce about how many heart-lung transplants he intended to do that year? 'Ten' he said. 'Fine', she replied, 'I'd like to be number ten after you've got your act together, and everything straightened out.'

Mary was forty-five with very high blood pressure in the arteries to her lungs - pulmonary hypertension and she was now end stage, a respiratory cripple. Medical treatment no longer helped and in the background she had been politically instrumental in pressuring for the introduction of cyclosporin. For her operation the brain-dead donor was brought to the adjacent theatre so that the organs could be removed and re-implanted with minimal ischaemic time. Everything went smoothly though onlookers were astonished to observe a patient with a completely eviscerated chest cavity.

There was just the gullet and aorta left, making their lonely way down to the diaphragm beside the vertebral column. And what a sight it was to see the collapsed airless donor lungs inflate like balloons again to fill the chest. As the heart filled with blood it took off like a train. New organs, new life. A scene that epitomised the sentence 'Those magnificent men and their heart-lung machines'. John Gibbon could not have predicted it. Walt Lillehei accomplished it by the end of his surgical career, but not successfully.

Mary was taken off the ventilator and had the tracheal tube removed on the second post-operative day. She could breathe freely for the first time in years. Acute rejection episodes occurred at ten days then twenty-five days post-operatively. On the first occasion this forced her to be put back on the ventilator. An increase in steroid dosage dealt with the problem and she was discharged from hospital after five weeks. Mary was alive and well five years later. Indeed four out of the first five Stanford heart-lung transplants were long-term survivors and Shumway described cyclosporin as 'an improvement of magnitude that I think we will never see again'. Unfortunately, until the dosage levels were better characterised it sometimes predisposed to cancer. When I mentioned to Dr Kirklin that I had assisted Roy Calne at the kidney transplant when cyclosporin was first used he simply gave me that so what look. It would be his son James who would carry the flag for heart transplants in Alabama.

Surgeons came to realise that cardiac transplantation was not just a relatively simple operation for superstars in the profession. The plumbing is the easy part. Rather it is a complex immunological challenge best managed by experts in the field. In England Terence English at Papworth Hospital and Magdi Yacoub at Harefield Hospital developed successful and productive transplant programmes in what used to be countryside tuberculosis sanitoriums. One of Yacoub's patients, John McCaffery, was thirty-nine when he received his donor heart in 1982, lived for a further thirty-three years, ran half marathons and raised considerable funds for the hospital.

In 1996 I obtained the vigorous young heart of a girl who was having a heart-lung transplant for cystic fibrosis at Harefield. On a quiet Sunday morning it was carried in a cool box to Oxford twenty-five miles away where we implanted it into an 8-year-old boy. He had been rescued from certain death by attaching him to an experimental 'Berlin Heart', dispatched to the John Radcliffe Hospital by Professor Roland Hetzer who pioneered transplantation and mechanical assist devices at the HertzCentrum there.

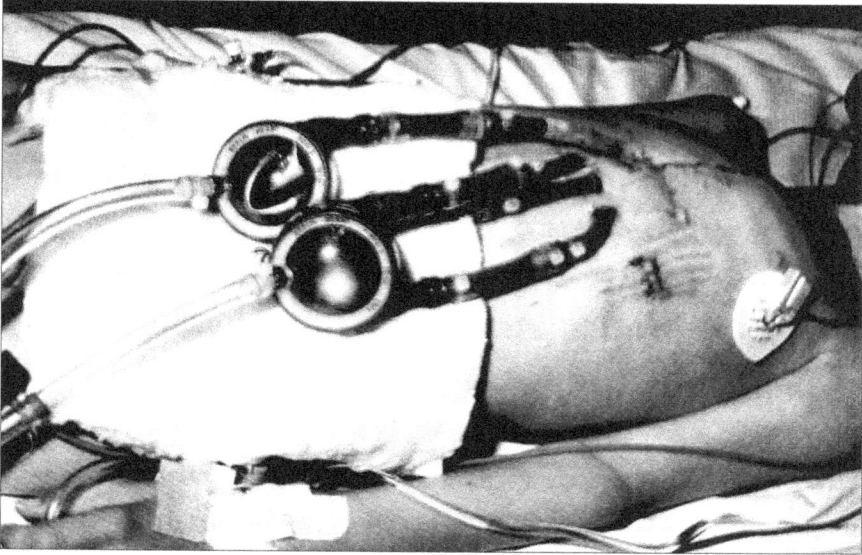

Fig 11.7 Child supported by the Berlin Heart in Oxford.

This was a carefully coordinated national and international collaboration to save a child's life. We were not a heart transplant centre in Oxford but the lad could not be moved. He is still alive twenty seven years later with the girl's heart beating away in his chest as he plays with his own children.

It was shortly before the boy's operation that I received an invitation to the 25th anniversary conference to commemorate Washkansky's transplant in Cape Town. Many of the pioneers were there but not Shumway and ironically I was invited because I was leading the charge for mechanical alternatives. Heart failure was common, but transplants were limited to patients less than 65 years of age who had to be fit enough to survive the immunosuppressive regime. That meant that some of the common complications of heart failure including kidney impairment and high pressure in the pulmonary artery were sufficient to rule patients out. Even in that young eligibility group only a fraction of those who wanted a transplant would ever be accepted onto the list. So many were assessed, rejected and left in misery. Moreover it was soon shown that in transplant recipients, immunosuppression predisposed to cancer. In 10% of patients by five years in fact, so we were driven to find an alternative.

By then Barnard's bright star had faded in South Africa. His pursuit of celebrity status with three wives and well-publicised extramarital affairs, lost him the respect of his colleagues. He told me: 'The unpopularity I have hurts because I have contributed so little to it.' Yet was that really the case? One of his much reported quips was: 'On Saturday I was a surgeon in South Africa, very little known. On Monday I was world renowned', and that was something he took great advantage of, at least in the early days.

Barnard retired as Professor of Cardiac Surgery at Groote Schuur in 1982 with an acrimonious dehiscence. He had expected a Rolex but received a hospital tie. Then tragically he lost his son, a paediatrician at the Red Cross Children's Hospital, found dead in the bath with a syringe. Chris had been a dynamic, hardworking and charismatic heart surgeon who excelled in the treatment of complex congenital heart problems. He could be difficult in the operating theatre but instilled tremendous confidence in his patients who loved him irrespective of race.

When I made that 50th anniversary program for the BBC those of his staff who were still alive spoke warmly about him. They vividly remembered the thrill of being called in from a fancy-dress Christmas party to help with what was thought to be the world's first heart transplant. But perhaps the most poignant comment of all came from Deirdre, Chris's daughter. She told us: 'We lost my father to the world. But he came home in the end.'

On Saturday 20th September 2001 Barnard was alone in Paphos, Cyprus on a business trip when he suffered a severe asthma attack in a swimming pool. Grappling for an inhaler he collapsed and died. A lonely man far from home.

Now Back to the Machines

The limits of the possible can only be defined
by going beyond them into the impossible.
—Arthur C Clarke

How can we distribute blood around the body with an implantable device that is equivalent to, or indeed outperforms, a donor heart? What are we trying to achieve here? We would need a machine that pumps 7,600 litres each day against the hugely different pressures in the blood vessels to the body and lungs. A system that allows an acceptable quality of life, responds to a change in activity, and is energy efficient. And above all with a pumping mechanism that is consistently kind to the fragile components that constitute human blood. For sure it's a tall order to mechanically mimic an exquisite organ that evolved over hundreds of thousands of years. Yet what should have been a story of bold ambition and high science would rapidly descend into a tale of intense rivalry marred by acrimonious deceit and subterfuge destined to rock the world's most prestigious health care system. And it was very exciting to be part of it!

My bold public interjection at the Barnard meeting declaring that 'no treatment that needed someone else to die first could ever prove mainstream', turned out to be realistic. Consider the well-worn phrase 'cardiac transplantation sets the gold standard for the treatment of heart failure'. Perhaps it did for the first fifty years but not now. There are more than seven million heart failure patients in both Europe and North America, ten percent of which are in the severely symptomatic category. A fifth of these are younger than 65 years of age amounting to 150,000 and 100,000 potentially transplant eligible patients respectively served by fewer than 2,500 heart donors per annum. The phrase 'epidemiologically trivial' has been applied to the operation because of this discrepancy, and increasingly borderline quality donor organs are used by centres as a result.

The logistics of cardiac transplantation can be a nightmare with long-distance procurement runs, emotional interaction with the donors' relatives, then doubts about the quality of the organ on harvest. The process is intensive and expensive irrespective of the fact that the acquired product is free. For the advanced heart failure patient the primary objective is to provide symptomatic relief from intolerable breathlessness, fluid retention and crippling fatigue. And given a probability of death amounting to 50% in two years, we want to significantly improve survival.

Consider a surprising statistic. Given the progressive improvements in drug treatment for heart failure, clear transplant survival benefit can only be demonstrated in patients who are already in hospital on life support and circulatory support devices. Records show that those put on a waiting list but resident out of hospital who do not receive a donor heart survive just as long as those who did. In one comprehensive study which includes thousands of patients transplanted in the last couple of decades the average survival was twelve years. Yet 58% had died within ten years and for those recipients the average lifespan was less than four years. Predictors of poor long-term outcome included factors that are closely associated with coronary artery disease such as diabetes, obesity, high blood pressure and kidney impairment. This suggests that a donor heart conveys only limited benefit for the commonest cause of heart failure. Given fewer than two hundred donor organs are made available each year in the UK in contrast to around 40,000 heart failure deaths in the under 65s age group, the bar is set low against a new gold standard. What's more, an off-the-shelf solution has the potential to supersede transplantation by a factor of 20:1. Are animal hearts an option? As Norman Shumway used to say, 'Xenotransplantation is something for the future – and always will be!' Certainly research in Britain and the United States tend to support that sentiment despite the recent noble efforts of Bartley Griffiths and his colleagues in Pittsburgh.

The goal for artificial heart protagonists was to design an effective mechanical substitute that could be taken from the shelf during normal working hours and implanted with the ongoing requirement of little more than an anticoagulant. That fantasy has always captured the imagination of cardiac surgeons, the media and those dying from heart disease. Then little by little the fantasy turned to reality.

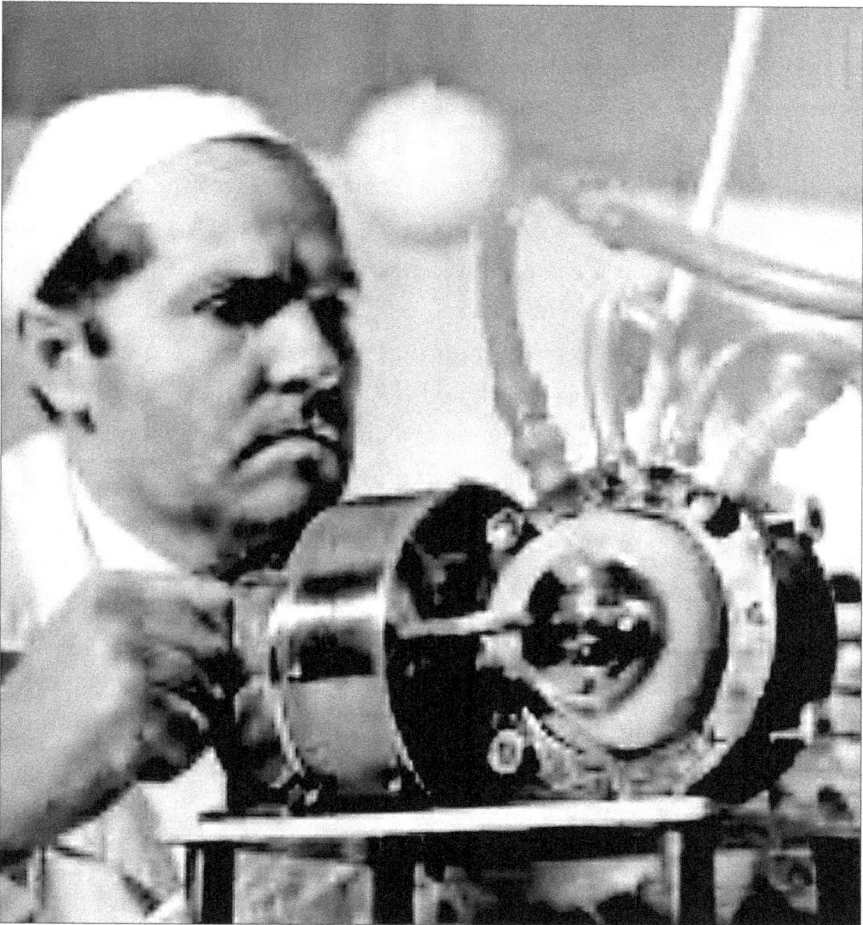

Fig 12.1 Vladimir Demikhov in Moscow.

The first concerted efforts were made by the visionary surgeon Vladimir Demikhov in 1930s Moscow long before Gibbon's heart-lung machine.

His device, about the same size as a normal adult heart, consisted of two membrane pumps fixed side by side which he primed with salt solution. Obviously these were intended to substitute for the right and left ventricles with inflow tubes inserted into the left and right atria and outflow conduits to the aorta and main pulmonary artery. The flexible rubber membranes were driven in pulsatile fashion by a drive shaft passing through the chest wall and powered by an electric motor. Animal implants began in 1937 with the longest survival being five hours. Yet the dogs' brains seemed to function and they continued to breathe. Unfortunately the blood was destroyed as if it had been poured into an egg whisk, but the concept was proven. The mammalian circulation could be maintained by a machine.

The University of Tokyo tried again twenty years later amidst a Buddhist culture that was never going to support transplantation. Kazuhiko Atsumi developed a hydraulically driven plastic heart which succeeded in supporting a dog for six hours, but he then moved on to a completely different roller pump concept with an electric motor that doubled the modest survival duration. Their main problem was blood clotting within the chambers which they attempted to avoid by changing to a dual chamber bellows pump lined with silicone rubber. Of course that didn't work either, but many of the complex problems which would compromise blood pump engineering were identified at this stage. One of the most important was the need for control systems sophisticated enough to respond to changes in recipient physiology. Though visionary and talented, the Japanese were poorly supported financially after World War II, and several of their artificial heart engineers were motivated to move to the United States. I guess they felt that a country equipped to develop an atomic bomb should be capable of constructing a blood pump. As the old song goes, 'Enola Gay, you should have stayed at home yesterday.'

The brilliant Willem Kolff who pioneered kidney dialysis using sausage skins in wartime Europe was now working on his own artificial heart at the University of Utah.

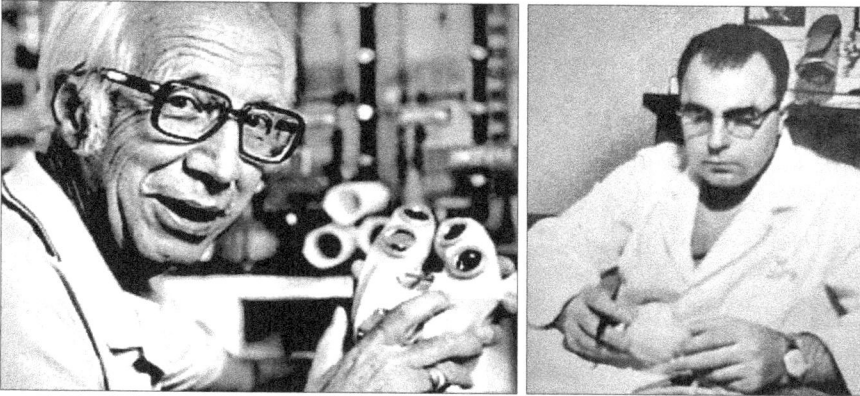

Fig 12.2 A. Willem Kolff. B. Domingo Liotta.

With him now were the engineers Tetsuzo Akutsu and Yukihiko Nose who between them developed a pendulum type of device whose two blood sacs emptied alternatively. In the laboratory the device maintained a dog's circulation with pressures greater than 80 mm Hg for two hours, after which the experiment was concluded. They also tested a roller pump design with outflow valves and by 1965 had developed a one-piece four-chambered heart which maintained the circulation of a calf for thirty-one hours. This was genuine progress in the field, so when cardiac transplantation became reality in 1967, the aim of the Kolff's team was to provide a short-term artificial heart to sustain dying patients who were waiting for a donor organ. In addition the initiative was well funded by the National Institutes of Health. The Kennedy administration in particular supported both artificial hearts and the race to the moon. Prestigious but difficult projects.

At the University of Cordoba in Argentina, Domingo Liotta with his brother Salvador constructed an implantable mechanical heart using plastics from an aeroplane factory owned by immigrant German generals. They obtained financial backing from the Cordoba Public Health Ministry and worked alongside Thomas Taliani, a retired Italian engineer and Director of the Archimedes Institute in Rome. After hundreds of laboratory implants into dogs and calves their third prototype appeared so effective that the Dean of the University persuaded Domingo to present the work at the American Society for Artificial Organs in Atlantic City. When Kolff listened to the presentation he immediately invited Liotta to join him at the Cleveland Clinic. But Michael DeBakey was also at the meeting and had an eye on the technology himself. When Kolff had difficulty in fulfilling Liotta's research needs, DeBakey offered both financial support and modern laboratory facilities at Baylor. So the plastic hearts relocated to Houston and would soon generate the most spectacular political fall-out in the history of surgery.

In turn the disillusioned Kolff was recruited to establish a programme at the University of Utah whilst the Cleveland Clinic appointed the innovative Japanese engineer Yuki Nose to keep them in the game. It was like King and Queen chess pieces moving around the board seeking advantage. Institutional prestige came to depend upon having an artificial heart in the making and the US were well ahead of the game.

It was 1961 when Liotta became the first assistant to William Hall, the Director of the Baylor cardiac assist programme. What he was unaware of was that DeBakey quite reasonably believed replacement of the whole heart to be too problematic and wanted his team to concentrate on support for the failing left ventricle. That was a more achievable strategy but it did not sit well with Liotta who wished to see his own life's work come to fruition. Denton Cooley was still working with DeBakey at the time, and together with Liotta, obtained a substantial grant from the American Heart Association to support the DeBakey ventricular assist device programme.

The concept was relatively simple. Blood entered the device from the left atrium and through a silastic tube reinforced with Dacron with a ball valve at each end. Surrounding this blood path was a second tube connected to an external power console and source of compressed air. Air was pulsed into the sleeve electronically in synchrony with the patient's own heartbeat as sensed by the electrocardiogram. The intermittent pulse pressure squeezed blood onwards through the pipes, which entered the circulation through a cannula in the descending aorta. A simple and effective concept.

In a first for circulatory support, this DeBakey left ventricular assist device, or LVAD, was found to function in animals for weeks, even months, without significant blood damage. It was able to pump around three litres of blood per minute, sufficient to sustain life in a human, and as such was stationed on standby within the operating theatre complex. The opportunity to use it arose on 19th July 1963. Stanley Crawford, the outstanding Baylor aortic surgeon, had implanted a Starr Edwards valve into a 42-year-old man with aortic stenosis and decompensated left ventricular function. Whilst the operation was uncomplicated he came out of the operating theatre with inadequate blood flow, then progressively deteriorated and suffered a cardiac arrest hours later. The sternum was reopened in the intensive care unit and frantic internal cardiac massage performed to return him to the operating theatre. In haste Crawford attached cannulas for the assist device to left atrium and aorta and the pump functioned well for the next four days. Unfortunately the early phase of resuscitation proved inadequate and the man never regained consciousness. Another great success, but the patient died.

With this encouraging start for his device DeBakey appealed directly to the government for funding with an appearance before the Senate Subcommittee on Health. Moreover, he had reasons to be optimistic. The chairman was Senator Lister Hill of Alabama, the son of the first American surgeon to close a cardiac stab wound. Baylor were keen to remain ahead of the game as rival developments were emerging in Europe, Japan and Russia. And others including Adrian Kantrowitz in New York and Dwight Harken in Boston were already working on their own circulatory support systems.

DeBakey's big reward finally came on the 8th August 1966. His extracorporeal pulsatile tube device was used successfully to salvage a 37-year-old woman who could not be separated from the heart-lung machine after aortic and mitral valve replacement for rheumatic fever. Again the pump was attached to the left atrium and aorta to maintain blood flow to the brain and body whilst her own right ventricle functioned well enough to support the lower resistance circulation to the lungs. This was an important detail. More often than not the right ventricle could look after itself if the failing left ventricle was offloaded. That said, there was an important learning curve for the recovery process.

Over the first few days several attempts were made to wean her from the system but her own left ventricle was simply not strong enough to cope. But they were patient and persisted. Supported by the device her kidney function improved, and they were finally able to switch it off completely on the tenth post-operative day. After an anxious wait and watch period, they re-opened the sternum and removed the cannulas, then three weeks later she was discharged from hospital, no longer oedematous and breathless.

Spurred on by the triumph, the team next used the device in October, this time on a 16-year-old Mexican girl, Esperanza del Valle Vasquez, who had been considered too sick for mitral valve replacement back home. Failure to separate from the heart-lung machine was predictable so the LVAD was held in readiness and deployed. Again blood entered the pump from a cannula in the left atrium but this time was returned to the major artery to the right arm. Fortunately the left ventricle recovered in days and her life was transformed by the Starr Edwards valve. Spectacular result.

This was a recurring theme in the days before adequate myocardial protection. The heart, temporarily deprived of its blood supply, would be too weak to take over the circulation again. Despite being potentially recoverable the patient would simply die on the operating table, then off to the mortuary leaving the grieving family behind. Staying longer on the bypass machine was not the answer. The longer the blood interacted with the extensive foreign surfaces in the oxygenator, the greater the likelihood of whole body inflammation and organ dysfunction. Yet a reliable temporary external circuit would probably save two thirds of those who would otherwise die. Autopsies suggested that, clinical experience eventually proved it.

Adrian Kantrowitz came up with a particularly interesting concept whilst studying the physiology of coronary artery blood flow with the distinguished cardiac physiologist Carl Wiggers, and his physicist brother, Arthur. Other organs receive their blood flow predominantly when the left ventricle contracts, ejects blood and raises the pressure in the arterial circulation. Yet this is not the case for the heart itself. Why? Because vigorous contraction of the muscle during systole, constricts the blood vessels in the heart wall. Then, as the heart muscle relaxes in the diastolic, or resting phase, blood flows more freely throughout the myocardium. However, the pressure in the aorta is much lower in diastole so in shock states, when it falls even further, blood flow to the heart itself is compromised. This vicious cycle precipitates heart rhythm disturbances and can lead to death if untreated. Heart attack with cardiogenic shock is the perfect example.

The Kantrowitz brothers' idea was simple enough. They designed a large sausage-shaped balloon which they positioned on the end of a catheter. This they introduced into a leg artery in the groin and fed upwards to the top of the descending aorta in the chest. When inflated rapidly in diastole the balloon would occlude the descending aorta and push blood backwards under pressure into the aortic root and coronary arteries. The technique was appropriately referred to as intra-aortic balloon pump counter pulsation and it worked well. Moreover the abrupt deflation of the balloon had the effect of sucking blood onwards through the aorta with a modest increase in cardiac output. Air and carbon dioxide were tested as the gas for inflation but were unsatisfactory. Success came with low viscosity helium gas rhythmically pulsed into a polyurethane balloon by an external electrocardiogram synchronised control console.

Kantrowitz was eager to test this temporary bedside device on a patient, and the opportunity presented itself on 29th June 1967. A 45-year-old diabetic woman was admitted in a moribund state after a heart attack. Once the cardiologists had deemed her shock irretrievable, Kantrowitz was given the hospital authority's permission to proceed. He made a puncture wound into the main artery of the left leg and threaded the stiff supporting catheter well up through the aorta towards the arch. When the rhythmically pulsating balloon was switched on it produced a pronounced pressure wave in diastole that exceeded that of the poorly contracting left ventricle, and sure enough given a better blood supply, the patient's heart function began to improve. The group were ecstatic when they managed to wean her from the device and though she required prolonged hospital care she was eventually discharged home. A triumph. Ironically having returned to normal activities, she died in a road traffic accident the following year. The intra-aortic balloon pump survived and is still in widespread use today.

Christiaan Barnard's transplant later in 1967 acted as a powerful stimulus for further innovation in Houston. Though he had helped to refine the left ventricular assist device at Baylor, Liotta was becoming increasingly frustrated. And so was his boss, William Hall, who resigned following an argument with DeBakey about disposing of laboratory animals to save money. From then on, Liotta had no research associate and the Baylor programme ground to a halt.

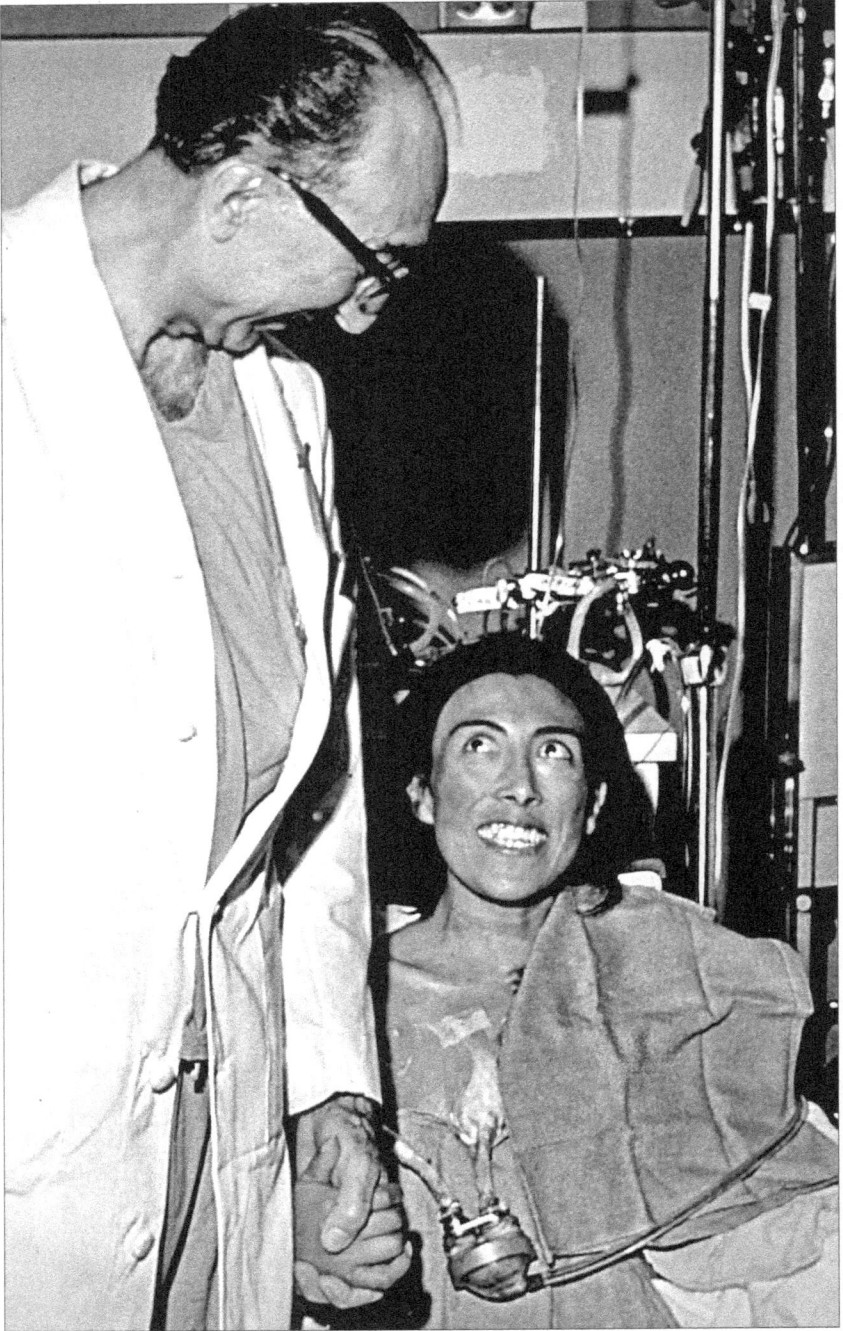

Fig 12.3 A. Michael DeBakey with Esperanza supported by the LVAD.

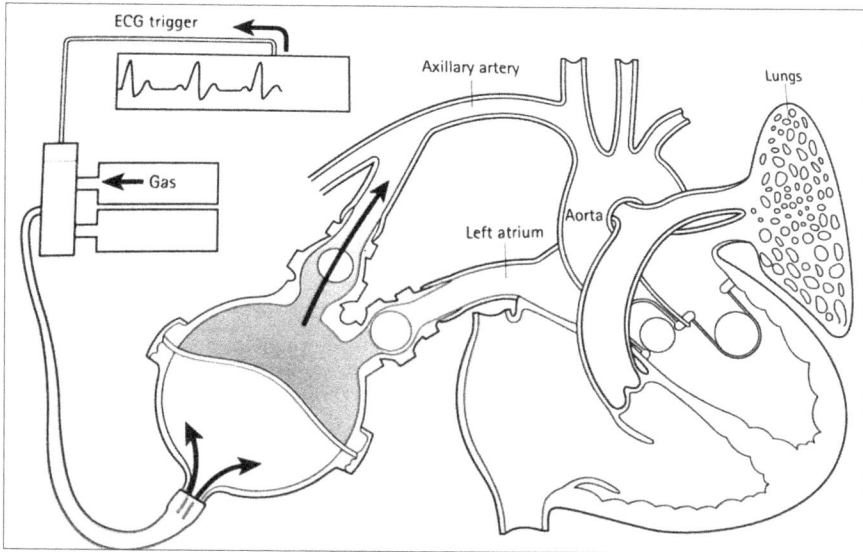

Fig 12.3 B. Diagram of the LVAD.

Until the transplants, the Cooley-DeBakey relationship had been amicable and mutually productive. Competitive yes, but certainly not malicious. Then Cooley effectively separated from DeBakey to set up his own Texas Heart Institute in conjunction with St Luke's Hospital down the street. This was shortly before Crawford implanted that first ventricular assist device. Henceforth, developments took place against a background of intense rivalry, fuelled by constant media attention and financial competition. Television crews parked outside of St Luke's and the Methodist Hospitals in anticipation of the next landmark events. And certainly Cooley's early entry into the transplant arena shifted the focus from DeBakey to him. Acrimony crept in rapidly.

In response to Cooley's first three transplants in rapid succession, DeBakey declared in *Medical World News* that the artificial heart would evolve as the better solution for cardiac replacement. Cooley replied, perhaps appropriately for the time, that the artificial heart was closer to science fiction than fact. Then, following the first Baylor transplant, in a complete about-turn Cooley announced that since donors were hard to come by he intended to build his own artificial heart. There was scheming behind that remark. Meanwhile Liotta sent monthly memoranda to DeBakey requesting more funds or at least a meeting with him to restore his total artificial heart research. He received no reply.

Cooley remained a full professor at Baylor at that stage and was aware of Liotta's frustration. Just before Christmas 1968, he invited Liotta to meet with him privately in his office at St Lukes. Domingo explained that his laboratory was at a standstill, that he needed both materials and animals for testing, but nothing at all was forthcoming from DeBakey. He felt let down. The prototype total artificial hearts he had brought with him from Argentina seven years before remained untouched and he was massively disappointed about that. Their enormous potential had been squandered by the boss.

Cooley asked the Argentinian how much he was willing to risk to have the facilities he needed. At this juncture Liotta realised where the exploratory conversation was heading. He responded that primarily he was a scientist and the artificial heart was his passion. He was therefore willing to risk whatever it took to achieve his ambitions. At that point his fate was sealed.

Liotta's device was an implantable total artificial heart (TAH) consisting of two flexible diaphragm type pumps constructed from Dacron-impregnated silastic with a reticular Dacron fabric lining. The mobile diaphragms were driven by carbon dioxide pulsed through tubes from an external control console. The system still needed one-way valves for unidirectional flow, so Cooley obtained the newly-developed Wada-Cutter disc prostheses, two for the inflow to the prosthetic ventricles and two for their outflow. The drive console was in need of more work and Cooley considered that a local company, Texas Medical Instruments, could help with that. Unfortunately their specialist in the field, William O'Bannon was the Professor of Engineering at Rice University and already a participant in Dr DeBakey's LVAD programme. Should DeBakey be informed of the initiative he would certainly block his participation. However O'Bannon was a large stockholder in Texas Medical Instruments, so Cooley, a firm believer in the persuasive nature of profit, convinced Liotta that an appropriate arrangement could be made.

It was Cooley who went to meet with O'Bannon at Rice University. He explained the design for an implantable TAH that could pump six litres of blood per minute, and temporarily keep a patient alive pending the availability of an organ donor. O'Bannon immediately expressed concern about conflict with the Baylor-Rice programme, but Texas Medical Instruments was in financial difficulty so Cooley's venture was commercially compelling. After consultation with David Hellums, Chairman of the Department of Engineering at Rice, it was agreed that O'Bannon could work on the power console in his own time. Accordingly, the project was undertaken in his garage at home and the stage was set for the greatest interpersonal conflict in the history of medicine.

On 30 January 1969 within weeks of the Cooley meeting, Liotta began a series of TAH implants in calves. Initially, there were problems with the bulk of the device and the inability to produce blood and airtight seals between biological tissue and plastics. These issues were all identified and eliminated during the first four calf implants. The fifth modification of the device, with its new Wada-Cutter valve system, resulted in a substantial increase in efficiency. The next calf implant proved more successful, until one of the rubber diaphragms ruptured, causing sudden failure and further redesign. Clotting on the lining of the prosthetic ventricles presented problems and sixty different fabrics were tested before a synthetic material with relatively low thrombogenicity was finally found. It then seemed that the last major problem had been solved. Cooley was becoming impatient. He knew of emerging competition and did not have the mind-set to come second.

On 5 March 1969, a prospective patient, Haskell Karp, was admitted to St Luke's Hospital with coronary artery disease, previous myocardial infarction and a large left ventricular aneurysm. On arrival he required an urgent transvenous pacing wire for heart block. The initial plan was to resect the left ventricular aneurysm, but because this was a high-risk operation Cooley considered using the artificial heart in the context of rescue bridging to cardiac transplantation. Karp consented to that approach but was unwilling to undergo transplantation as a primary procedure. Accordingly, O'Bannon delivered the filing-cabinet-sized control console with two cylinders of carbon dioxide attached. The white silastic heart was immersed in water in a stainless steel sink to test the system which functioned well for three days. So far, so good. The anticipation was building, the outcome predictable.

On Wednesday 2 April Cooley asked Henry Reinhard, the Chief Executive Officer of the Texas Heart Institute, to produce a special consent form for Karp's aneurysmectomy followed by mechanical heart implantation and cardiac transplantation should the need arise. On the afternoon of the 3rd April Cooley explained the plan to Mr and Mrs Karp and obtained written consent. Predicting the extent of the media interest, Liotta, Cooley and Reinhard prepared the following answers to predictable questions.

Q1. Which individuals are to be credited with the design and development of the device?

Answer: The intrathoracic pump was developed by Dr Liotta and Dr Cooley at Baylor. The control system was developed by off-duty engineers, Hardy Bourland and Bill O'Bannon of Rice University in conjunction with the company Texas Medical Instruments and Mr John Maness.

Q2. How long did it take to develop this particular model of the heart device?

Answer: The device was the product of many years of research by investigators throughout the world; the accumulated knowledge was shared at meetings of such organisations as the American Society for Artificial Internal Organs. The model used was constructed and tested over a four-month period by Dr Cooley and Dr Liotta.

Q3. When did research on this particular device being?

Answer: The device is a refinement of a prototype described by Dr Liotta in 1959 from his research in Argentina.

Q4. What institution or company is credited with the development of the equipment?

Answer: The intrathoracic device was constructed at Baylor University College of Medicine. The control console was designed by Texas Medical Instruments.

Q5. Where was the intrathoracic device built?

Answer: At Baylor and the control console at Texas Medical Instruments.

Q6. To what extent has this device been tested in animals?

Answer: The present device was the result of years of testing of many different designs and models.

Q7. How long did it sustain life in an animal?

Answer: The post-operative problems of maintaining an animal after implantation of the device are considerably more complex than in a human being. For this reason one should be cautious about assigning too great a value on the length of animal survival. This particular device had sustained a calf for 47 hours at the end of which time the device was functioning adequately when the animal was sacrificed.

Q8. Where were the animal experiments carried out?

Answer: Baylor University College of Medicine.

Q9. Is the artificial heart in any way similar to the left ventricular bypass pump used previously by the DeBakey team?

Answer: The device was built on an entirely different concept.

Q10. How is the artificial heart attached to the patient?

Answer: The intrathoracic device is attached in the same manner as a transplanted human donor heart. The device is connected externally to the control console by two polyethylene tubes through which carbon dioxide is pulsed to supply the pumping action.

On the evening of 3rd April Cooley met with Liotta and O'Bannon to make final checks on the equipment and with the operating room nurses, Barbara Lichty and Gwynn Baumgartner, to explain the likely sequence of events. Karp's operation was scheduled for around midday on Good Friday, 4th April, after six other cases.

The next day the surgical team comprised the anaesthetist, Arthur Keats, the perfusionist, Euford Martin, and two surgical assistants, Robert Bloodwell and Bruno Messmer. Liotta was to stand in as third assistant. When Keats went to premedicate Karp before lunchtime that day, he was alarmed to find him struggling for breath and already cold and blue. So much so that Cooley was called and together they pushed him directly round to the operating theatre. As candidates go for an artificial heart poor Karp was ideal. On opening the pericardium Cooley knew that the excision of an enormous full thickness scar from the left ventricle would never work but he followed the consent agreement and went through the motions. What was left of the scarred chamber would not separate from the bypass machine. Accordingly, the native heart was excised and replaced with the mechanical TAH.

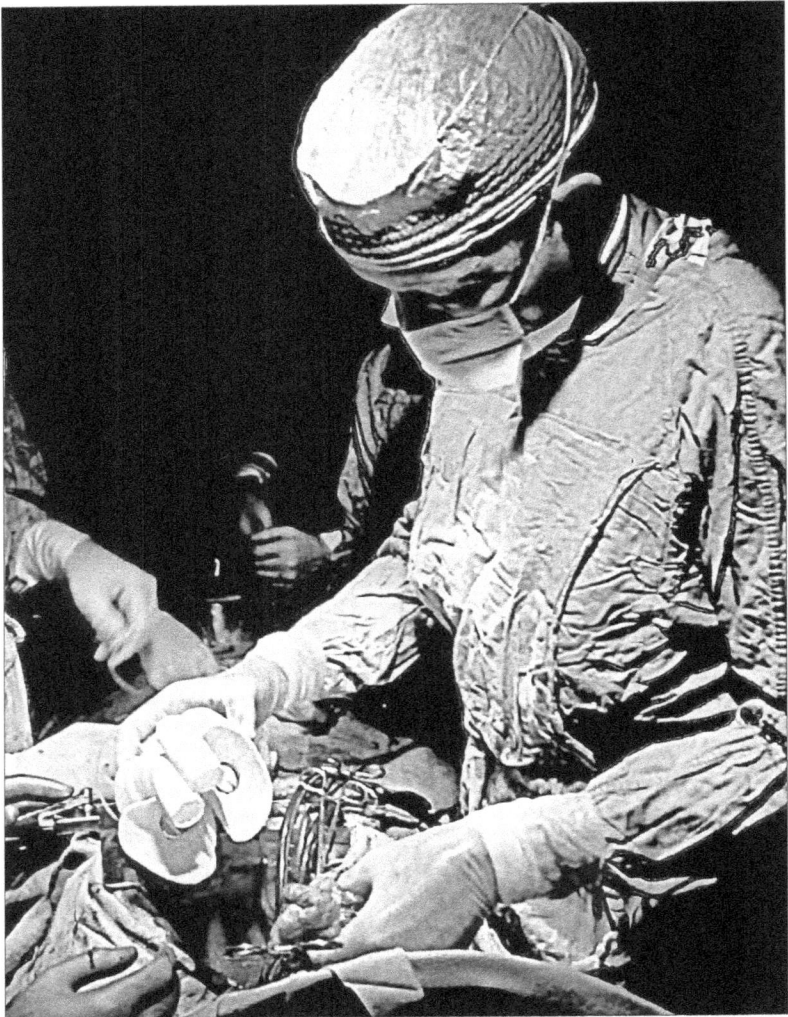

Fig 12.4 A. Denton Cooley implanting Liotta's total artificial heart.

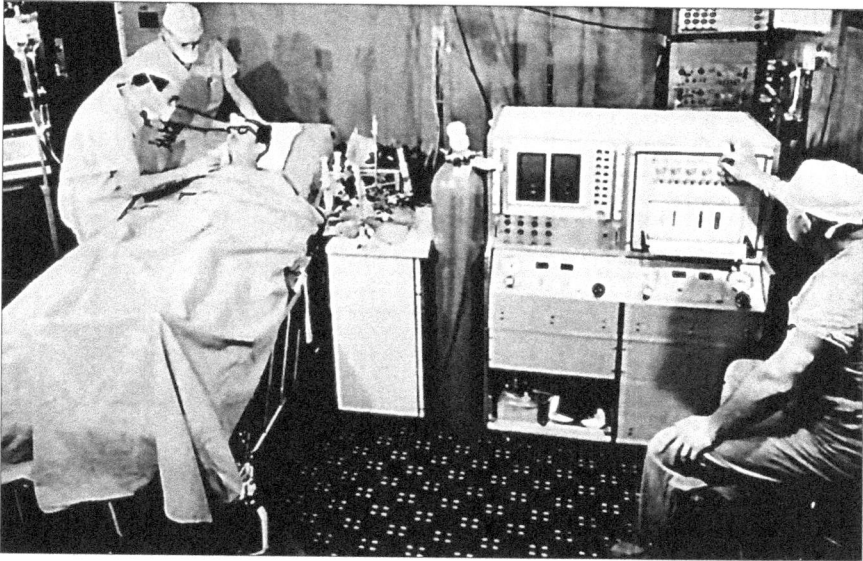

Fig 12.4 B. Haskell Karp supported by the machine in the recovery area. The tracheal tube was removed for just ten minutes to take the picture.

There were technical difficulties sewing the friable atrial tissues to the Dacron sewing cuff of the mechanical parts but with Cooley's exceptional skill, these were overcome. With both the prosthetic sacs of the artificial heart pumping at 6 litres/min, Karp was successfully weaned from the bypass machine. The world's first TAH implant was complete and the clock was ticking. Almost immediately the team began the search for a transplant donor. Why the haste? Because the device was already causing haemolysis – the destruction of red blood cells through constant mechanical pounding, and free haemoglobin released into the plasma was causing the kidneys to fail rapidly.

Ironically, Michael DeBakey had left his office at 4.30 p.m. the same afternoon to attend an artificial heart meeting at the National Institutes of Health in Washington DC. He was informed of Cooley's epic procedure by Ted Diethrich, then a staff surgeon at the Methodist Hospital. Meanwhile Karp was kept within the operating room, but regained consciousness and was taken off the ventilator in the early evening. There were immediate, though bizarre, referrals of transplant donors that same night in response to the frantic media coverage. One of the first was a 31-year-old housewife who suffered catastrophic amniotic fluid embolism during childbirth. She had been dead for at least thirty minutes when the body arrived by ambulance at the emergency room of St Luke's Hospital.

In the meantime, Karp's kidneys had stopped producing urine and he was becoming anaemic due to haemolysis. By Easter Sunday, 6th April, his lungs had filled with fluid requiring re-ventilation. There was a further offer of a local donor, but the still conscious Jehovah's Witness dying from uterine bleeding was considered too controversial to accept. The same day, DeBakey's team in his absence, performed a lung transplant at the Methodist Hospital but Karp was knowingly denied the donor's heart. At 3.00 p.m. the same afternoon, a female patient in Massachusetts was declared brain dead after a cerebral haemorrhage during electroconvulsive therapy for depression. The patient's relatives requested that she should be kept on a ventilator and considered as a donor for Karp.

A Lear jet was despatched from Houston to collect the ventilated body, together with the woman's eldest daughter and the referring physician. They set off for the return journey at 12.25 a.m. but ninety minutes into the flight as the donor's condition deteriorated progressively, the aircraft's hydraulic system failed and the plane lost altitude. The pilot was forced to make an emergency landing at a closed Air Force base near Shreveport, Louisiana, without breaks or flaps. Almost simultaneously the woman's ventilator ran out of oxygen. An oxygen cylinder was provided by the base infirmary and fifteen minutes later a second Lear jet arrived to continue the journey.

During the transfer between Houston's airport and St Luke's Hospital the donor suffered ventricular fibrillation with cardiac arrest but was defibrillated. The transplant began at 07.00 with cardiopulmonary bypass established from Karp's groin vessels. The mechanical heart was easily removed and, since Cooley had already performed nineteen cardiac transplants, the operation went smoothly. Unfortunately the organ was already compromised by the resuscitation efforts and thirty-two hours later on Tuesday 8th April, it failed and Karp died. Liotta's precious device died with him. He was a broken man.

This was the beginning of the most extensive series of investigations and litigations the medical profession had ever witnessed. Cooley and Liotta's claim was that they had independently built and comprehensively tested a new TAH using private funds and the help of Texas Medical Instruments. DeBakey's stance was that Cooley had made secret arrangements to obtain a duplicate of the device being developed under the NIH grant in his laboratory at Baylor. DeBakey, backed by the Central Judiciary Committee of the American College of Surgeons, claimed that Cooley had deliberately planned to use the Baylor designed TAH prior to Karp's operation and had actively participated in immediate and extensive publicity afterwards. Cooley countered by insisting that the device was developed exclusively by himself and Liotta and was used as an emergency bridge to transplantation in a patient who would otherwise have been lost on the operating table.

The dispute was fuelled by incessant media coverage, prompting Cooley's resignation and removal from Baylor. During the same week, the American College of Surgeons voted to censure Cooley but simultaneously invited him to present the Karp case at their annual congress attended by Barnard and Shumway. Then in August 1969, Cooley was invited to a private audience with Pope Paul VI, whilst operating in Rome. The Pope is said to have favoured the artificial heart in preference to human organ donation because of the difficulty in defining brain death. Other religions concurred, making transplantation impossible in many countries.

This and other controversies were addressed in Cooley's own biography by Harry Minetree, an ex-patient with a thoracic aneurysm. In the *Hospital Tribune* of 14th July 1969, Kolff wrote: 'The implantation of an artificial heart in Houston, Texas, on April 4th was a step forward in medical history. Dr Denton Cooley, Dr Domingo Liotta and others kept a patient alive for sixty-four hours with a mechanical heart before he received a natural heart transplant. While the patient eventually died of complications from having the second operation, the important fact is that the Houston doctors proved that an artificial heart can indeed replace a natural one in man.' But given the vicious political backlash it would be twelve years before Cooley tried again.

Away from the cauldron that was Houston, Kolff persisted with his efforts towards an air-driven system with silastic blood sacs. In one design a diaphragm compressed the prosthetic ventricles during systole then returned to the filling position through springs in both. Electronic timers were developed to govern the pulse rate but despite the sophistication, survival rates in calves were abysmal. Excess blood clotting on the silicone rubber surfaces frequently caused uncontrolled bleeding, so the programme was going nowhere. That is until Kolff persuaded a bright young man, Robert Jarvik to join his team.

Jarvik's interest in medical engineering stretched back to high school years but he changed focus to medicine after his father died following surgery for an abdominal aortic aneurysm. That said, he never did practise. By the time Jarvik arrived in Utah, Kolff had already switched from electrically driven to pneumatically powered blood pumps. One of the persistent issues in testing was the poor fit between the stiff walls of the device and the anatomy of the recipient animal. This frequently led to distortion of the calf's blood vessels with obstruction to flow and thrombosis. Failed implant.

Jarvik's role was to overcome these issues and by 1977 the group achieved reproducible 60-day day survival with rhythmically air pulsed blood sacs replacing the calf ventricles.

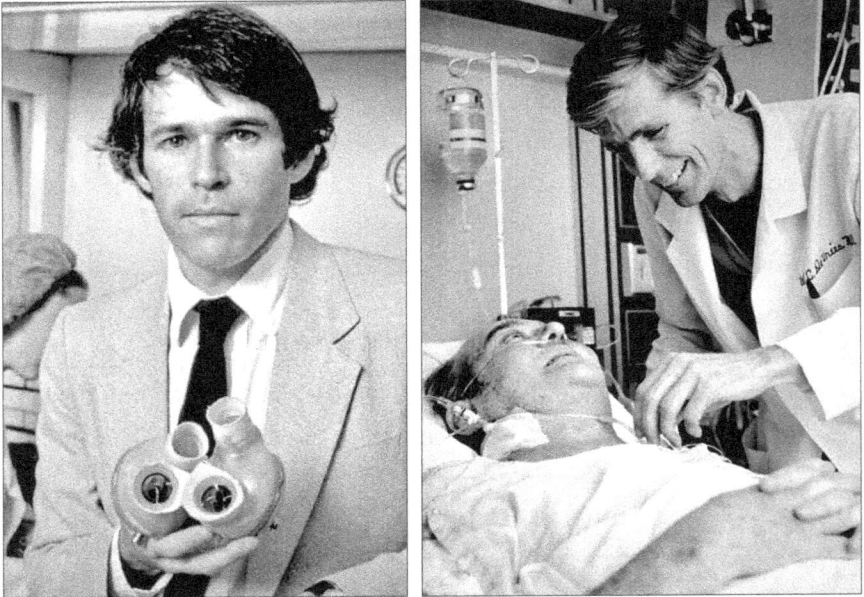

Fig 12.5 A. Robert Jarvik with the Jarvik 7 artificial heart.
B. William DeVries with Barney Clarke.

With further design modifications and improvements in the synthetic materials used, survival increased fourfold so that the animals outgrew their prosthetic hearts. The reiterations were numbered over time and by model 7 the laboratory outcomes had greatly improved.

The Jarvik 7 TAH comprised two polyurethane ventricles supported on an aluminium base. Rings of polycarbonate secured Bjork-Shiley tilting disc valves at the inflow and outlet of the air driven polyurethane sacs. For the implants the native ventricles and valves were cut away and polyurethane cuffs sewn to each of the atrial remnants, the transected aorta and the main pulmonary artery. The process essentially mimicked biological cardiac transplantation, but with a mechanical replacement. Separate prosthetic right and left ventricles were then snapped onto the polyurethane cuffs and connected to the external drive console by means of tubes traversing the chest wall. Finally the outflow of each blood sac was joined to the large arteries.

In the longest surviving animal the pulsatile device sustained growth from a weight of 200 lbs at implantation to more than 350 lbs several months later. The pump did not cause life-threatening blood damage and the calf could walk on a treadmill for an hour even though it was twice the size of a prospective human recipient. In January 1981 Jarvik wrote about the encouraging progress in *Scientific American*. Towards the end of the article he states: 'How long will it be before total artificial hearts are routinely implanted in human beings? The devices themselves, the surgical techniques and the post-operative care have all been highly developed but the pneumatically powered artificial hearts are not portable. The animal is confined to a cage, tethered to a large drive system and exercised only on a treadmill. Such conditions would be unacceptable for human beings.' Then the crux of the article. 'If the artificial heart is ever to achieve its objective, it must be more than a pump. It must be more than functional, reliable and dependable. It must be forgettable.'

Of course that meant it should be patient friendly enough to allow for good or even acceptable quality of life when used on a bridge to transplant basis until a donor heart came along. Yet Karp's experience had been nothing less than diabolical.

In the USA, Congress allocated funds for artificial heart development under the guidance of the National Heart Lung and Blood Institute, and needless to say there were guidelines. First the device had to be small enough to fit within the chest without compressing the lungs. Next it must not damage the blood or be prone to thrombosis or stroke risk. And finally there should be the facility to vary the rate of pump flow according to metabolic requirements including exercise.

Because of the complexity of the physiological responses to activity, the National Aeronautics and Space Administration (NASA) was formally asked to participate whilst working towards the first moon landing. And given the tethering aspect that Jarvik alluded to, even the US Atomic Energy Authority were brought into the discussions. High science was the order of the day, but not in the UK's National Health Service where there was no interest whatever. This 'envy of the world' health system was focussed on cost containment not ambitious achievement.

There was already a programme to develop nuclear-powered pacemakers in the US but their energy requirement was miniscule in comparison to the artificial heart. Kolff with his Japanese associate Tetsuzo Akutsu looked into it carefully. They encapsulated radioactive plutonium-238 of around 50 gram weight within a hermetically-sealed pod of tantalum after which the radioactive decay caused the walls surrounding the enclosed isotope to heat beyond 500°C. This turned water to steam, and drove a piston to pump blood. Ingenious. It was like a tiny nuclear steam engine with a lifespan of at least ten years; but bloody dangerous too. The fuel cell produced so much radiation that cancer was a likely complication both for the patient and those around him. Even more so than immunosuppression for transplantation so the project was abandoned.

In the merry-go-round that was artificial heart research, Akutsu also abandoned Kolff for Cooley's team, and designed what could best be described as a biventricular polyurethane, hemispherical diaphragm blood pump with Bjork-Shiley valves. Again the prosthetic ventricles were air-driven by an external electrical power console but with a sophisticated monitoring system. Measured inflation pressure then vacuum were applied separately to each ventricle but with a controlled common rate and duration of systolic ejection. In addition a separate battery-powered backup was available in case of emergency. Again it looked promising.

Years after his controversial first effort, Cooley implanted this second TAH into a post-operative coronary bypass patient on 23rd July 1981. As usual the circumstances were far from ideal. The patient had required an in-tra-aortic balloon pump and powerful drugs in the struggle to wean him from cardiopulmonary bypass but deteriorated inexorably in the intensive care unit. Ventricular fibrillation prompted early re-entry of the chest for internal cardiac massage until he could be taken back to the operating room and supported by the heart-lung machine. No one could have criticised Cooley for deploying an artificial heart in his attempt to save the man. Or could they?

The fibrillating heart, bypass grafts and all, was chopped out and Akutsu's model III machine sewn in. No one could do this better. When asked in a medical liability trial whether he considered himself the best heart surgeon in the world, he quickly responded to confirm that. When the judge suggested that he was somewhat immodest, Cooley replied, 'Perhaps, but I am under oath'. Barnard once watched him operate and stated: 'It was the most beautiful surgery I had ever seen in my life. No one in the world could equal it. What's more his skill was matched by grace and kindness.'

Akutsu's device maintained a blood flow of around four litres per min-ute and at first the kidneys continued to produce urine. But there was a serious technical problem. The bulk of the prosthetic ventricles pressed on the veins from the left lung causing congestion and oedema. So an urgent appeal was made for a heart donor.

On the morning of Friday 24th July I learned about the implant from excited residents during the early morning intensive care ward round in Birmingham. Birmingham Alabama that is, not Warwickshire. Late that evening I speculatively caught the red eye to Houston and purely by chance met Dr Cooley at 06.30 a.m. in the reception hall of St Luke's. Barnard's 'grace and kindness' description shone through from the start. After I ex-plained that we had both trained at the Brompton with Oswald Tubbs, Cooley personally gave me the Texas Heart Institute tour and showed me his patient struggling on the device.

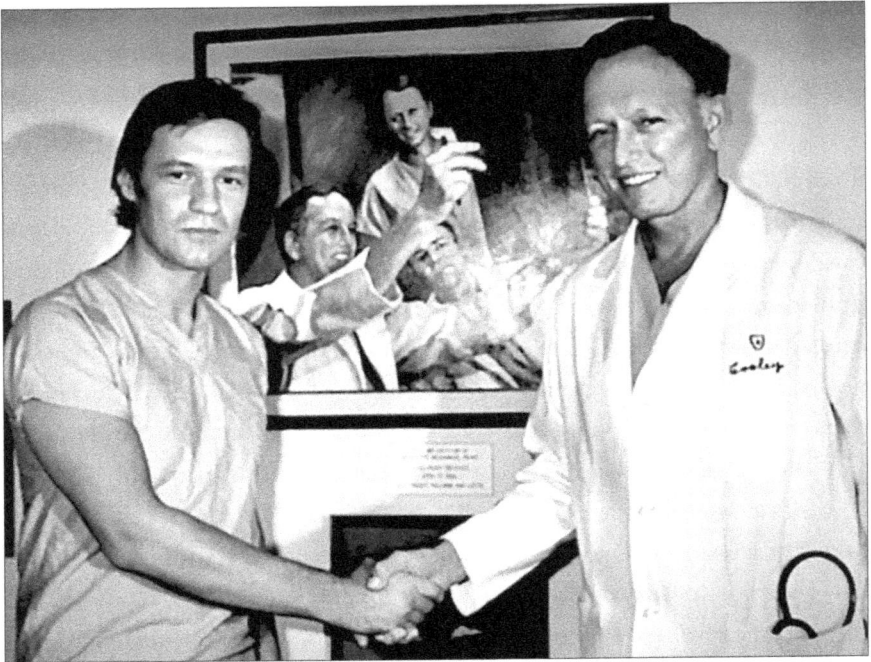

**Fig 12.6 Dr Cooley with the author in 1981
following his second total artificial heart operation.**

A new circulatory support system called extracorporeal membrane oxygenation was needed to keep the man alive by then because his lungs were full of fluid. And the dwindling urine was red with haemoglobin through bashed and smashed red blood cells. The pumps hissed and grunted but the patient was doomed.

That night I received a call in from the hotel to watch the transplant, a landmark in my own career. It wasn't the best donor-recipient tissue typing match but beggars can't be choosers. The following day, I flew back to Birmingham fuelled by the pioneering spirit, remembering my grandfather's miserable death and wanting to get involved. Eventually I did, but by the following weekend the patient was dead. Terminated by infection and multi-organ failure that destroyed any chance of life for the donor heart.

Again Cooley was subject to criticism, this time from the Food and Drugs Administration whose permission should have been sought before using Akutsu's device. It had not been approved for human use. Dr Kirklin said that the whole enterprise was premature, and of course he was right. Whenever was he not right? Both Liotta's and Akutsu's artificial hearts may have functioned for a while in animals but were beset by problems. And a huge distance from being patient friendly even on a short term basis.

In December 1982, after more than $160 million in Federal funds had been invested in artificial heart research, Kolff's team in Utah embarked upon the first permanent implant of a TAH in a patient not suitable for transplantation. The patient, 61-year-old Barney Clarke, was a dentist and lifelong smoker with chronic bronchitis. After developing what is known as idiopathic dilated cardiomyopathy he lapsed into end-stage heart failure made worse by uncontrollable rhythm disturbances. After multiple hospital admissions for medical stabilisation he had finally reached a decompensated state close to death. His abdomen was distended with fluid. His legs and feet were grossly oedematous, having gained 10kg in weight despite maximal medical therapy. Already deemed too sick for conventional heart transplantation he was just the candidate Kolff and his colleagues had been waiting for. When taken to see the calves in the laboratory with a Jarvik 7 he remarked: 'Those cows look far more comfortable than I feel. Go ahead and give me one of those things.' And to give Clarke due credit he wanted others to learn from the experience, regarding himself as another experiment.

In an effort to avoid the abuse publicly aimed at the Houston team, Clarke's surgeon William DeVries put together an elaborate consent process. Clarke was interviewed by a panel of hospital administrators and heart failure specialists. Next he was asked to read an eleven-page form that listed everything that could possibly go wrong, then to go through it again the following day. Moreover DeVries was told by the intrusive hospitals ethics committee that he should only go ahead when death seemed imminent, a factor that substantially increased the risk of failure.

After repeated practice in the laboratory the technical aspects of the implant went smoothly. Once in place the drive system delivered regular bursts of compressed air through the percutaneous drive lines to pulse the polyurethane diaphragm within each prosthetic ventricle. Inflation ejected blood through the aortic and pulmonary disc valves, after which passive filling occurred through the mitral and tricuspid valves. Collapse of the pulsatile diaphragm forced air back through the controller unit for measurement and computer analysis. So far so good, but so bulky was the machine that the chest could not be closed over it. Within minutes the highly stressed mitral disc valve malfunctioned requiring replacement of the whole chamber. In the end Clarke was supported by the heart-lung machine for more than four hours and it was 7a.m. in the morning before he could be transferred to the intensive care unit.

Irrespective of the difficulties, Clarke regained consciousness within three hours, moved all limbs on command and could communicate with his family. He is said to have told his wife, 'I want to tell you that even though I have an artificial heart, I still love you.' Difficult to know how he said that with a ventilator tube through his vocal cords, and his sternum held open but that's what the romantics would have us believe. The chest was eventually wired together the following day when some of the reactionary swelling had abated. Then he was taken off the ventilator after a diuretic-boosted urine output had cleared fluid from his waterlogged lungs.

There was more misery to come. The substantial pressures needed to inflate Clarke's lungs caused surface cysts to rupture and leak air into the right chest cavity. This needed a further operation to ligate them, but in the meantime his air-filled subcutaneous tissues inflated like the proverbial Michelin Man. By day four the urine turned red through damaged red blood cells and as always, large amounts of free haemoglobin in the plasma caused the kidneys to fail. The response of the intensive care doctors was to increase pump blood flow to an excessive twelve litres per minute in an attempt to produce more urine. But what the high flow actually did was to trigger epileptic convulsions the treatment of which caused coma for the next couple of weeks. Apart from that everything was fine and the power system pulsed on like a steam train. It was hardly the 'forgettable implant' that Jarvik had advocated in his journal article.

On post-operative day thirteen the abrupt onset of haemorrhagic foam pouring from Clarke's mouth and nostrils heralded pulmonary oedema through an overt fracture of the Bjork-Shiley mitral valve. Rushing back to the operating theatre the valiant DeVries established cardiopulmonary bypass and re-replaced the prosthetic left ventricle again. This was a difficult time for the 35-year-old surgeon who had not yet developed Cooley's resilience or immunity to media intrusion. Journalists were constantly lurking in corridors and making their own way to the intensive care unit. So much so that the police were called to guard the entrance. The developing human tragedy was at risk of disintegrating into farce.

There were periods of stability amidst further misadventures and even a television interview was filmed for public consumption on March 2nd. It was not an inspiring watch. With the device churning away like a washing machine in the chest, he showed only brief periods of lucidity amidst the confusion. That said, lack of sensibility must have been a blessing for Barney in the most part.

Attempts to reverse Clarke's frail cachectic state with 3000 calories per day delivered intravenously again caused fluid overload and lung oedema. Then bacterial pneumonia, soon followed by a fungal infection warranted aggressive antibiotic treatment, which damaged his large bowel. Pseudomembranous colitis is the medical term for this, a miserable and dangerous condition manifest by diarrhoea and projectile vomiting. Soon things progressed from bad to worse. With circulatory shock through fluid loss, poor Clarke was placed back on the ventilator on the 109th post implant day. Sadly he died just three days later. With the family at their wits' end DeVries switched off the machine himself. The world's first permanent artificial heart implant was at an end, to the great relief of everyone involved.

Again the professional response was harsh. DeBakey emphasised Clarke's universally dismal quality of life on the Jarvik 7. Shumway deemed it a clot machine certain to kill patients with strokes. Cooley stated: 'The artificial heart is not ready for planned permanent use and certainly can't approach the expectations of cardiac transplantation.' DeVries had taken a risk in the public eye but it hadn't paid off. Nor was the University of Utah prepared to pay for further cases, given the public and professional abuse aimed at the project.

In contrast, the private Humana Hospital in Louisville, Kentucky offered to support no fewer than a hundred implants at their hospital, so naturally DeVries moved. The next operation took place on 25th November

1984, in another patient who had been declined transplantation. Bill Schroeder was 54 and cachectic through severe end stage coronary artery disease, diabetes and kidney impairment. Much had been learned from Barney Clarke's operation and on this second occasion everything went according to plan. Schroeder was able to get out of bed and stand during the first week though he would always remain tethered to the large noisy power console by the transthoracic tubes. But then came the first stroke so his anticoagulation had to be increased. Next were infections around the rigid tubes emerging from the skin which constantly prevented any chance of true healing. Drive line infection would persist as the Achilles heel of artificial hearts because sepsis releases inflammatory toxins in the blood, which in turn promote clotting, thrombus formation and stroke.

There was some encouraging quality of life however. Three months postoperatively Schroeder participated in a rehearsal for his son's wedding in the hospital chapel. Emotionally the family felt that justified his bravery in embarking on the adventure. Then the highlight of his new life came when he was escorted on a fishing trip supported by a portable pump driver attached to the back of a wheelchair. Sadly soon afterwards, came a massive stroke from which he never recovered. Shumway's prediction was proven correct. It was a clot machine unless something could be done to improve matters.

DeVries performed just two more of those hundred potential procedures. One patient died ten days afterwards, whilst the next survived for more than a year. For one brief period the three Humana patients all lived together in one, albeit noisy, hospital apartment. Jarvik made the best of it celebrity wise, appearing frequently on news bulletins and having his life story told in *Playboy* magazine. And whilst DeVries's efforts came to a full stop, the Jarvik 7 was used in other cardiac centres throughout North America and Europe. Most of the 160 cases were implanted on a bridge to transplant basis. With improved anticoagulation protocols a third of them survived beyond twelve months with the machine and two thirds received a donor heart.

The leading French surgeon Christian Cabrol had the largest series in Paris, where one woman with difficult transplant cross match characteristics was supported for 620 days. Ultimately the Food and Drug Administration called a halt to Jarvik 7 implants through inadequate record keeping by the parent company. Perhaps the criticisms should be put in perspective by the comments of Barney Clarke who had given up fishing years before his operation. 'I cannot stand watching the fish gasping for breath on the dock like I do.' Severe heart failure patients are desperate for help, vanishingly few are eligible for transplantation; thus work on an alternative was entirely justified. This was just the beginning.

Think Big – But Small!

Is there any way you can be of help in this
operation – other than by leaving the room?
—Michael E DeBakey, 1908-2008

There was general consensus amongst cardiac surgeons that permanent replacement of the whole heart with a machine was just too problematic. It
would never allow satisfactory tether-free quality of life, and the risks of
stroke were too great. Indeed many non-transplant eligible patients who
were offered the opportunity actually declined it, preferring to die peace-
fully. The question was then asked, 'Do we really need to replace both right
and left ventricles?' Just because a heart transplant of necessity did that it
didn't mean that a mechanical substitute had to. Dr DeBakey's left ventricular assist device suggested that offloading of the congested lungs with
a pump produced spontaneous improvement in right ventricular function,
and showed that dysfunctional heart muscle had the propensity to recover.
So focus switched to conceptually simpler LVADs both on a temporary and
long-term basis.

In 1969 Dr Cooley established the Cullen Cardiovascular Research
Laboratories at the Texas Heart Institute intending to eclipse the Baylor
mechanical circulatory support programme. The Cullen team first devised
an air-driven polyurethane bladder within a titanium housing. This utilised silicone rubber valves to direct flow from the apex of the left ventricle
through the diaphragm to the aorta within the abdomen. The pump itself

was positioned within the belly, to avoid compression of the lungs. Only the inflow tube in the apex of the left ventricle sat within the chest.

Cooley implanted the assist device on February 9th 1978 for a patient dying from low cardiac output state following aortic and mitral valve replacement. Despite the left ventricular support, gross distension of the right ventricle still prevented chest closure. When they went back to theatre to attempt sternal wiring two days later both ventricles were markedly dilated and non-functional, so the patient was being kept alive by the pump alone. Kidney failure ensued, yet desperate to make a success of the endeavour Cooley decided to transplant both the heart and a kidney. By then the LVAD had sustained life for five days with just passive flow through the non-contractile right ventricle. Cooley made the analogy with congenital hypoplastic right heart syndrome where infants are born without a functional right ventricle. As a result he was firmly convinced that right ventricular replacement or support was unnecessary and henceforth they should concentrate on the long term LVAD concept. The Texas Heart Institute persisted with the encouraging first model which was used in twenty-two adults in Houston and seventeen children in Boston. Three of Cooley's own patients were subsequently weaned from circulatory support in what were the first examples of mechanical bridge to myocardial recovery.

By 1980 heart transplantation had reached a watershed. At least one third of the highly selected patients under sixty years of age died whilst on the waiting list. A male patient weighing more than 200 lbs would wait an average of 595 days for a donor heart which was longer than many would survive after receiving an organ. In the longer term, outcomes were determined by the side-effects of immunosuppression, including opportunistic infection and cancer together with accelerated coronary artery disease in the transplant itself. This last problem required re-transplantation in a remarkable 40% of cases by six years. That year the National Heart, Lung and Blood Institute invited applications for funding towards the development of a tether-free electrically powered LVAD that would allow unrestricted freedom of mobility for the patient. The major objective was mechanical reliability with durability beyond two years. In other words, this was to encourage implantable left heart replacement on a long-term basis.

THINK BIG — BUT SMALL

Two innovative pump engineers, Peer Portner and Victor Poirier were awarded grants. They established the successful companies Novacor and ThermoCardio Systems whose LVADs came to be used widely in the bridge to transplantation arena.

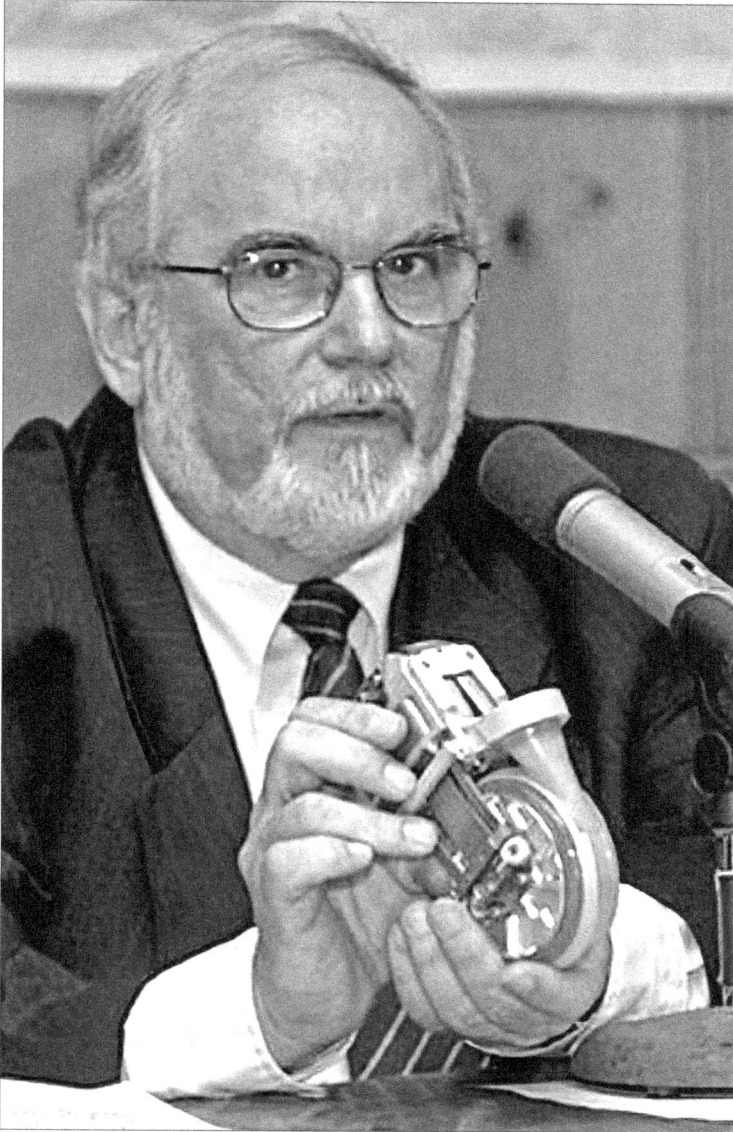

Fig 13.1 A. Peer Portner.

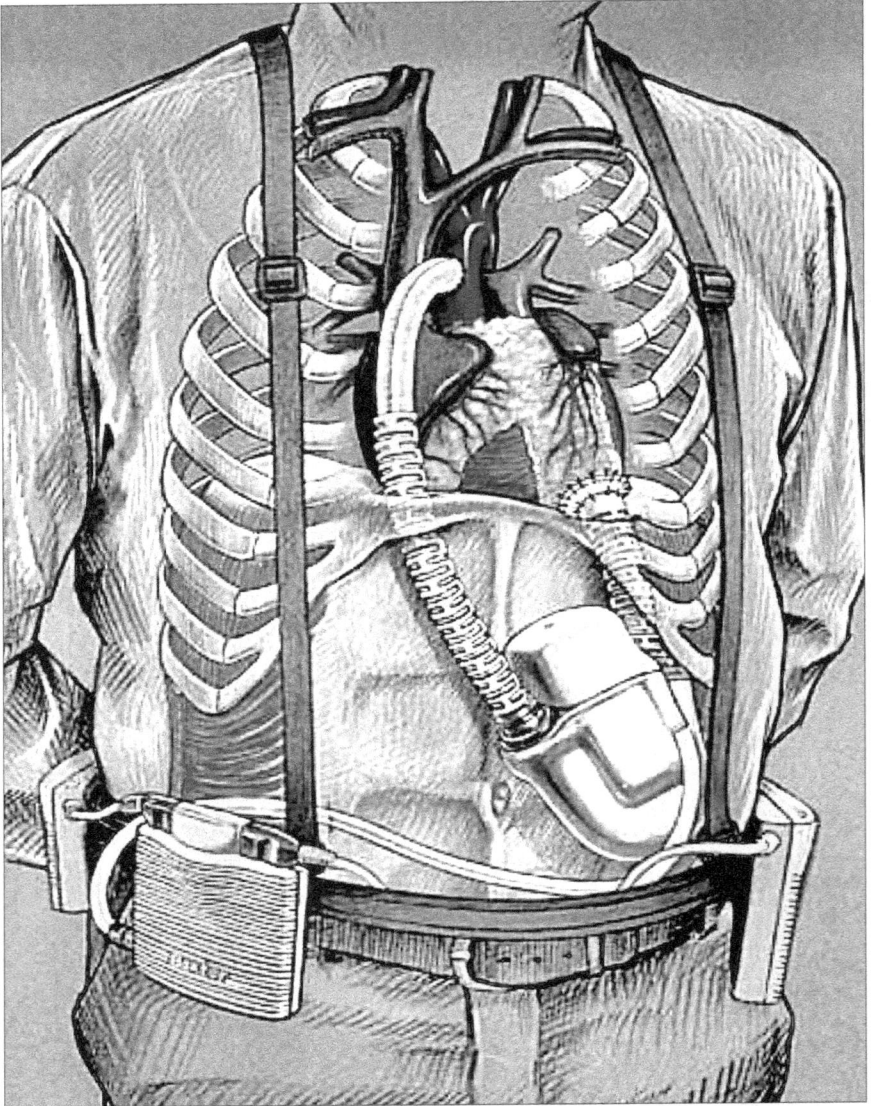

Fig 13.1 B. Diagram showing an implanted Novacor LVAD.

Cooley's Baylor-trained colleague Bud Frazier collaborated with Poirier to develop an air-driven externally vented pusher plate LVAD with a portable power source. Venting was necessary to compensate for continuous fluctuations in air volume within the device and build-up of negative pressure behind the pumping diaphragm. The first model was attached to a 73lb external drive console which the patient could push on a cart, but this was considered a serious limitation. Poirier overcame this by developing an electrically powered version with a 900g portable battery pack small enough to be worn by the patient. A percutaneous drive line incorporating the vent exited the abdominal wall to connect with the power source.

There was one more innovation in what would become the HeartMate LVAD. As usual the most daunting challenge was to avoid blood clotting on synthetic surfaces followed by embolic stroke. Clotting was frequently initiated by white blood cells aggregating on imperfections or flaws on the pump lining. These tiny biological aggregates would propagate to form clots and if these broke free they would occlude arteries to the brain. Frustration with the inability to refine synthetic pump surfaces eventually led to a new concept. As the New York Surgeon Mehmet Oz explained: 'After years of trying to overpower Mother Nature the tack was changed and we said "Let's allow blood cells to coat over a rough surface instead. A surface so rough that once your blood sticks to it, it can't come off again".' So the HeartMate engineers produced a lining that encouraged the blood cells to deposit and form a biological coating so adherent that clots would not break free. And sure enough the strategy worked. The pulsatile HeartMate LVAD eventually proved safe without warfarin anticoagulation with a very low stroke rate.

In contrast, Portner's pusher plate LVAD was electrically driven from the outset and reached the clinical arena first. On 5th September 1984, Shumway's colleague Philip Oyer at Stanford implanted the Novacor system into a dying 51-year-old man with coronary artery disease who was waiting for a transplant. The pump kept him alive for nine days until a suitable donor became available and after a stormy post-operative course this became the first successful bridge to cardiac transplantation with an implantable LVAD. It wasn't until two years later that Poirier's air driven ThermoCardio Systems Heartmate LVAD gained Food and Drugs Administration approval for bridge to transplantation and of the first 164 patients supported 106 survived to receive a donor heart. When the improved electrical version was finally approved Bud Frazier began a series of highly successful implants at the Texas Heart Institute.

Bud is a remarkable character who served as a front-line trauma surgeon on assault helicopters in the Vietnam War.

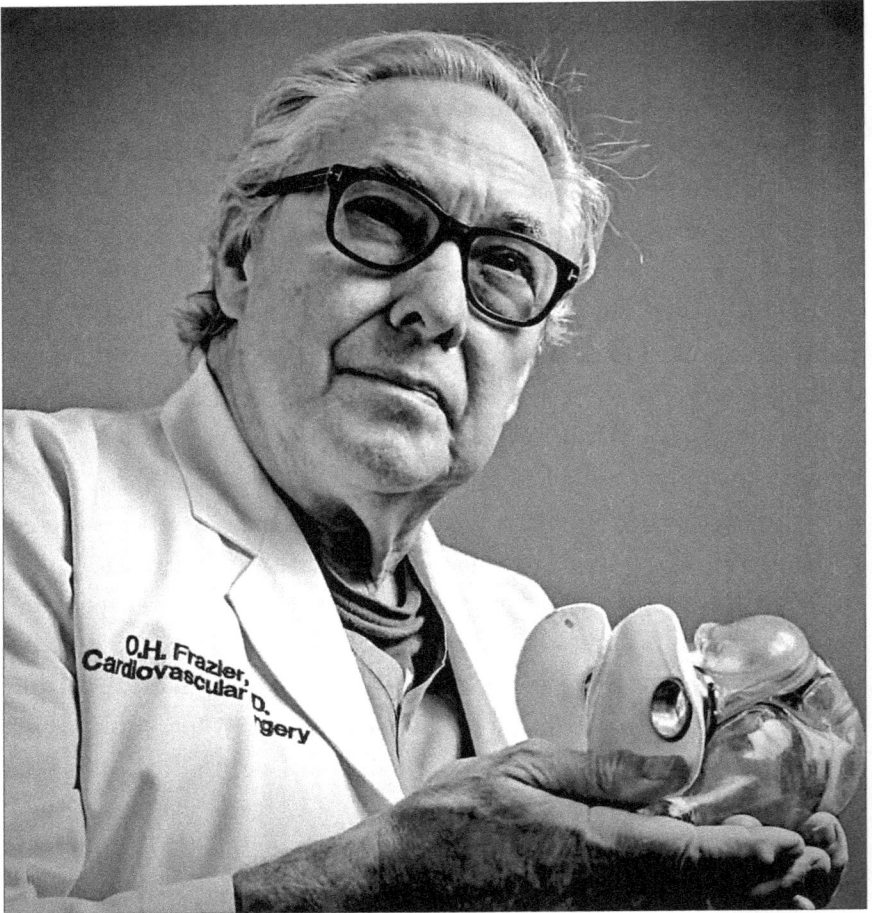

Fig 13.2 A. Professor O H (Bud) Frazier.

Concerned about the significant mortality amongst his army medical colleagues he was informed that to have a flight surgeon on the front line was good for the men's morale. To that point, Frazier glibly responded that Marilyn Monroe would be even better. On 3rd September 1991 he implanted the electric Heartmate LVAD into a sick young man with cardiomyopathy who was supported successfully for 505 days. Because of his dilated poorly-functioning ventricles and a history of blood clots to the lungs he was anticoagulated with warfarin. Within a month the chronic heart failure disappeared and he was able to return to near normal activity. However, under the terms of the Food and Drugs Administration investigational agreement the patient had to be kept in St Luke's Hospital, who kindly employed him in computer work. Unfortunately isolated as he was from his girlfriend and family he descended into depression, and without informing anyone stopped taking his medication. Without the warfarin he suffered a massive stroke and was deemed irrecoverable. Yet when the pump was switched off his own heart took over generating the same blood pressure and cardiac output. Mechanical offloading had rested his own left ventricle over time and allowed the muscle to recover. When the LVAD was removed at autopsy it was found to have that important layer of cells lining the blood foreign surface interface and no other clots were found.

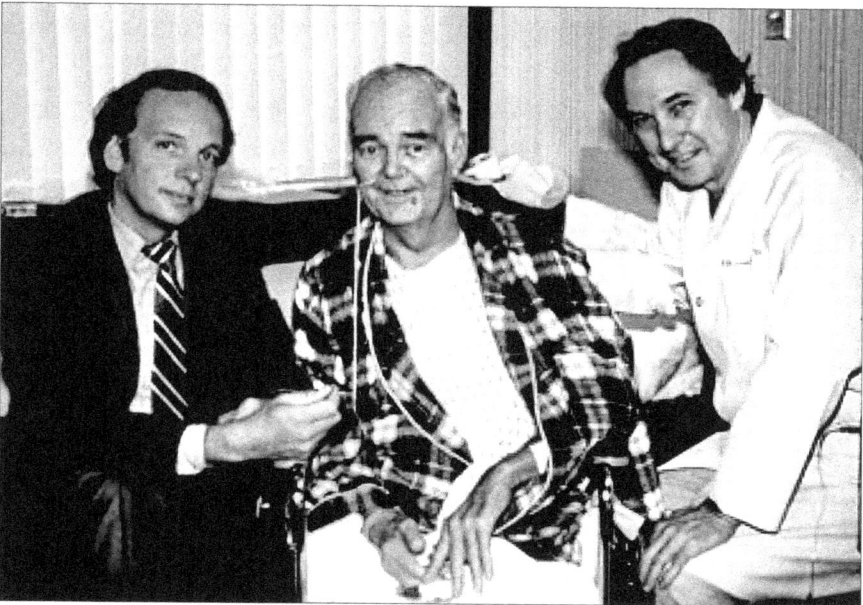

Fig 13.2 B. Wampler with his Hemopump patient.

There was a much more important discovery when the heart muscle was examined under the microscope. The cells which enlarge in dilated cardiomyopathy and heart failure had reverted to a normal size. What's more much of the fibrous tissue had gone. This was true bridge to recovery at cellular and molecular level, pointing towards a new LVAD strategy.

Within months of introduction the implanted HeartMate and Novacor LVADs were associated with dramatic physiological rehabilitation and significant reduction in death rates for patients awaiting transplantation. Disappearance of fluid retention, kidney and liver failure improved the patient's physical state and quality of life and allowed them to be moved out of intensive care units whilst they waited for their donor organ. Soon it became apparent that survival after transplant was improved as a result. Despite the more complex re-operation to remove the LVAD together with the native heart, the recovery was much faster afterwards. And worryingly some hearts that were substantially, if not completely, recovered from their pre-LVAD state were thrown away.

Estimates at the time suggested that between 40,000 to 60,000 heart failure patients below the age of sixty were dying each year in the USA with fewer than two thousand donor hearts available. What's more virtually any significant heart failure complication ruled out being placed on the transplant waiting list. With LVAD patients now surviving for more than two years should these patients be denied the chance of a longer and more comfortable life with a pump? It seemed so. The Food and Drug Administration would not allow Frazier or any of his American colleagues to use either the Novacor or HeartMate LVADs for the treatment of non-transplant eligible patients. So Houston came to Oxford.

I was appointed to develop a new regional cardiothoracic centre for Oxford in 1986, the year the HeartMate LVAD received FDA approval. Prior to my arrival all patients needing cardiac surgery were sent to London or Birmingham. Once in post the cardiologists stopped referring patients away so I was inundated with work yet still had to share intensive care beds with trauma, medicine and all other surgical specialities. I was given no dedicated ward facilities or staff, so had to be innovative. We changed anaesthetic techniques and, with the bypass machine being less damaging than it used to be, we elected to remove patients from the ventilator in a fast track cardiac recovery area in the operating theatre complex. As a result they returned to the hospital ward on the day of operation. This cardiac surgery without intensive care initiative undertaken by experienced critical care nurses caused reverberations throughout the specialty. Most patients were fit enough to leave hospital on the third or fourth post-operative day, having avoided many hours of unnecessary sedation and ventilation in an intensive care bed. The strategy was proven safe and effective with profound cost-saving implications.

The next step was to replace the junior doctors and general surgical trainees with advanced surgical nurse practitioners. These were initially trained to harvest the veins for coronary bypass grafts. I was well familiar with this practice from Alabama but it caused massive consternation in Oxford and the Dreaming Spires. The Royal College of Surgeons threw a fit and the College of Nursing said it couldn't happen. But it did, and again the practice proved very successful.

With the introduction of congenital heart surgery, major aortic surgery, off-pump coronary bypass operations, then a mechanical circulatory support programme, Oxford soon evolved from the smallest to the second largest unit in the country. At one of the meetings addressing cost containment in cardiac surgery I became reacquainted with the Texas Heart team, and Frazier asked whether I was interested in collaborating with them? When he recognised my enthusiasm to do so the question became more specific. 'Would you consider using the HeartMate LVAD in non-transplant eligible patients if we provided the technical support? We're not allowed to do it here in the USA.'

We went ahead with the project, eventually gaining permission to implant the LVAD on a permanent basis in patients who were close to death and previously declined transplant wait listing. The first thing I learned was that the patients and their families were desperate for help. Being referred for transplantation, assessed and then turned down had been a dreadful experience for them. In the aftermath many could be described as having post-traumatic stress disorder. Severely and constantly symptomatic with only death to look forward to. If we could help them why wouldn't we?

Bud Frazier brought his team to Oxford for the first operation. With his expert assistance I joined the outflow graft from the pump to the ascending aorta, went onto cardiopulmonary bypass then cored out the apex of the dilated fibrotic left ventricle to insert the inflow cannula. We implanted the HeartMate itself in the left upper quadrant of the abdomen with a thick, stiff power cable emerging through the skin of the right flank. It was noisy but the patients soon became accustomed to it. Their terrible breathlessness was gone when they awoke from the anaesthetic. The abdominal swelling and ankle oedema disappeared in days, and in weeks they went home. Exercise tolerance returned to virtually normal.

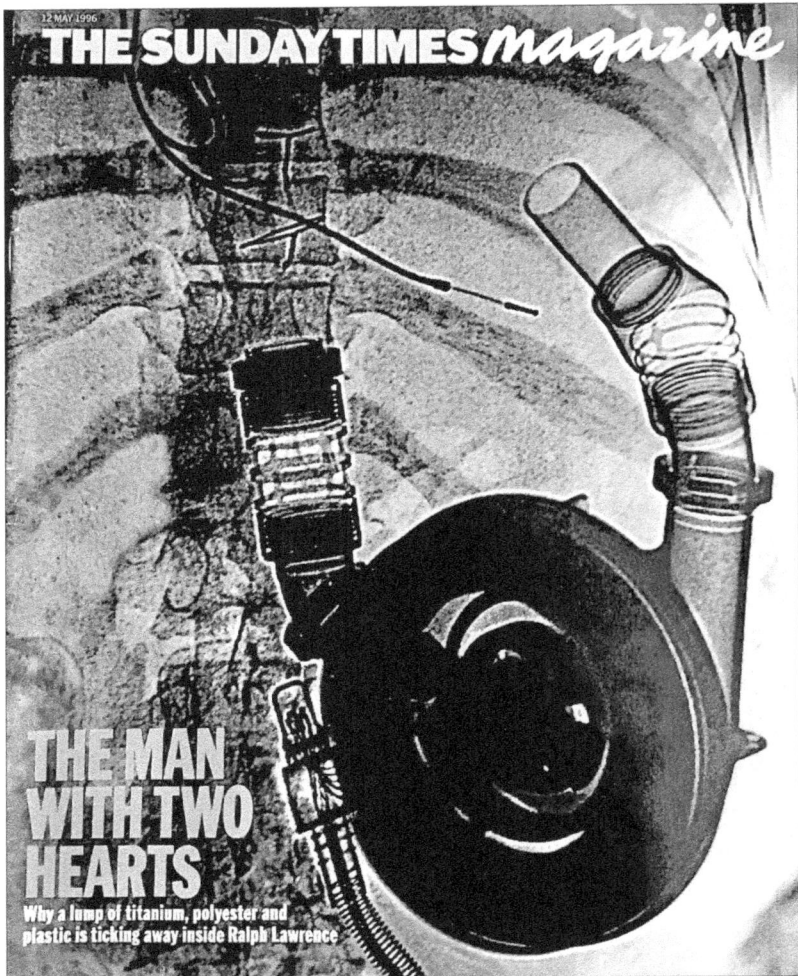

Fig 13.3 A. Sunday Times front page showing the ThermoCardioSystems LVAD implanted as a permanent artificial heart in Oxford.

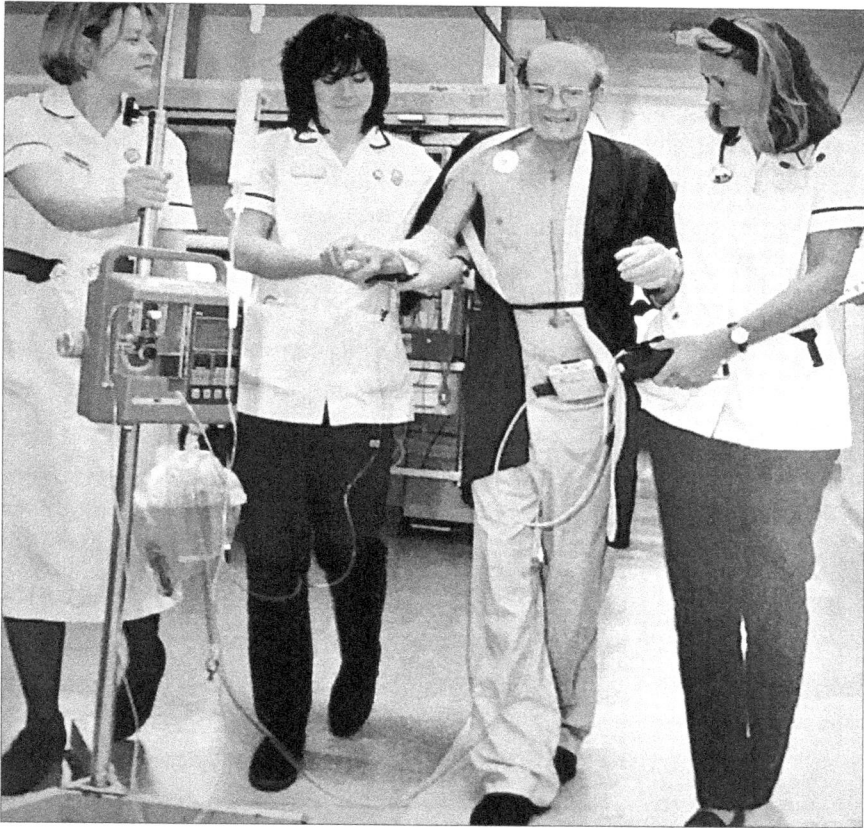

Fig 13.3 B. The patient with his carers.

Then came the problems. The first candidate had a debilitating stroke, and others developed infection around the power cable needing antibiotics and surgical revision. Eventually all of them succumbed to septic complications. Disappointing, but it became clear that bulky pulsatile LVADs with transcutaneous drivelines and portable batteries would not provide long-term survival. Nor could they be regarded as patient friendly. That said, the initiative opened the doors to an off-the-shelf alternative for the many thousands of patients discarded by the transplant system.

Some years later a landmark clinical study, the Randomised Evaluation of Mechanical Assistance for the Treatment of Congestive Heart Failure trial, known as REMATCH, tested HeartMate LVAD implantation against continued medical treatment in twenty hospitals in the USA. Survival at one year was 52% with the LVAD versus 25% on continued drug therapy, though this fell to 23% and 8% respectively by two years. REMATCH told us two things; firstly that heart failure had a worse prognosis than most cancers; and second that LVADs have the capacity to relieve symptoms and prolong life.

The implantable pulsatile LVADs launched the possibility for long-term mechanical circulatory support but their shortcomings were readily apparent. Their size was based on the premise that they had to mimic human physiology. All mammalian hearts produce pulse in the circulation so it was widely assumed that substitute left ventricles must rhythmically empty and fill too. As a result the bulky pulsatile LVADs could only be used in patients of sufficient size to accommodate them. This effectively excluded most women, teenagers and children. To date therefore, both TAHs and LVADs were discriminatory. A men-only thing, so something had to change.

Perhaps the first scientist to challenge the pulsatility dictum was Richard Wampler who argued: 'When you go to the doctor he can feel the bounding pulse in your radial artery, but when the blood reaches the capillary bed where gas exchange takes place, the pulsatility is totally dampened. So really in the most important part of the circulation the flow is continuous.' Of course that is correct. Where the cells and plasma of the blood interact with the cells of the tissues there is no significant pulse pressure.

Given that insight, Wampler designed a temporary catheter-based circulatory support device akin to an Archimedes screw for insertion through the aorta and aortic valve into the left ventricle. The concept was similar to the intra-aortic balloon pump but with continuous flow rather than a pulsatile propulsion mechanism. The screw rotated at high speed drawing fluid in at one end to be pushed out of the other. And when the animal experiments looked positive, Wampler approached Frazier who was keen to test the concept. A heart transplant patient at the Texas Heart Institute was struggling with life-threatening rejection and provided the perfect opportunity. Another nothing to lose case where the so called Haemopump took the load off the failing left ventricle for several days pending recovery. Happily the man survived. Success breeds success so other cases followed rapidly. Frazier said of a particularly joyful outcome: 'I had one little boy who lived for three days without any pulse at all. He was very small so this little pump could sustain his whole circulation. He woke up, he ate popsicles and he did very well until his own heart had recovered enough to start beating.' This was another case of mechanical bridge to recovery which avoided transplantation.

Aside from the apparent safety and efficacy of continuous non-pulsatile flow, the main surprise was that a pump spinning at speed like an egg whisk, did not traumatise the protein and cells of the blood more than it did. Even so the Haemopump could only be used in the relatively short term by the bedside because it needed a continuous infusion of glucose solution to lubricate the moving parts. Robert Jarvik then suggested that blood might be sufficient lubricant in itself. Remember the statement: 'It must be more than functional, reliable and dependable. It must be forgettable.' Jarvik was already working on that concept, but he wasn't going to get there first.

The big breakthrough came when Michael DeBakey performed a heart transplant on an expert in fluid dynamics. David Saussier was referred to the Methodist Hospital after an extensive heart attack that he was fortunate to survive. He just happened to be a National Aeronautics and Space Administration (NASA) engineer whose job was to design the huge turbopumps that feed liquid hydrogen propellant to the space shuttles' main engines. Whilst Saussier was recovering DeBakey, in the light of Wampler's work, asked if he would help design an implantable rotary pump for blood. When Saussier was delighted to be given the chance, DeBakey proceeded to approach NASA directly. Not only was the organisation an ideal source of financial support but their space shuttle engines were already fed by axial flow pumps carefully engineered so as not to damage the fuel.

NASA agreed to collaborate with Baylor but handling blood was going to be different. Turbulence and shear stress had to be minimised to prevent smashing the red cells. As the NASA scientist Bob Benkowski pointed out: 'Pumping blood is like pumping a whole bunch of water-filled balloons that are suspended in liquid. You're trying to pump these things without having them rupture.' The small prototype pump had just one moving part, an impeller powered through the use of magnets within the blades themselves. A coil in the pump housing created a magnetic field around the impeller causing it to spin at thousands of rotations per minute, drawing the blood in and ejecting it with continuous flow.

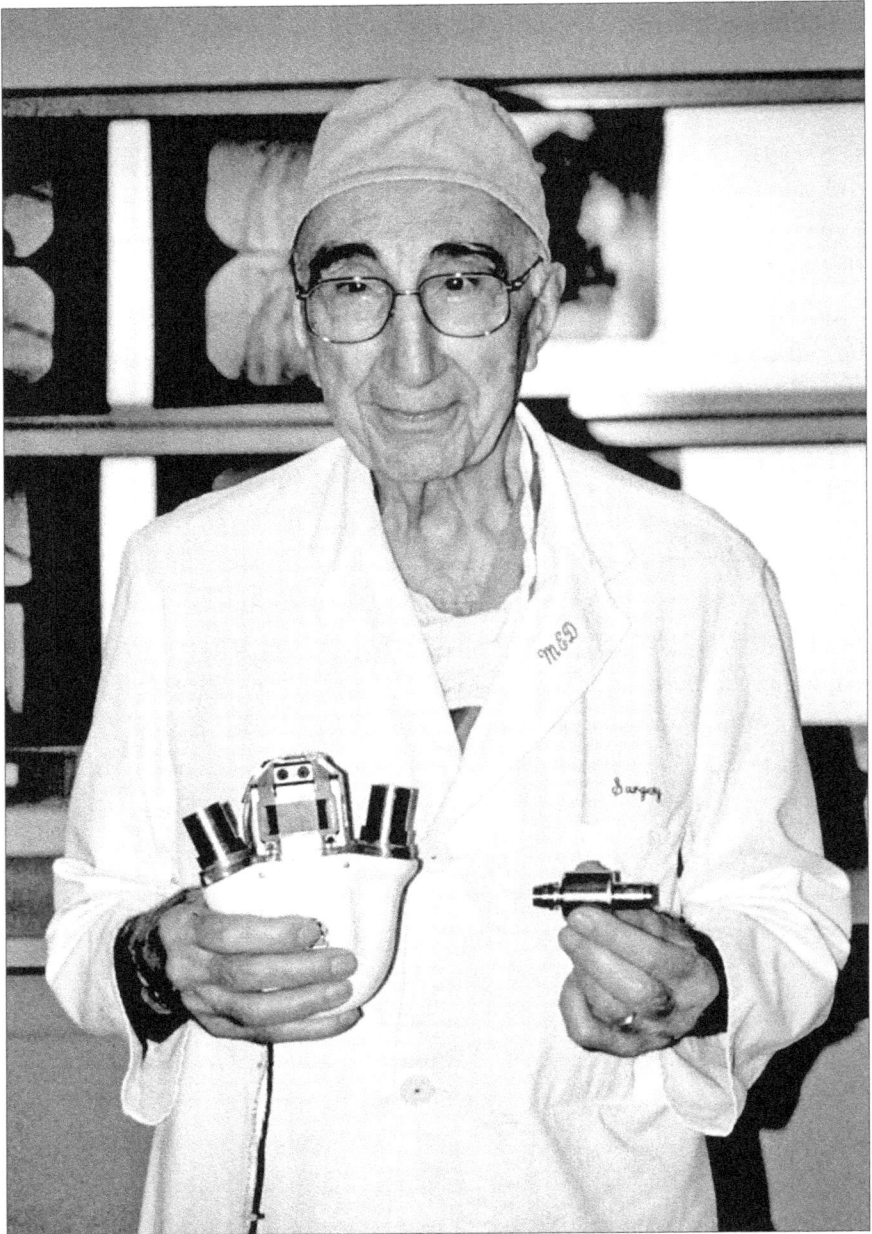

Fig 13.4 Michael DeBakey with Novacor and NASA LVADS.

The NASA team allocated to the project went to extraordinary lengths to minimise haemolysis, using their Cray super-computers to model the flow fields. What they showed was that the tolerance around impeller and blade shape was minimal. Changes in geometry amounting to ten or twenty thousandths of an inch could create highly destructive pressure changes within the blood path, but eventually the engineers were satisfied. The magnetic blades rotated so fast that the red cells whizzed straight through. As Frazier put it: 'It's sort of like passing your finger through a candle flame, if you go fast enough it won't burn you.'

The final DeBakey VAD was manufactured from titanium by the MicroMed Technology Company. Weighing less than four ounces, the inflow cannula was inserted into the apex of the left ventricle whilst the body of the pump ejected blood through a Dacron graft to the ascending aorta. It fitted easily within the chest cavity. This was a complete revelation in comparison to the pulsatile pumps. It still needed a power cable exiting through the skin to the controller and batteries but again this was smaller and less intrusive. So were the portable components.

The colourful Rob Jarvik moved to New York City setting up his company office and laboratory in a Manhattan skyscraper. I met him completely by chance at the 1996 Society for Thoracic Surgeons meeting in San Antonio, Texas, when a cardiovascular company asked my opinion on one of his inventions intended to boost blood flow through obstructed leg arteries. At the conclusion of those conversations Jarvik took me aside, opened his briefcase and produced a thumb-sized titanium cylinder. Within the housing was a torpedo-shaped rotor. When he plugged the device into an electric socket and placed it in a sink of water it went whoosh. Six litres of flow per minute through a pump no larger than a small carrot. I said: 'That's a great pump for water but it will damage the red blood cells'. I was unaware of the emerging DeBakey VAD at the time so opportunistically I followed up with: 'But I would love to test it in my lab in Oxford.'

The only group collaborating with Jarvik on his axial flow pump were Cooley and Frazier at their animal facility in Houston. As usual they were in stiff competition with DeBakey in their efforts to pioneer long-term circulatory support, and this was my opportunity to join the race. Cambridge were pursuing pig hearts, I would work towards a mechanical alternative. It was like the boat race but first things first. I didn't have a laboratory in Oxford. I would have to establish one and quickly.

Bud Frazier was at the conference in San Antonio so Jarvik asked him to take me on the short hop to Houston and show me the device in a calf. Sure enough it was very impressive. A miniaturised blood pump directly inserted within the cavity of the left ventricle and with its rotor spinning at 8000 revolutions per minute without significant blood damage. Magic. One problem was that the calves rapidly grew into cows too large to be kept in pens. That limited the duration of pump use. Whilst not wishing to operate on animals, it occurred to me that full-grown sheep would be an alternative.

The unique aspect of what became known as the Jarvik 2000 was that the body of the titanium cylinder was held within the apex of the left ventricle by a cuff so there was no inflow graft between heart and pump. Blood entered the orifice and encountered the rapidly-spinning rotor directly. It was propelled into a short Dacron graft which I chose to join to the descending aorta in the back of the chest. What's more, I could perform the whole operation through the left side of the chest without needing the heart-lung machine so the sheep recovered quickly. Some survived for a year with completely pulseless blood flow and maintained normal organ function. So the brain, kidneys, liver and gut of a large mammal seemed fine with this intriguing physiology. Wampler was correct in his hypothesis. And I was wrong about the egg whisk effect and haemolysis. An LVAD the size of my thumb was sufficient to sustain life, and I soon felt sufficiently confident to try it in a patient.

Other lifesaving technology found its way to Oxford whilst the Jarvik research was ongoing. In 1998 Richard Clarke, the Chief of Cardiac Surgery at the National Institutes of Health in Washington, retired and came for a year's sabbatical with me in Oxford. Richard had been involved in the development of a new continuous flow LVAD for temporary use in heart attack patients and those who couldn't be weaned from the heart-lung machine. Permission had been granted to use it on an investigational basis in the USA but the first patients in Pittsburgh had not recovered, so after three consecutive deaths the programme had stalled.

In February that year I had been invited to Washington by the FDA to discuss my experience with the HeartMate LVAD as a transplant alternative. Clarke was at that meeting. He took me aside to show me the new AB180, a spinning blood pump the size of a bicycle bell, weighing just half a pound. It had one moving part, a six-bladed turbine that had been developed over five years in the laboratories of George Magovern, the Chief of Cardiac Surgery at the Allegheny Hospital in Pittsburgh. Like Wampler, Magovern argued that when blood passes through tiny capillaries one cell thick, there is no pulse pressure. This should allow smaller less traumatic pumps to be used in salvage situations. But Magovern and Clarke wanted a system that could support the patient for as long as six months, arguing that many hearts take much longer to recover than a couple of days.

Richard arrived in Oxford with his wife on 7th August and brought an AB180 with him. From skyscrapers to dreaming spires made for some stark contrasts. From the world's best-funded health care system to the struggling NHS. Yet something remarkable was about to happen. The call came at 02.00 a.m. on the 9th August. It was a cardiologist at the Middlesex hospital in London who had been following our circulatory support adventures. She was caring for a 21-year-old student teacher at an Oxford College who was at home for the vacation. Julie had initially complained of flu-like symptoms but within days became listless and short of breath, sweating but cold, and not passing urine. Dying in fact. The district hospital recognised this and passed her rapidly on to the cardiac unit of the London teaching hospital.

The cardiologist diagnosed viral myocarditis with very poor residual left ventricular function, so placed her on a ventilator and inserted an intra-aortic balloon pump. That was the best treatment on offer but simply didn't help. What's more it occluded the main artery to the leg which was cold, blue and pouring out lactic acid. The caring doctor stayed by Julie's bedside and eventually considered an LVAD as the last chance saloon. 'Did we have one,' she asked? 'I'm not sure', I responded 'but send her up and we'll see what we can do.' Then I called Richard.

Julie arrived just before 04.00 a.m. by which time her blood pressure was not measurable and her kidneys and liver had failed. We had the operating theatre ready with the heart-lung machine primed. By the time I ran the scalpel down her chest, there was no bleeding and the electrocardiogram was slowing to a stop. Only minutes later would have been too late. Once on the bypass machine black blood drained into the oxygenator and turned red again. Peace reigned. I knew Richard was preparing his pump so I simply asked: 'How do we implant this thing?'

First there was a stiff inflow tube for insertion into the left atrium. This would drain oxygenated blood from the lungs into the centrifugal pump, which in effect became her new left ventricle. Then there was a flexible vascular graft to convey blood to the aorta. Simple. The device itself would sit in the right side of the chest between lung and heart, and given the rigidity of the inflow cannula versus the fragility of the atrial wall I sewed on a length of human aorta to aid safe removal. We kept donated human valves and segments of blood vessel in the operating theatre fridge for emergencies like this. Spare parts, pickled and preserved, thanks to the Homograft Department.

With the plumbing complete Richard threw the switch and the pump started spinning. As we reached five litres blood flow per minute Julie's own right ventricle began to beat again, but there was no blood pressure trace on the monitor. No systole nor diastole, just a flat line. We had continuous blood flow from the centrifugal pump spinning at 4000 rpm. Counterintuitive physiology that the first three patients did not survive. Would Julie? Only time would tell, but for now things were looking good. She was in the intensive care unit by 08.00 a.m. with the team wondering how to monitor a patient without pulse or discernible blood pressure. The arterial line in her wrist read 70 mm Hg, but her feet were pink and warm. Was pressure more important than flow? Not at all. This was similar to being on the heart-lung machine.

Kidney dialysis was needed for a couple of days then her own urine began to flow and the jaundice disappeared. In fact all parameters of organ function returned to normal within a week. At 07.00 a.m. on the 11th I was called to the phone at the intensive care nurses station. Someone with an American accent wanted to speak with me, but the responder didn't get the name. It was George Magovern calling from Pittsburgh well after midnight local time. Richard had contacted him with the encouraging news and he wanted to congratulate us personally. His engineering team were still out in the city celebrating. I said that we would celebrate when Julie left hospital.

13.5 Julie Mills on the cover of *Readers Digest*.

Within a week the cardiac echoes showed considerable improvement in the contractility of Julie's own left ventricle. We had started the search for a donor heart but now we didn't need one. With the AB180 we had saved Julie's own heart which still supports her twenty-five years later. Hers was a momentous case for one specific reason. In the 1990s any patient who received an LVAD in the USA was committed by law to a cardiac transplant. We had achieved bridge to recovery which had to be the preferred approach for Julie's viral myocarditis and many other forms of shock.

Just before Christmas 1998 the Pittsburgh engineers and researchers who'd worked on the AB180 filed into a conference room for a special party arranged by Dr Magovern. No one knew what the occasion was – until Julie walked in. 'The girl without a pulse' was instantly recognisable from photographs pinned to the bulletin board and from magazine covers after her ground-breaking survival. Magovern shook her hand saying: 'You being here is the best Christmas present any of us could have had.' And he was right. The company not only survived but thrived and the device was modified so it could be used as an assist device in the catheter laboratory without opening the chest. Now called the Tandem Heart it is used worldwide for the treatment of shock.

Julie's case gave us confidence regarding the use of continuous non-pulsatile blood flow in humans if only for a short period. Now we needed to explore longer-term support but the sheep were looking good after several months.

Just as for the HeartMate LVAD, DeBakey had to bring his NASA pump to Europe for testing. This was done in Berlin and Vienna on a strictly bridge to transplant basis in 1998. Pump rotor speeds between 9000 and 11000 rpm generated flows of up to six litres per minute without significant haemolysis. And longer term pulseless patients seemed to be fine as Wampler implied. The same improvement in organ function occurred as for pulsatile LVAD patients so this was a major breakthrough. Then given the European success, DeBakey's colleague George Noon performed the first implant as a bridge to transplant at the Methodist Hospital in 2002. Sadly Saussier didn't live long enough with his donor heart to see the Houston operation. He died in 1996.

Early in 2000 the Jarvik Heart gained FDA approval for a series of bridge to transplant implants at the Texas Heart Institute, and generously Dr Cooley included me as part of the surgical team for the first implant. Sadly it was a desperate case, a bridge too far, that Dr Frazier was keen to help. The young man in his early twenties already had a HeartMate LVAD afflicted by drive line infection which had extended along the cable to the pump itself. To replace the infected mess with the Jarvik 2000 was a tall order.

Scrubbed around the operating table were Drs Frazier, Cooley and me but as we sawed through the sternum we soon encountered pus and bleeding. To keep the lad alive cardiopulmonary bypass was established via the blood vessels in the groin. Having done so we managed to remove the HeartMate inflow cannula and replaced it with the Jarvik 2000, but he lapsed into septic shock and died hours later. Perhaps that outcome was predictable but it epitomised one important fact. Bud was much more interested in helping his patients than trumpeting his own reputation.

On April 10th Frazier implanted the Jarvik 2000 into Lois Spiller, a bedridden 52-year-old woman with cardiomyopathy. This time the patient and her operation were both straightforward. The pump worked perfectly and she was successfully transplanted 79 days later. Great but because these devices cost the same as a high spec Ferrari, I was persuaded that they would be better used as a long-term solution for non-transplant eligible patients. Otherwise they were being thrown into the bin just weeks or months later when a donor appeared. No one would do that with an expensive car, not even in Formula One.

Then came another landmark case. Peter Houghton had suffered a viral chest infection followed by myocarditis, not dissimilar to Julie. This left him with an enlarged flabby heart, a leaking mitral valve, and regular rhythm disturbances so debilitating that he gasped for breath on the slightest exertion. And coincidentally he was a psychologist working with terminally ill cancer patients at the Middlesex Hospital so he had heard of Julie's case.

After many hospital admissions for escalation of heart failure treatment, Peter's cardiologist referred him to a surgeon who specialised in mitral valve repair. But at the outpatient visit the man was dismissive stating that it was far too risky and Peter should organise a transplant referral. That was disingenuous given the one functioning kidney that was failing. He was in fact assessed at two transplant centres and was discarded on both occasions. Why? Because he was too sick. The correspondence described him as grossly fluid overloaded, breathless and exhausted on minimal exertion, unable to lie flat and only able to sleep propped up on pillows or sitting in an armchair. That was exactly how I remembered my own grandfather in Scunthorpe. He received the same advice. 'Nothing can be done.' In other words, 'Go away and die without making a fuss.'

Peter appeared at my office door on a warm summer's morning in June 2000. The knock was tentative, almost apologetic as his large swaying frame filled the doorway. Out of pride he had refused to be pushed through in his wheelchair. Yet weeks before he had received the last rites during an acute downturn. Now he stood head bowed, lips blue and sweating profusely, held up by his foster son. His belly bulged with an engorged liver and fluid, ascites. His legs were swollen, ulcerated and purple. He wore oversized sandals with socks stretched tightly over massively swollen feet. I felt he might die any minute but that fitted the bill.

Both my own hospital's ethics committee and the UK Medical Devices Agency had insisted on independent verification that the first patient to be given a Jarvik 2000 on a permanent basis must be terminally ill with very short life expectancy. Personally I had serious doubts that he could survive an anaesthetic but he had clearly suffered enough. So I told him that it would be a great privilege if he would allow us to help him and that if he decided to go ahead, the first pump was his.

There followed a look of astonishment. A religious man, he expected another rejection and was resigned to the fact. When asked about the odds of surviving the surgery I simply guessed at 50:50. My own back was up against the wall being forced to operate on absolute end-stage patients and Peter worried about suffering brain damage if things didn't go well. I reassured him, if that's the right word, that any misadventure would definitely result in his death. The operation would either help him with symptomatic relief or amount to euthanasia. He was content with that.

I showed Peter the remarkably small pump and probed as to whether he would cope with 'life on a battery'. He would have to carry the controller and batteries in a shoulder bag at all times, and there was an alarm which sounded when the power was low or disconnected. The batteries needed charging twice each day but at night he'd plug into the mains electricity at home. That was all straightforward. No more taxing than taking immuno-suppressive drugs and he would need much less medication overall.

The next explanation came as a surprise. Between us, Jarvik and I had worked out a revolutionary new method to deliver electrical power into the body aiming to avoid those power line infections that had terminated my HeartMate patients. The issue with cables that emerged from the abdominal wall was that the interface between stiff foreign body and skin frequently broke down. Movement at the site allowed bacteria to enter the subcutaneous fat until eventually the pump itself was infected. And in addition chronic infection promoted blood clotting in the pump and stroke. So reducing drive line infection risk would also combat the likelihood of other device complications.

What we planned was to screw a metal plug into Peter's skull. Why? Because the scalp skin is virtually fat free and has a generous blood supply. Also with the titanium bolt firmly fixed in bone there would be no movement between power line and skin thereby avoiding disruption to the healing process. In essence, Peter would have an internal cable from the pump itself, up through the chest and neck to the bolt. Then a separate external cable to batteries and controller. The first real Frankenstein's monster. Appropriately Peter asked whether I had done this before. I told him no one had ever done it before, but I had drilled holes in heads for trauma and would try to avoid that in his case.

I warned Peter that other doctors or nurses that he might encounter would not be able to feel a pulse, or take his blood pressure. The impeller would simply push blood through his body continuously like water through a pipe. Moreover, the pump was completely silent within his body, a huge blessing compared to the incessant noise from pulsatile LVADs or total artificial hearts.

Peter was curious to know whether pulseless circulation was compatible with life in the long term. All I could say was that I believed it to be. And the sheep never complained. They seemed perfectly content and were well cared for. Then another penetrating question. If he lost consciousness out of the hospital without a pulse would anyone know whether he was alive or dead? That was moving away from my comfort zone, so I sidestepped with a speculative response. But he was right to ask. Months later over the winter one of my Jarvik 2000 patients fell and banged his head at home. He was found some hours later, cold and pulseless and taken to the mortuary.

Two days after the meeting, Peter confirmed in writing that he wished to go ahead. Now I needed Professor Philip Poole-Wilson, Europe's leading heart failure cardiologist, to agree our choice of patient. There was no time to waste. Peter could die at any time. Phillip was in Europe when I contacted him but kindly agreed to come to Oxford on his way back to London on June 19th. Confident as to what his conclusion would be I planned the implant for the 20th. That gave just a few days for Jarvik, Frazier and the technicians to fly in.

On the evening of the 19th we brought Peter to our cardiac recovery room where David Pigott the anaesthetist inserted monitoring lines. Our chief nurse Sister Desiree Robson shaved the left side of Peter's head in preparation for the skull pedestal incision. The Professor arrived from Heathrow at 22.30, talked at length with Peter and emerged just after midnight to give us the go ahead. As my Oxford cardiology colleague Professor Adrian Banning said: 'Houghton was functionally dead. All he had left was a mind full of frustration. Once you have fallen off the threshold for transplantation, medicine has nothing to offer. Every cardiologist has clinics full of these poor people, unable to work, just hanging on waiting to die.'

We all arrived in the anaesthetic room of operating theatre 5 at 07.30. As usual Frazier appeared in Stetson and cowboy boots. Normal for Texas, less so in Oxford. Once Peter was asleep we positioned him left side up on the operating table with the side of his head and neck exposed. I marked the site of the prospective surgical incisions with an indelible black marker pen, then the first step was to insert the cannulas into the blood vessels of the groin to attach him to the bypass machine. I had hoped we didn't need to use it but the blood pressure was sagging already. Usually a stimulating cut with the scalpel helps irrespective of the anaesthetic, so I began to open the left chest between the fifth and sixth ribs. This gave easy access to the apex of his grossly enlarged left ventricle at the front of the incision, and the aorta at the back. But the first priority was to insert the power cable and skull pedestal securely, allowing us to switch on the LVAD quickly in the event of cardiac arrest.

To negotiate the neck and side of the head with the cable was challenging. We made a C shaped incision above and behind the left ear and raised a flap of scalp away from the bone.

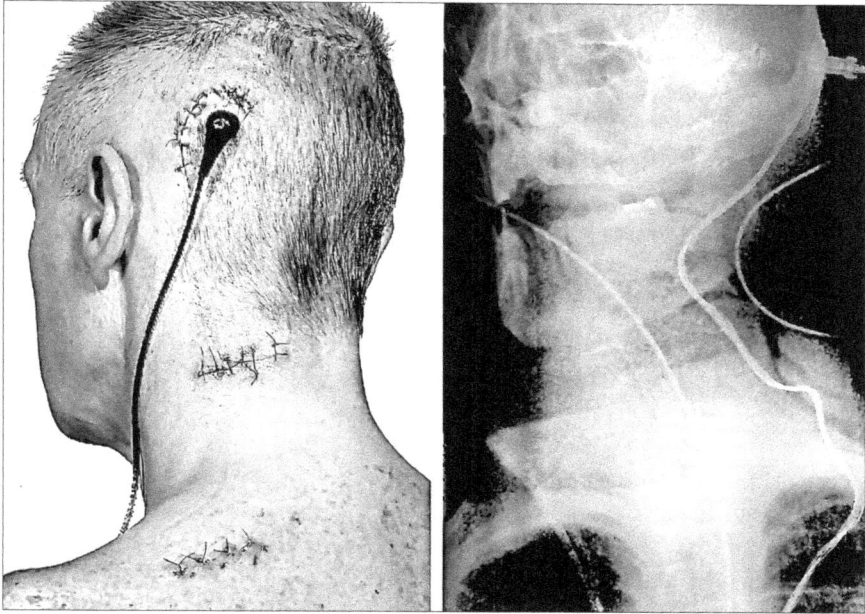

Fig 13.6 A. Recently implanted skull pedestal power delivery.

The small plug at the end of the internal power line was then inserted through the titanium pedestal which we secured to the skull with six tiny screws. A trifle worrying without specialised instruments but we just got on making the exit hole and plugged him in to the batteries.

Next came the join between the Dacron outflow graft to the descending aorta. The length had to be right – a smooth curve around the diaphragm – but otherwise just routine vascular stitching that mustn't leak. Moving on swiftly I slit open the pericardium around Peter's huge heart, which appeared more fibrous tissue than muscle. It barely moved, quivering being a better description than beating. Still hoping to avoid the bypass machine, I began to sew on the restraining cuff and from this moment on, Peter's dismal heart would never bear sole responsibility for his circulation.

Henceforth his life was permanently reliant on technology, a leap into the unknown.

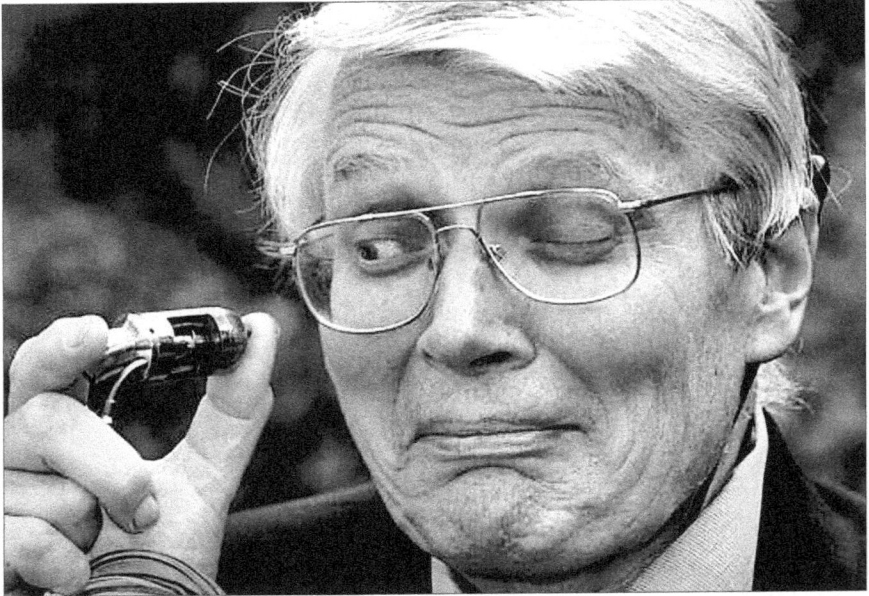

Fig 13.6 B. Peter Houghton the first permanent Jarvik 2000 LVAD patient.

All that remained was to core out the plug of heart muscle within the cuff then insert the pump. But the first cut made the sick heart fibrillate. No problem. We simply went onto cardiopulmonary bypass to maintain the circulation. What's more he desperately needed that help. With consistently poor blood flow the lactic acid in his bloodstream had risen to dangerous levels. One more minute, and the LVAD was in. 'Switch it on', I said, 'and as soon as the blood gases have improved let's slide off bypass.'

With the pump speed set at 10,000 rpm, the flow probe around the outflow graft registered four and a half litres per minute. When we cut back on cardiopulmonary bypass flow, allowing Peter's own heart to fill, the LVAD output increased accordingly, 'Come off then', I said hopefully.

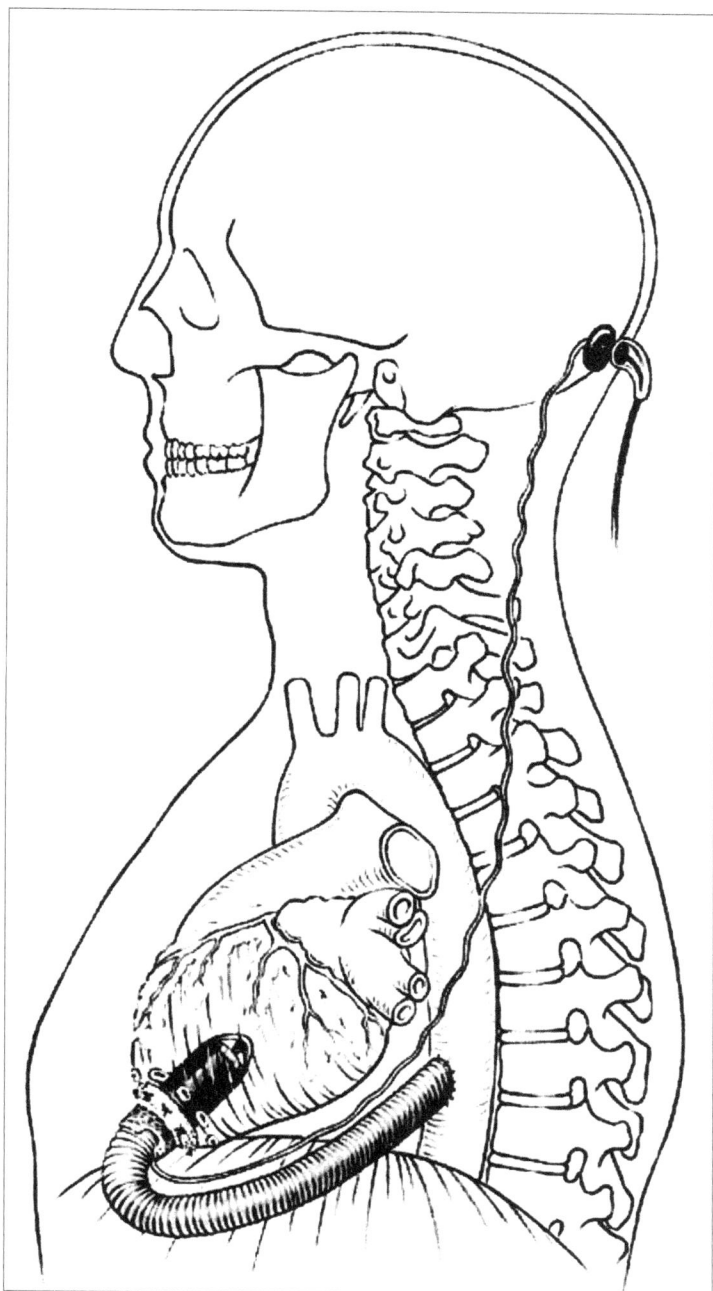

Fig 13.7 Diagram showing the Jarvik 2000 LVAD in situ.

All eyes were fixed on the monitor screen. Peter's arterial pressure trace was an absolutely flat line registering around two thirds of normal human blood pressure. But the pressure in the veins was low, he needed more blood in the circulation topped up from the reservoir in the bypass circuit. It was vital to keep Peter's own left ventricle well filled otherwise the powerful turbine could suck it empty causing an obstruction. Such details mattered in this great pulseless adventure.

The remaining and most troublesome issue was to stop the bleeding. Every cut surface and needle hole was oozing blood because Peter's distended liver had not been making clotting factors. We needed donor clotting factors and bags of concentrated platelets, the small cells that plug leaks and initiate clotting. Meanwhile the device was operating on seven Watts power consumption and we could literally turn up or turn down Peter's blood flow by turning a knob. And counterintuitively when his blood pressure surged as he began to wake up, pump flow decreased because the impeller was having to work against greater resistance in the circulation.

We had assembled an elite nursing team to supervise this baffling physiology post-operatively. Some had helped with the sheep and knew what to expect. Equally they were excited and proud to see the flat-line patient with a revolutionary new type of artificial heart on a lifetime basis. We hoped it would provide an off-the-shelf alternative for those like Peter who would never be given a human heart. As we have said, you need to be pretty fit to undergo transplantation except from a pig, that is.

Peter left hospital eleven days after the surgery when we were satisfied that he was in full control of his own equipment. Life on a battery is not exactly normal existence but the relief to be free of breathlessness more than compensates for the tedium of battery exchange and plugging into the mains overnight. His exercise capacity increased progressively to virtually normal for a man of his age. His belly began to shrink and his huge legs became slim again. His only medications now were the anticoagulant warfarin and a pill to consistently keep his blood pressure down. And now his engaging personality began to shine through. He'd shifted from inexorable fear and bewilderment to undisguised pleasure at avoiding death at fifty-nine. Until his hair grew back around the pedestal, children would approach him and ask why he had a bolt in his head – was he a robot, or Frankenstein's monster?

Out shopping one day he felt a sharp and painful jerk at his head. A would-be thief had snatched the shoulder bag containing the controller and batteries, thinking it contained an expensive camera. The skull pedestal plug was avulsed and his pump stopped – a potentially lethal event. When the pump alarm sounded the juvenile dropped the bag and ran off. Peter managed to retrieve the equipment but was passing out. He urgently beseeched a passing old lady to plug him in again after which the pump started promptly, resurrecting him.

Not all my Jarvik patients were as lucky. One went out Christmas shopping without a spare battery. When the low power alarm warned him of problems he tried to get home but didn't make it. Pump off, life's end. Desperately sad because he was so fit, yet his own ventricle was too badly damaged to sustain him. Peter came close with a similar incident. He was in the middle of having a tooth filled at the dentist when his battery alarm went off. The anxious dentist had to stop drilling and drive him home expeditiously.

The new miniaturised high speed rotary blood pumps were a great advance. For every one I implanted I was forced to pay for it using charitable funds as the NHS wouldn't contribute. Peter travelled the world to spread the word. In Washington he helped us to gain permission for destination therapy – or transplant alternative – with improved LVADs. On the fifth anniversary of his operation, my team including Jarvik and Frazier were given a reception at the Prime Minister's residence, 10 Downing Street. At that gathering the lack of affordability of the American devices was raised and the laser physicist Professor Marc Clement suggested we develop a British equivalent. We have achieved that with the company Calon CardioTechnology, producing an original device that has great blood handling.

Peter was in great form in Downing Street. He was already by far the longest artificial heart survivor ever, and went on for almost three more years. Ironically having recovered from heart failure he was offered the opportunity to be transplant wait listed in his own city. He pointedly refused to discuss it. Why should he go that route when he felt perfectly well? As well as fund raising to buy pumps for others he took a job helping the homeless and deprived. And having interacted widely with the US health-care system he became a harsh critic of the NHS who he considered had abrogated all responsibility for him. 'Second-hand shop health care', he called it.

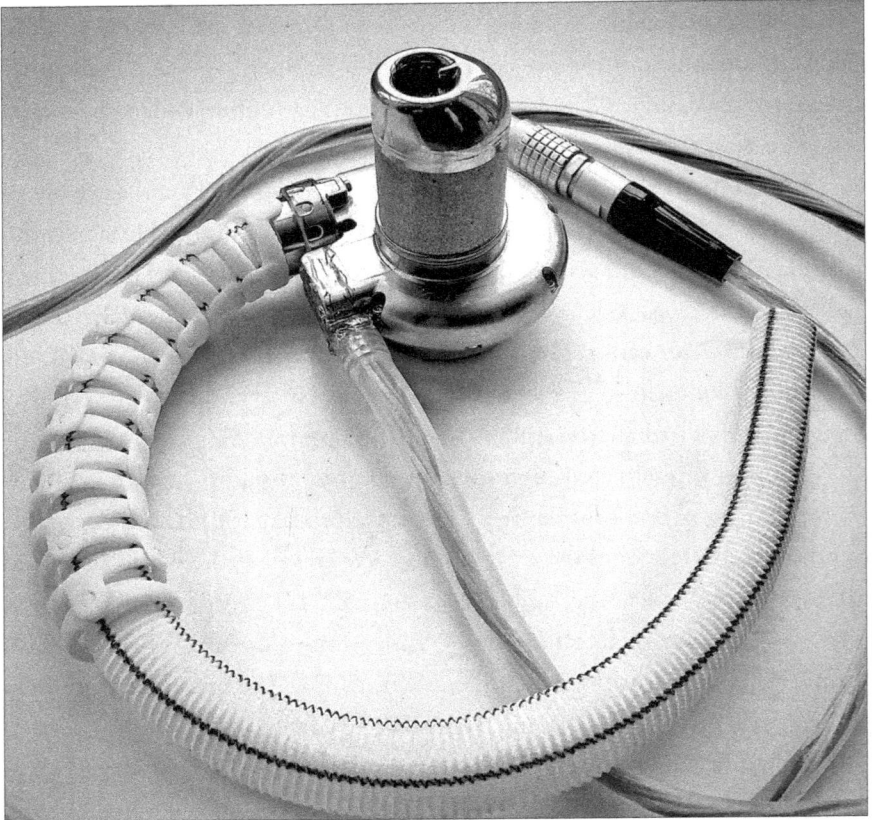

Fig 13.8 CalonCardioTechnology LVAD.

Eventually, having had no strokes or infection on his skull pedestal he suffered a prolific nose bleed. And of course warfarin didn't help. His single kidney stopped producing urine whist I was away at a conference in Japan. The teaching hospital close to home declined to dialyse him because of the pump and pulseless circulation. The kidney could have recovered so I considered it a totally unnecessary death. Yet Peter left an important legacy.

His extra life, more than 10% of his overall lifetime, confirmed the huge potential of LVAD technology. And no one else had to die first.

There are few ethical dilemmas with an LVAD. Those that need them otherwise have short wretched lives. As I've said, if you could help them why wouldn't you, yet in the NHS, twenty-five years after we began Oxford's lifetime circulatory support programme, heart failure patients may only be considered for an LVAD on a bridge to transplant basis. Fewer than a hundred are used each year because of the paucity of donor hearts, little influenced by the presumed consent laws that allow organs to be taken without the family's permission.

This is a cost-containment strategy not compassionate healthcare. Moreover it is false economy. Advanced heart failure patients require masses of medication and multiple hospital admissions that could be offset by a symptom-relieving device which provides an economically productive life in the younger age groups. Moreover, sick hearts spontaneously improve when offloaded. Some recover completely. We should have pacemakers for heart rhythm problems and LADs for pump failure. Why the difference?

What is the status of LVAD technology at the time of writing? Much of what we know comes from comprehensive data banks, the principal of which is the International Society of Heart and lung Transplantation Registry for Mechanically Assisted Circulatory Support under the direction of my friend and co-worker, James Kirklin at the University of Alabama. The registry records pre-operative patient information, device details and follow up on post implant clinical events. Hugely important details that eventually determine which LVADs are safe and effective and should remain in the market place. Or not! The Third Annual Report in 2019 encompassed more than 16,000 LVAD patients from 24 centres. The data showed centrifugal blood pumps such as the HeartMate 3 to outperform axial flow pumps like the Jarvik 2000, in respect to the incidence of gastrointestinal bleeding and haematological adverse events, though the incidence of stroke was similar.

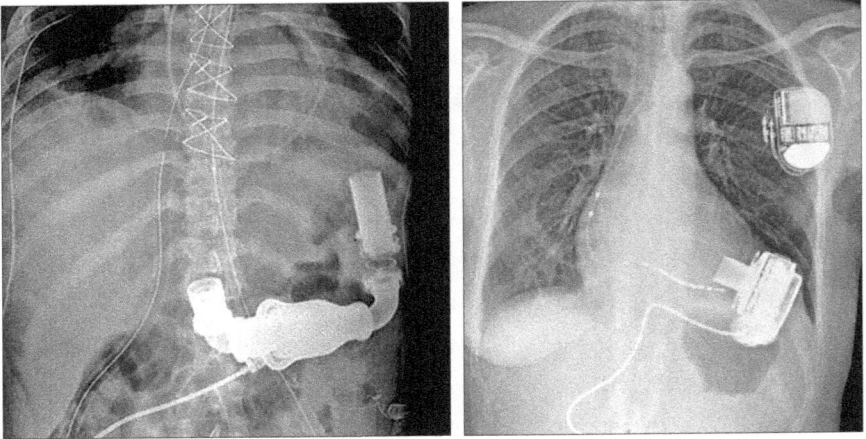

**Fig 13.9 A. Chest X-ray showing the HeartMate11 LVAD in situ.
B. HeartMate111 and an implanted pacemaker.**

The past decade has witnessed rapid evolution in the design and durability of centrifugal flow blood pumps that can be implanted at low surgical risk. Whereas the original pulsatile LVADs and some of the first-generation high speed rotary devices were plagued by prohibitive rates of pump thrombosis, stroke and gastrointestinal bleeding, contemporary blood pumps exhibit superior haemocompatibility and far fewer adverse events when properly managed. Infection where the power cable exits the skin remains problematic but new methods to pass energy into the body without a drive line are in development. We call that transcutaneous energy delivery.

In the best-case scenario, contemporary survival for advanced heart failure patients is less than two years with persistently dreadful symptoms. In contrast patients implanted with the bearingless magnetically levitated HeartMate3 device manifest an average survival exceeding five years, and remain symptom free with an active life. Originating from Poirier's ThermoCardiosystems and now owned by Abbott, many HeartMate patients have already lived for more than ten years and other innovative LVADs are in the pipeline.

One last word from the author's perspective. The finding that the patient's own heart improved during LVAD support was an important one. Some hearts with dilated cardiomyopathy recovered sufficiently for the device to be removed. But those with scarring after myocardial infarction didn't. Once established scar tissue has always been seen as permanent and as we have said, scar stretches causing the heart to fail.

One theory to explain 'bridge to recovery' with an LVAD was that the process of resting the ventricle whilst simultaneously improving its blood supply caused proliferation of the small number of adult heart muscle cells that remain capable of replicating. Some studies show that targeted drug therapy may also promote recovery. Coincidentally I had operated on a number of babies born with congenital coronary artery anomalies which caused them to suffer extensive life-threatening myocardial infarction during their first months of life. If diagnosed in time we could provide normal coronary blood flow by surgically rearranging the anatomy of these tiny vessels. Nonetheless we expected scarring to remain unchanged. In fact it didn't. After following the children into teenage years when they were able to tolerate magnetic resonance imaging we found something quite remarkable. The scar had largely disappeared and their heart contractility was restored. Of course we published this optimistic observation in the medical literature but exactly how did it happen?

Our hypothesis was that, with greatly improved blood supply, the embryonic stem cells which ordinarily survive for just months after birth had divided to produce new heart muscle cells and in turn regenerated the myocardium by removing scar tissue. This made me wonder whether these biological mechanisms might be genetically engineered to help adults with myocardial infarction.

At the time our LVAD development company Calon Cardio Technology was based in Wales where I learned of the ground-breaking discoveries of the Nobel Laureate Professor Sir Martin Evans at Cardiff University.

Sir Martin was the first to isolate and culture embryonic stem cells from mice and had developed methods to genetically modify and transplant them into other animals and indeed humans. Having employed the techniques to help patients with cystic fibrosis and breast cancer we discussed the possibility of applying the science to rescue the scarred left ventricle in heart failure patients.

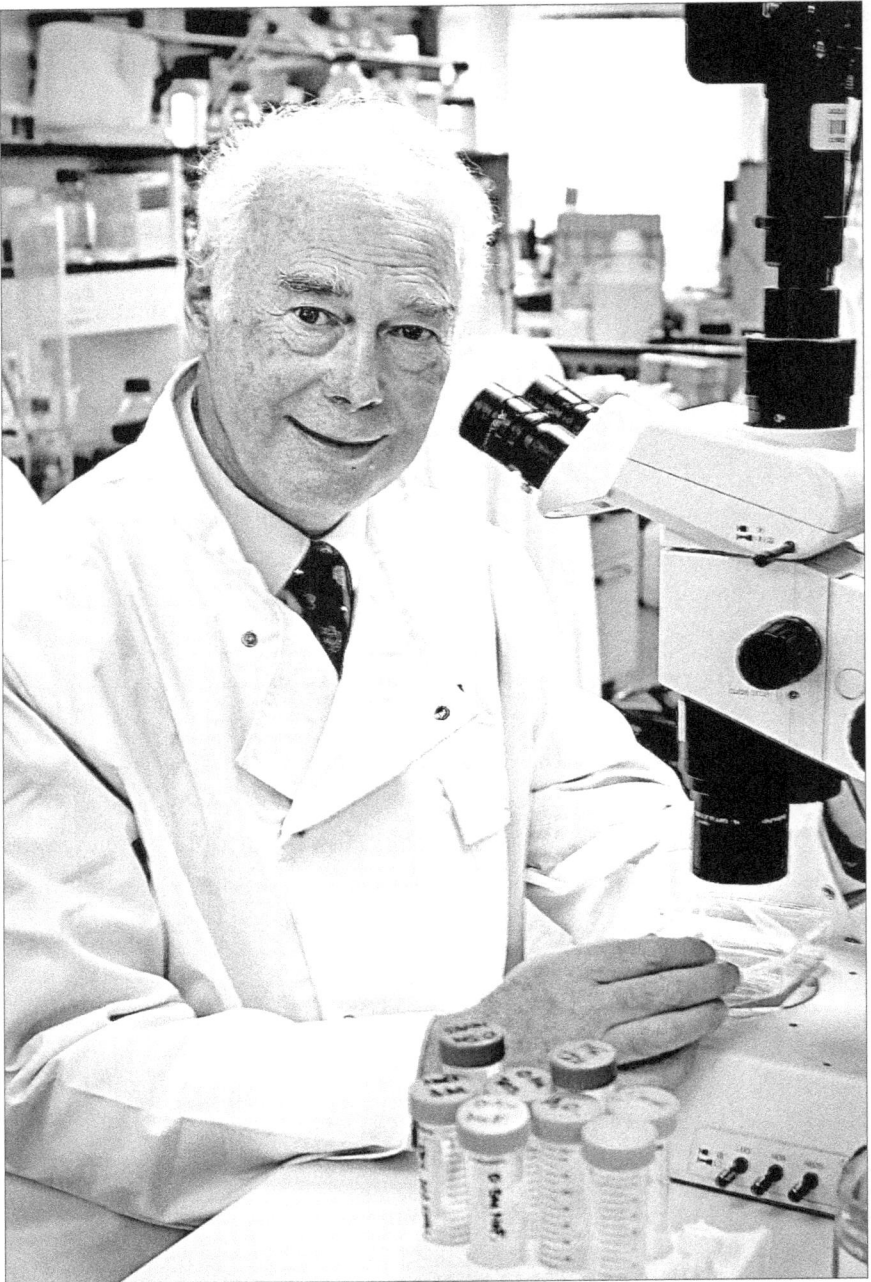

Fig 13.10 Professor Sir Martin Evans.

Evans went on to isolate immunomodulatory progenitor cells from the bone marrow of healthy volunteers which could be transplanted into others without generating an inflammatory rejection response. We wondered whether these might evolve into new muscle cells if injected into the scarred wall of the left ventricle of patients with coronary artery disease.

To address the controversy surrounding first clinical use in humans I suggested that we begin with dying patients who required salvage with an LVAD on a bridge to transplant basis. With that scenario we could examine the treated organ when it was subsequently removed and would have nothing to lose should an unexpected complication occur. Their lives depended upon the LVAD not their own muscle contractility. Could I do that in Oxford? The project was rejected out of hand if for no other reason than the NHS would not supply the life-saving technology and my research funds were exhausted. So I took the project to some of my distinguished trainees in Greece who were beginning a mechanical circulatory support programme. In short there were no adverse reactions to the injected cells so we progressed to treating myocardial infarction patients with substantial areas of scar who were undergoing coronary bypass surgery.

What we discovered was unexpected and remarkable. The patients recovered well and in a matter of months a significant amount of the heart's scar tissue had disappeared. As much as forty percent in several of them. Whilst the results needed to be confirmed in a larger study the revelation that bone marrow cells can be isolated, modified and reproduced to target a specific need contributed another vital step towards the 'keep your own heart' strategy. A safer bet than pig hearts I suspect. The history of heart surgery has been characterised by the interaction between bold intrepid surgeons and men of science. Occasionally the two come together in one individual, though less so these days with increased focus on restricted duration of training. Things have certainly moved on since those magnificent men and their heart-lung machines just seventy years ago. What a privilege to have been part of it all.

Postscript

> Open heart surgery is now part of a typical life
> experience for many people. Folks talk casually
> about having a stent put in as if they had their
> tyres rotated.
>
> —Roger Ebert

Thanks to those magnificent men and their heart-lung machines, structural heart disease became safely and reproducibly treatable during the second half of the twentieth century. This was an epic period in the history of healthcare and for me the timing was perfect. From inheriting Lord Brock's boots at the Royal Brompton Hospital to meeting Lillehei at Culzean Castle; through training under Kirklin in Alabama then working with Cooley and Frazier in Texas; and then those friendships with Barnard, Bentall, Ross and others. When writing *Landmarks in Cardiac Surgery* for the surgical profession, I received many priceless contributions from the likes of Dwight Harken, Charles Bailey and Viking Bjork, who by then were elderly but proud for their stories to be told. Great characters who made monumental contributions so what happened to them?

Russell Brock was knighted in 1954 and became President of the Royal College of Surgeons in 1963. During his professional life he was said to give 'the impression of perpetual disappointment at the unattainability of universal perfection'. He operated with 'watch spring tension' and was a difficult boss to please. Made a Life Peer in 1968, he retired from the NHS and became Director of the Department of Surgical Sciences at the Royal College. But he was a strong advocate of private medicine, continuing to operate in independent hospitals and becoming Chairman then President of the Private Patients Plan. Baron Russell Claude Brock of Wimbledon was described as a 'gracious guide to the House of Lords, masterfully elucidating its place in history'. He died in 1980 at the age of seventy-seven.

The American surgeons Dwight Emery Harken and Charles Philamore Bailey were both born in 1910, Harken in Osceola, Iowa, where his father was a physician and Bailey in Wanamassa, New Jersey. Professionally they were rumoured to detest one another, often fighting like wild dogs at surgical conferences. Harken became Chief of Thoracic Surgery at Peter Bent Brigham Hospital in Boston and with nurse Edith Heideman established one of the world's first intensive care units to support his heart valve surgery. His citation for the Texas Heart Institute Ray Fish Award included his contributions to the development of heart valves, the heart-lung machine, the direct current defibrillator, his stance against the dangers of smoking and the importance of animal research. He was widely recognised for rendering the heart 'surgically accessible' when others were afraid to touch it.

Bailey became Professor and Chief of Thoracic Surgery at Hahnemann College, Philadelphia in 1948 where he wrote *Surgery of the Heart*, a compendium of all aspects of the specialty, published in 1955. He then moved to New York City and St Barnabas Hospital in the Bronx for ten years before a radical career change. In the early 1960s Bailey was sued in four cases of medical malpractice though all patients had survived their operation. Two of them involved very substantial awards of $25,000 and $50,000 against him. Bewildered by the fact that the attorneys could reasonably justify the actions, Bailey decided to study law himself. This he did at Fordham Law School at night whilst performing heart surgery during the day. 'In my abrupt fashion', he wrote, 'I decided to go to law school so that I could understand what was happening, and what to do about it.' This was the era when medico-legal work took off in the USA and by 1973 Bailey had become a licensed lawyer of New York State. He later considered medical malpractice insurance an easier option and became a full-time member of the Physicians Reliance Association in Georgia. A radical change from his pioneering days at the operating table.

Having been born in the same year, Harken and Bailey died within days of each other in 1993, both aged 83. Harken's surgeon son Alden commented that Bailey had preceded his own father on the Obituary page of the New York Times, by just two days.

Clarence Walton Lillehei was born in Minneapolis in 1918 where in his early twenties he completed a three-year medical course in just two years at the University of Minnesota. Most of his ground-breaking career was spent in his home town after overcoming the aggressive cancer in his neck at the age of thirty-one. He showed determination, persistence and courage to perform the incredibly audacious cross circulation operations, develop the first successful bubble oxygenator, and introduced haemodilution and cooling techniques to improve the safety of cardiopulmonary bypass. Lillehei left Minneapolis for New York in 1967 where as Chairman of the Department of Surgery at Cornell University Medical Centre he undertook a series of thoracic organ transplants before his life began to unravel. With deteriorating vision caused by radiotherapy he was obliged to stop operating at the age of fifty-five. By then he had trained more than one hundred and fifty cardiac surgeons including Christiaan Barnard. Perhaps losing the obsession with work was at the root of his flamboyant, if not reckless, personal life that followed. What should he do but return to Minneapolis where he remained well respected as a writer, lecturer and consultant. It was a privilege to spend those hours with him, sipping whisky whilst listening to his stories and exchanging anecdotes about our cases. He was clearly a generous and compassionate character much loved by his patients. And at the end of the day, who doesn't want to side-step the tax man, or make out with a beautiful woman? Who amongst us is blameless in this high pressure environment?

There was huge rivalry between Lillehei and John Kirklin, at the Mayo Clinic in Rochester, yet they had great mutual respect for one another. Kirklin's father was the first specialist radiologist at the Mayo Clinic before becoming Professor and Chairman of the department there. John attended Harvard Medical School and was ranked first in his class of one hundred and fifty for four consecutive years. Dr Elliot Cutler wrote of him, 'This is the brightest medical student I have ever seen.'

One of the most fascinating insights into those pioneering days comes from an account by the master himself when reflecting on his early career. 'In 1951 I did a closed pulmonary valvotomy on a man with pulmonary stenosis. He had thickening of the heart muscle below the valve and died two days after the operation. At autopsy the valve was opened but the muscle hypertrophy beneath was enormous. The patient could not have survived without relief of the obstruction. My co-worker Dr Earl Wood, a great physiologist, and I went back to his office and decided that we would either have to be content with cardiac surgery as a minor specialty, limited to passing instruments into the heart, or we would need a heart-lung machine. It's the oxygenator that's the problem', said Wood. Then we visited John Gibbon in his laboratories in Philadelphia and Forrest Dodrill in Detroit to learn about the mechanical pump oxygenator. The Gibbon machine had been developed commercially by International Business Machines Corporation and looked quite a bit like a computer. Dodrill's heart-lung machine had been built for him by General Motors and looked a great deal like a car engine. We came home and decided to try to persuade the Mayo Clinic to let us build our own pump-oxygenator similar to Gibbon's. Of course a number of visitors came to our laboratory to see what we were doing. Dr Ake Senning from Stockholm was one of them. I still remember the day he was there and one of the connectors came loose. We ruined his beautiful suit as well as the ceiling by spraying blood around the room.'

The electrifying day came in the spring of 1954 when the newspapers carried an account of Walt Lillehei's successful open-heart operation on a small child. Of course I was terribly envious and yet I was admiring at the same moment. That admiration increased exponentially when a short time later I visited Minneapolis and observed an operation with controlled cross circulation. Walt then took us on rounds and it was absolutely exciting to see small children recovering from these miraculous operations.

In the winter of 1954 and 1955 we had nine surviving dogs out of ten cardiopulmonary bypass runs. With my paediatric cardiologist, Dr Jim DuShane, we selected eight patients for intracardiac repair and planned to go ahead with all of them even if the first seven died. We did the first on a Tuesday in March 1955 and four of the eight survived. By then Walt and I were on parallel but intertwined paths. I witnessed a similar situation between Dwight Harken and Charles Bailey in the first days of closed mitral valve surgery. I felt, and, I hope you will forgive me, that their interactions were somewhat demeaning to themselves and to the scientific progress of cardiac surgery. Therefore I am extremely grateful to Walt Lillehei and very proud for the two of us, that during the twelve to eighteen months when we were the only surgeons in the world performing open intracardiac operations with cardiopulmonary bypass, we continued to communicate and argued privately in nightclubs and on aeroplanes rather than publicly over our differences.

In 1966 Kirklin was recruited to the University of Alabama School of Medicine where his operating theatre sessions were disciplined and highly regimented. Nothing was left to chance. He often compared going on, and weaning from cardiopulmonary bypass to taking off and landing a commercial airliner. He had checklists which the anaesthetist read off to him during those procedures. He also liked to draw analogies between cowboy gunslingers and heart surgeons. During one tedious situation when faced with continuous oozing of blood after coming off the heart-lung machine, one of his assistants, Claude, kept probing him with tedious questions. Why was he not using a certain drug to stop the bleeding and so on?

Finally Dr Kirklin became weary of the dialogue and said, 'Claude, let me tell you a story. There was this old gunfighter who had killed many men, but was sick of it and didn't want to fight anymore. He came to this town and there was a young punk who was bothering him and trying to provoke him into a fight. Finally the lad who was trying to make a name for himself aggravated the old gunfighter so much that the two of them went out into the street and drew their guns.' He then said, 'Claude do you know what happened next?' Claude said, 'No Dr Kirklin, what?' And he said, 'Well the old gunfighter drew first and shot the punk through the heart. Do you understand the significance of that story, Claude?'

Soon Kirklin had the best surgical results for every congenital heart defect, publishing over seven hundred medical and scientific articles, a handful of which I had the privilege to co-author during my time in Birmingham. Just after the end of my training there he relinquished the Chairmanship to Al Pacifico, and his son James, a brilliant clone later became the head of transplantation. The great man himself continued to operate until the age of seventy-two in 1989 with the same obsessive focus on perfection.

When I left Alabama, Dr Kirklin gave me one of his famous 'blue books' of patient management protocols. Clear directions on how to manage virtually every situation in cardiac surgery.One of my proudest moments was when I received a manuscript acceptance letter from Dr Kirklin when he was editor of the *Journal of Thoracic and Cardiovascular Surgery*. He ended with the personal note '....and I heartily congratulate you on your spectacular career'. I kept that document framed on my office wall in Oxford. Dr Kirklin died on April 21st 2004. He will be remembered as the most influential cardiac surgeon of all time.

If Kirklin was the brain, Cooley was the hands. Harry Minetree, Denton Cooley's biographer, described their first meeting before his aortic aneurysm operation. 'Dr Cooley was three hours late for our appointment and looked as if he had just stepped out of a band box. As he held a stethoscope to my chest I said, "I've been waiting for you for three hours". Shhh!' He responded as he listened to my chest again. 'Now, what did you say?'

I said: 'Its eight o'clock. You're three hours late.' His stare was then edged with arrogance. 'I did six open-hearts today; what did you do?'

The man was tall and tanned in a grey silk suit and two tone shoes. I said: 'You sure don't look like it.'

'Some folks relax playing golf', said Cooley. 'I like to operate on people's hearts. Okay?' He winked, I smiled. 'You've got an aneurysm in there as big as a grapefruit and it's about to burst. But you're a big strong boy and I'm the best surgeon in the world, so if this had to happen, we've got the best possible odds.'

Cooley was the antithesis of Dr Kirklin. On the subject of humility he was also known to remark, 'A successful cardiovascular surgeon should be a man who, when asked to name the three best surgeons in the world, would have difficulty in deciding on the other two.'

Drs DeBakey and Cooley did not communicate for forty years after the artificial heart debacle which graced the front page of *Life* Magazine. Cooley referred to the short distance between their offices as a demilitarized zone.

Dr De Bakey was ninety-nine and recovering from emergency surgery for aortic dissection, when the reconciliation finally came. Cooley was eighty-seven. After all that time, DeBakey explained in an interview that he refused to testify against his rival in the litigation that followed. He actually did not want Cooley to be found guilty. 'Much as I regretted what he did', he explained, 'I didn't think vengeance would solve anything.' Nonetheless 'He disappointed me with his ethics and poor judgement which was a little childish.'

Dr Cooley's response was that he was 'justified in what he did. That he was performing many more heart operations than anyone else, and so considered himself 'the appropriate person to perform the first implantation of an artificial heart'. I guess all this seems arrogant but in the real world he was a very nice man.

The actual coming together was instigated by Cooley just a few days after Dr DeBakey received the highest civilian award in the USA from Congress – the Gold Medal in recognition of a host of towering achievements. Included in the citation was the fact that he had helped create the mobile army surgical hospitals, or MASH units during World War II and was instrumental in developing the Veterans Administration medical system.

At a special ceremony at the Cooley Cardiovascular Surgical Society at St Luke's Hospital on October 27th 2007 Dr DeBakey accepted a Lifetime Achievement Award.

I was there at the time. Dr Cooley stepped down from the stage and shook hands with his old boss who sat head bowed in a motorised mobility scooter. There was rapturous applause from an appreciative audience who had wanted this to happen for many years. Kneeling reverently beside him the ever modest Denton joked: 'It must be a heavy burden for one person to be honoured by a Congressional Gold Medal and membership of the Cooley Society all in one week.'

Dr DeBakey replied that since the Congressional medal was pure gold he hoped the Cooley Award was the same. 'It's 14 Karat' came the response. The ice was broken, the feud over. Subsequently DeBakey said of Cooley,

'I never considered him a rival because I had all the patients I could handle and all the honours I could take care of. He kind of suffered from the fact that I was considered more prestigious than he was.' Great Texan egos heading up two of the world's top cardiac surgery centres on the one street.

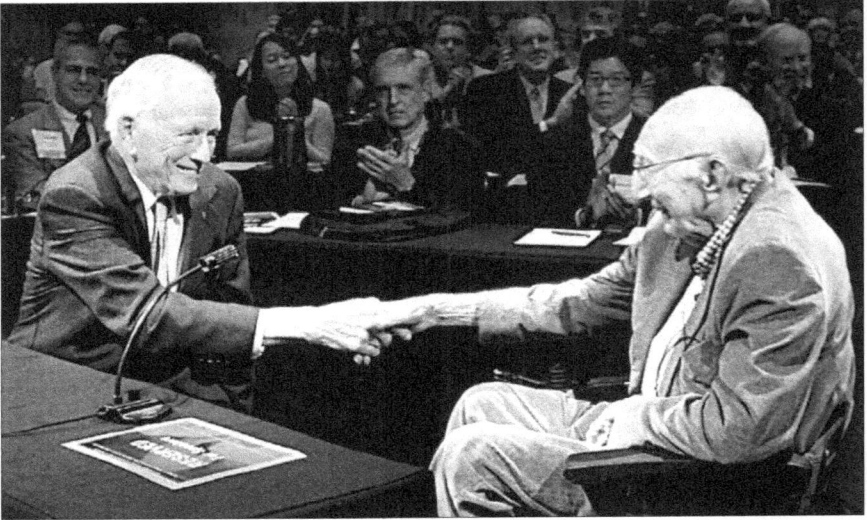

Postscript Fig 1. The reconciliation.

The following spring the DeBakey Society reciprocally honoured Dr Cooley who said: 'I believe both of us were relieved and comforted that peace had finally been declared and we could enjoy our remaining days without animosity towards each other.'

But what was it that prompted an end to the hostilities? Cooley had read the astronaut Gene Cernan's autobiography *Last man on the moon*, which described the competitive space race between the USA and Russia. Cernan had been a patient at Texas Heart, and wrote of the unnecessary animosity and mutual hostility between rival spacemen. In the book he admitted that the Russians were 'regular guys who just drank more vodka so why seek to discredit them? They couldn't be held to account for their political leadership. Perhaps the same applies today.

A further meeting was planned to celebrate Dr DeBakey's hundredth birthday but sadly he died on July 11th 2008 before it could be held. That was the year Dr Cooley presented me with the Texas Heart's 'Ray Fish Award' for my work towards long-term mechanical circulatory support as an alternative to transplantation. Given previously to pioneers such as Mason Sones, John Kirklin and Norman Shumway this was a tremendous honour for an English surgeon and memorable for more than one reason.

At the reception which followed at Cool Acres, Dr Cooley's ranch on the Brazos river, my wife Sarah took a step backwards in long grass to take a photograph of the two of us in rocking chairs on the ranch house veranda. Abruptly she stood still like a pillar of salt. Brought up in Kenya Sarah immediately recognised the rustling sound. It was a coiled rattlesnake ready to strike only inches behind her legs. That would certainly have spoiled the party. Dr Cooley died at home in Houston on 18th November 2016 aged ninety-six. Great cardiac surgeon, great character, never to be forgotten.

Bud Frazier was with us at Cool Acres. Bud and George Noon who bravely repaired Dr DeBakey's dissected aorta, went on to carry the torch for transplantation and circulatory support at the Texas Heart Institute and Baylor respectively. I remember visiting Bud's office for the first time. It had no windows, just a couch, a desk and threadbare old rug. Home from home where he spent days and nights with a television that was never switched off. It was always illuminating to hear him reminisce about the old days and how his fascination with artificial hearts began.

Whilst a medical student in Houston an Italian teenager was sent to Methodist Hospital for an aortic valve replacement by Dr DeBakey. Later that evening the lad suffered a cardiac arrest and had his chest reopened in intensive care as part of the resuscitation process. Frazier was beseeched to relieve the weary surgeon performing internal cardiac massage so for the first time he took a fibrillating heart into his hand and frantically pumped the blood. As he did so the lad woke up and raised a pleading hand to his rescuer's face. By all accounts it was at that agonising moment, just before they let him die, that Frazier understood his life's calling. He thought to himself 'if my hand can keep this kid alive, why couldn't we make a machine to do the same?' Melodramatic perhaps, but a true story told to me by Bud in a pub in Oxford.

He went on to assist with the development of numerous LVADs including the HeartMate, Jarvik and HeartWare pumps, and incredibly came to implant more than a thousand of them. He personally performed more than 1300 heart transplants.

During the official celebration of his one thousandth LVAD implant at the Texas Heart Institute. Bud said: 'I began this journey during the idealistic Kennedy era which had the goals of flying to the moon, curing hunger and poverty, and creating a realistic artificial heart. Except for reaching the moon, these laudable goals have remained elusive.' Perhaps that was a little pessimistic given his spectacular track record in mechanical circulatory support. Now in his eighties he retains that curious office and his secretary at St Luke's still spending many hours in the hospital and laboratory. Happily he remains a living legend.

In many respects my London mentor Donald Ross was a legend too. Ross graduated from the University of Cape Town in 1946, in the same class as Barnard, Rodney Hewitson who assisted in the first heart transplant, and Alf Gunning who preceded me in Oxford. It was Ross who took the medical school Gold Medal and was regarded as the brightest of the bunch. He became a Fellow of the Royal College of Surgeons in 1949 and was working in chest surgery in Bristol when Ronald Belsey first brought him to London to watch Russell Brock replace an aortic valve. Brock then employed the enthusiastic young South African at the Brompton Hospital just when Cooley took over Oswald Tubbs practice. Small world.

Undoubtedly the connection with Barnard and Cooley made it certain that Ross would attempt the first heart transplant in the UK. Years later I trained with him at the nearby Middlesex Hospital, learning much from his calm and relaxed manner during difficult cases. And he was a gentleman who invariably thanked his nurses and surgical assistants when leaving the operating table. Ross helped immeasurably in the progress of cardiac surgery in many countries and received numerous international honours. Out of the hospital he bred and rode Arabian horses. He died in 2014, aged ninety-one.

Rob Jarvik revelled in the media attention that artificial hearts generated. So much so that he elected to make television commercials for the cholesterol-lowering drug Lipitor manufactured by the pharmaceutical company Pfizer. In the first of these, he was depicted as an accomplished rower sculling out on beautiful Lake Crescent in Washington State. But the *New York Times* revealed that Jarvik was not a rower and it was someone else in the boat. A stunt double as they called it. As Frazier commented 'He's about as much an outdoors man as Woody Allen. He can't row!' In the commercials, Pfizer heralded Jarvik as the inventor of the artificial heart which upset his old colleagues in Utah. In a letter to the company in 2006 they made clear that specific accolade belonged with Kolff and Akutsu.

In another commercial Jarvik stared directly into the camera and announced, 'I'm glad I take Lipitor, as a doctor and a dad. Lipitor is one of the most researched medicines. You don't have to be a doctor to appreciate that.' At that point a Congressional Investigation was convened to examine Jarvik's credentials and it transpired that, though he had a medical degree, he had never been licensed to practise medicine in the USA. A distinguished scientist with a Masters in medical engineering – yes. A physician – no. He was not allowed to prescribe drugs. It was regarded as an ethical issue not that he had ever claimed to be a physician. He was simply reading from the script; for which he was apparently paid $1.34 million. As the journalist Katie Watson wrote in the *Chicago Tribune*, 'Robert Jarvik's ads for Lipitor were an important source of patient education about a terrible disease – physician addiction to drug money.' Rob still lives in a tower block in Manhattan. A number of his staff at Jarvik Heart came to work on our British LVAD. He wasn't happy about that.

After ending his own career in commercial mode Christiaan Barnard gave an interview with *Time Magazine* in which he confessed, 'The heart transplant wasn't such a big thing surgically. The point is I was prepared to take the risk. My philosophy is that the biggest risk in life is not to take the risk.'

In fact the whole development of cardiac surgery depended upon taking risks, but then the pioneering spirit died. The truth is it was effectively killed off. Charles Bailey saw it coming when he abandoned surgery for law. In the 1980s the US Health Care Financing Administration began to collect, but declined to publish, individual surgeons' death rates in New York State. But then a newspaper sued for the information and placed it in the public arena. Obviously it was the best surgeons who were repeatedly referred the sickest and highest risk patients who recorded the highest mortality rates. This may seem a rather obvious conclusion but the media seemed to lack that insight. The media's objective was to name and shame the surgeons. Some lost their careers and the whole profession became risk averse. In consequence the high-risk patients, through age or associated disease profiles were turned away. Those surgeons wanting to top the league tables and boost their private practices simply stuck with low-risk cases. Fewer were prepared to try something new and risk their reputation.

Cardiologists struggled to place patients with associated co-morbidity with a suitable surgeon. Attempting to stratify patients according to risk was not the solution. The public had little knowledge of the significance of risk algorithms. When surgeons were polled confidentially to ask whether publishing surgeon specific mortality information had affected their decision making, the vast majority said yes. So the days of pioneering were over.

Needless to say the UK's own NHS decided to follow on irrespective of the negative aspects of the process being widely discussed in the USA. The difference was that we already had to struggle to maintain low death rates in outdated facilities with inconsistent teams and without the rescue circulatory support systems that we had previously pioneered in Oxford. The NHS simply refused to fund those devices that kept patients alive until their own hearts recovered after surgery or heart attack. Therefore those still prepared to operate on the sickest patients would inevitably experience unnecessary deaths. Technology is expensive, death is cheap. And soon our cardiologists could show that patients in shock after a heart attack were less likely to receive an emergency coronary angioplasty. Why be associated with a death if you can avoid it?

If the aim of public outcome reporting was to increase transparency, it instead produced conflicts of interest, and a downturn in applicants for cardiac surgical posts. Because of the name and shame culture, previously respected individuals were found to have manipulated their outcomes for self-preservation. It was the death of innovation, the birth of mediocracy, and an invitation for catheter-based techniques to take over.

When we carefully analysed the causes of death after cardiac surgery in Oxford, we discovered one important fact. Very few were related to the surgeon's performance in the operating theatre. Most occurred through failure to rescue. The inability to cope effectively with a common complication in the post-operative period through mistakes or issues with staffing and equipment. I published the findings but the damage to the profession had already been done. When they recognised the implications of failure to rescue North America moved away from reporting individual surgeons' results. Instead they resorted to a Hospital Star Rating system using unit specific outcome measures and other relevant quality indicators. Should the same level of scrutiny be applied to NHS hospitals it would be a profound embarrassment. This is widely known now as the system struggles to overcome the consequences of the Covid pandemic. Patients with heart disease and cancer deteriorate inexorably on life-threatening waiting lists. The risks increase accordingly but the surgeons take the blame. Something has to change.

Undoubtedly the prevailing political climate held profound influence over my decision to retire from surgery at the age of sixty-eight. By then I had a severely deformed right hand. A form of Dupuytren's contracture where the instruments had smacked into my palm for forty years. I needed surgery to open the hand and couldn't face a dismal return to the NHS for retraining after the three months recovery period. The operation was scheduled at a different hospital on a Monday morning. The preceding Friday afternoon I walked out of the operating theatre and turned right to the car park instead of left to the office. I never went back. Much as I loved my team I didn't want them to know it was my last operation and make a fuss. No sycophantic handshakes, no gifts, no leaving parties where everyone would prefer to be at home. Just welcome relief to walk away from the crippling bureaucracy and finally lock the gates on that graveyard in my mind.

On the centenary of Cutlers first closed mitral valvotomy and seventy years after Gibbon's operation with his radical new machine, more than two million open heart operations are performed each year. In the USA alone, this number exceeds 900,000 though interventional cardiology now competes with open chest surgery thanks to the efforts of Dotter and Gruntzig. These days both aortic and mitral valves can be treated with a catheter, aneurysms repaired and there are more coronary angioplasties than bypass operations. Could those "magnificent men" have achieved their monumental advances in the current era? Absolutely not. Faced with constant scrutiny and an intrusive regulatory environment there would have been no cardiac surgery.

A Note on the Author

Operating on both adults and children, Professor Stephen Westaby is recognised worldwide as one of the most technically skilled and innovative surgeons of his generation. As a young trainee in the USA with a degree in biochemistry he identified the molecular mechanisms and root cause of the damaging effects of the heart-lung machine.

In 1986 Westaby was appointed to create a new cardiothoracic centre in Oxford. With restricted facilities Westaby initiated the internationally acclaimed 'cardiac surgery without intensive care' programme. As a result the unit rapidly expanded from the smallest to become the second largest cardiac centre in the UK.

His quest to find a mechanical alternative to scarce donor organs led to the longest survivor with any type of artificial heart following an operation performed in Oxford. High speed rotary blood pumps are now accepted as a solution for terminally ill heart failure patients.

Westaby has produced twelve surgical textbooks and more than three hundred peer reviewed papers in medical journals. He has trained numerous surgeons around the world on and has received honours from the USA, China, Russia and Japan.

In 2019 he was the first Western doctor learn about Covid when on a visit to Wuhan.

He lives outside Oxford.

www.ingramcontent.com/pod-product-compliance
Lightning Source LLC
Chambersburg PA
CBHW031426180326
41458CB00002B/461